SEXUAL BOUNDARY VIOLATIONS IN PSYCHOTHERAPY

SEXUAL BOUNDARY
VIOLATIONS IN
PSYCHOTHERAPY

SEXUAL BOUNDARY VIOLATIONS IN PSYCHOTHERAPY

Facing Therapist Indiscretions, Transgressions, and Misconduct

EDITED BY

Arlene (Lu) Steinberg
Judith L. Alpert
Christine A. Courtois

 AMERICAN PSYCHOLOGICAL ASSOCIATION

Published by
American Psychological Association
750 First Street, NE
Washington, DC 20002
https://www.apa.org

Order Department
https://www.apa.org/pubs/books
order@apa.org

In the U.K., Europe, Africa, and the Middle East, copies may be ordered from Eurospan
https://www.eurospanbookstore.com/apa
info@eurospangroup.com

Typeset in Charter and Interstate by Circle Graphics, Inc., Reisterstown, MD

Printer: Gasch Printing, Odenton, MD
Cover Designer: Beth Schlenoff Design, Bethesda, MD
Cover Photo: "Atmosphere.Blue.1," © Donna Bassin. All rights reserved.

Library of Congress Cataloging-in-Publication Data

Names: Steinberg, Arlene, editor. | Alpert, Judith L., editor. |
  Courtois, Christine A., editor.
Title: Sexual boundary violations in psychotherapy : facing therapist indiscretions,
  transgressions, and misconduct / edited by Arlene Steinberg, Judith L. Alpert,
  and Christine A. Courtois.
Description: Washington, DC : American Psychological Association, [2021] |
  Includes bibliographical references and index.
Identifiers: LCCN 2020048768 (print) | LCCN 2020048769 (ebook) |
  ISBN 9781433834608 (paperback) | ISBN 9781433837180 (ebook)
Subjects: LCSH: Psychotherapists—Sexual behavior. | Psychotherapy patients—
  Sexual behavior. | Psychotherapist and patient. | Psychologists—Professional ethics.
Classification: LCC RC480.8 .S47 2021 (print) | LCC RC480.8 (ebook) |
  DDC 174.2/9689—dc23
LC record available at https://lccn.loc.gov/2020048768
LC ebook record available at https://lccn.loc.gov/2020048769

https://doi.org/10.1037/0000247-000

Printed in the United States of America

10 9 8 7 6 5 4 3 2 1

Contents

Contributors

Alexis A. Adams-Clark, MS, Department of Psychology, University of Oregon, and Center for Institutional Courage, Eugene, OR, United States

Judith L. Alpert, PhD, Department of Applied Psychology, New York University, and New York University Postdoctoral Program in Psychotherapy and Psychoanalysis, New York, NY, United States

Tyson D. Bailey, PsyD, ABPP, Private Practice, Lynnwood, WA, United States

Kori Bennett, PsyD, Columbia Health, and Private Practice, New York, NY, United States

Laura S. Brown, PhD, ABPP, Private Practice, Seattle, WA, United States

Linda Campbell, PhD, University of Georgia, Center for Counseling and Personal Evaluation, Athens, GA, United States

Andrea Celenza, PhD, Boston Psychoanalytic Society and Institute and Harvard Medical School, Boston, MA; NYU Postdoctoral Program in Psychoanalysis, New York, NY; Private Practice, New York, NY, United States

Elizabeth Clark, PsyD, Counseling and Psychological Services, Fordham University, Bronx, NY, United States

Christine A. Courtois, PhD, ABPP, Private Practice (retired), Washington, DC; Christine A. Courtois PhD, PLLC, Bethany Beach, DE, United States

Goldie Eder, LCSW, BCD, Private Practice, Cambridge, MA, United States

Drew Edwards, MS, EdD, Neurogenesis Project, Jacksonville, FL, United States

Mark S. Gold, MD, Washington University in St Louis, School of Medicine, St. Louis, MO, United States

Jennifer M. Gómez, PhD, Department of Psychology, Merrill Palmer Skillman Institute for Child & Family Development, Wayne State University, and Center for Institutional Courage, Detroit, MI, United States

Elizabeth Goren, PhD, Private Practice, New York, NY, United States

Sue Grand, PhD, Private Practice, Teaneck, NJ, United States

Philip Hemphill, PhD, Tulane University, School of Social Work, New Orleans, LA, United States

Linda Knauss, PhD, School of Human Service Professions, Widener University, Chester, PA, United States

Stephen B. Levine, MD, Private Practice and Case Western Reserve University, Cleveland, OH, United States

Lauren Meaux, MA, Department of Psychology, University of Alabama, Tuscaloosa, AL, United States

Laura K. Noll, PhD, Department of Psychological Sciences, Northern Arizona University, Flagstaff, AZ, United States

Alexis Polles, MD, Professionals Resource Network, Fernandina Beach, FL, United States

Kenneth S. Pope, PhD, ABPP, Independent Practice, Norwalk, CT, United States

Frederic G. Reamer, PhD, School of Social Work, Rhode Island College, Providence, RI, United States

Monique N. Rodriguez, PhD, The University of New Mexico, Albuquerque, NM; body-centered Gestalt therapist in Private Practice, Albuquerque, NM, United States

Gary R. Schoener, MEq, Walk-In Counseling Center, Minneapolis, MN, United States

Arlene (Lu) Steinberg, PsyD, Ferkauf Graduate School of Psychology, and Private Practice, New York, NY, United States

Pratyusha Tummala-Narra, PhD, PhD Program in Counseling Psychology, Boston College, Chestnut Hill, MA, United States

Amy Wenzel, PhD, ABPP, Main Line Center for Evidence-Based Psychotherapy, Bryn Mawr, PA, United States

Janet Wohlberg, Therapist Exploitation Link Line (TELL) Founder, Williamstown, MA, United States

Foreword

We've long needed the book you hold in your hands or see on your screen. This comprehensive source thoughtfully covers the history, research, laws, and ethics of sexual boundary violations committed by psychotherapists and clergy and also offers practical guidance.

The curious history of this topic shows the need for a guide to help us—as individuals, institutions, and organizations—avoid both sliding down a slippery slope ourselves and holding back as guilty bystanders when we see others at risk or already heading toward harm that we could try to prevent. This volume fills that need. It shows us that although nonsexual boundary crossing may be helpful or hurtful depending on the situation, sexual boundary crossings (e.g., therapist–patient sex) are always boundary violations, and the responsibility for refraining from victimizing a patient in this way always falls on the shoulders of the therapist or clergy.

Much of what this book discusses was dragged kicking and screaming from a history of willful blindness, moral disengagement, institutional betrayal, and active resistance of a profession that too often professed ignorance. A brief bit of this history follows as context for the information and guidance presented in the chapters.

The ethical prohibition against engaging in sex with a patient stretches far back into history. Brodsky (1989) pointed out that the rule predates the 2,500-year-old Hippocratic Oath: The ancient code of the Nigerian healing arts contained this prohibition. As discussed in this book, it was not until 1977 that the American Psychological Association's (APA; 2017) *Ethical*

Principles of Psychologists and Code of Conduct (hereinafter, APA Ethics Code) included an explicit statement that sexual involvement with clients was unethical. However, 3 years earlier, Hare-Mustin (1974) noted that APA's 1963 code already contained standards that, taken together, prohibited therapists from engaging in sex with their clients. She wrote that "we must conclude from a review of principles relating to competency, community standards and the client relationship that genital contact with patients is ethically unacceptable" (p. 310). Similarly Holroyd testified that APA's 1977 revision codified but "did not change the standard of practice. The standard of practice always precluded a sexual relationship between therapist and patient" (*In the Matter of the Accusation Against: Myron E. Howland,* 1980, pp. 49–50).

Violations of this ethical prohibition and turning a blind eye to those violations also stretch back into history. This book names more than a handful of transgressors who are well-known as prominent pioneers of "the talking cure." The ethical prohibition was clear, but a not-insignificant number of the field's leaders and others were violating the standard according to anonymous surveys of therapists reviewed in this book. Yet the field strongly resisted admitting that violations occurred.

Here are two examples reflecting the resistance to recognition. The first survey of violations in the United States occurred in the late 1960s. The Los Angeles County Psychological Association and the Los Angeles Society of Clinical Psychologists granted Bertram Forer authority to conduct an anonymous survey of their memberships.

The results shocked both organizations. Psychologists had reported a relatively high rate of sexual involvement with their patients. The Board of Directors voted on October 28, 1968, to censor the findings, prohibiting disclosure at professional meetings and in journal articles, reasoning that it was "not in the best interests of psychology to present it publicly" (Forer, 1980).

Also in the 1960s, Greenwald (as cited in Shepard, 1971) urged collecting data on the scope and consequences of psychologists' sexual involvement with their clients:

> I just raised the questions . . . intending, as a clinical psychologist, that it be studied like any other phenomenon. And just for raising the question, some members circulated a petition that I should be expelled from the Psychological Association. (p. 2)

The tendency to resist recognizing violations was still so pervasive that in 1977, Davidson called the phenomenon "psychiatry's problem with no name."

Attempts to hide data and retaliate against researchers began to fail once newspapers started shining a light on the profession's silence on this issue and the effects of that silence (e.g., Bass, 1989). Patients sued their therapists and wrote books that gave voice to their experiences (e.g., Bates & Brodsky, 1989; Freeman & Roy, 1976; Noel & Watterson, 1992; Plaisil, 1985; Walker & Young, 1986), and anonymous surveys of therapists appeared in print. These books and the surveys began to highlight the topic and to help usher in new legislation and case law.

The profession turned to a new form of resistance, an approach commonly used by many organizations facing the fallout of their own wrongdoing, especially wrongdoing by those in positions of leadership, power, and authority. DARVO, which stands for Deny–Attack–Reverse Victim and Offender, a term coined by Freyd (1997; see also Freyd & Birrell, 2013; Harsey et al., 2017) is a clever and often successful maneuver perpetrators use to switch roles with their victim, a strategy also used by organizations. Wrongdoers deny having done anything wrong and launch an attack on their victims, painting themselves as the true victim and their victims as the real offenders. Discussions of DARVO not only appear in the professional and law review literature (e.g., Cantalupo, 2020; Chen & Chen, 2019; Gould, 2019; Javed & Gerrard, 1998; Lubit, 2016; Melville-Wiseman, 2016; Shepp et al., 2020) but have found their way into news articles (e.g., de Moraes, 2017) and popular entertainment (e.g., an episode of *South Park* titled "It's Called DARVO"; Parker & Stone, 2019).

The profession's deployment of DARVO portrayed female patients as the real offenders victimizing innocent, ethical male professionals. This was made clear in the first article accepted for publication in *American Psychologist*, APA's journal of record, that reported and discussed systematically collected data on the topic of therapist–client sex, published in 1971 (Brownfain, 1971). The author analyzed insurance carrier data for malpractice suits filed against psychologists over a 10-year span. He summarized his interpretation of the data by concluding that

> the greatest number of [all malpractice] actions are brought by women who lead lives of very quiet desperation, who form close attachments to their therapists, who feel rejected or spurned when they discover that relations are maintained on a formal and professional level, and who then react with allegations of sexual improprieties. (Brownfain, 1971, p. 651)

He mentioned no instance over the 10-year period in which a woman who sued her therapist for therapist–client sex was *not* considered to be making it all up because the therapist refused to have sex with her.

The attributions about the feelings and motivations women who sue psychologists that were stated in the *American Psychologist* article reflected a more general view about women prevalent among the legal and mental health professions. The 1970 edition of Wigmore's authoritative text

Evidence in Trials at Common Law, which U.S. Supreme Court Justice Felix Frankfurter (1963) wrote (of the previous edition) was "unrivaled as the greatest treatise on any single subject of the law" (p. 443)—presented this view as a settled matter:

> Chastity may have a direct connection with veracity, viz. when a woman or young girl testifies as complainant against a man charged with a sexual crime— rape, rape under age, seduction, assault. Modern psychiatrists have amply studied . . . girls and women coming before the courts in all sorts of cases. Their psychic complexes are multifarious, distorted partly by inherent defects, partly by diseased derangements or abnormal instincts, partly by bad social environment, partly by temporary physiological or emotional conditions. . . . The unchaste (let us call it) mentality finds incidental but direct expression in the narration of imaginary sex incidents of which the narrator is the heroine or the victim. . . . No judge should ever let a sex offense go to the jury unless the female complainant's social history and mental makeup have been examined and testified to by a qualified physician. . . . The reason I think that rape in particular belongs in this category is one well known to psychologists, namely, that fantasies of being raped are exceedingly common in women, indeed one may almost say that they are probably universal. (Wigmore, 1934/1970, pp. 745–746)

About a decade and a half after Brownfain's (1971) *American Psychologist* article and Wigmore's 1970 edition, Wright (1985), relying in part on his extensive experience chairing the APA Insurance Program, addressed those cases, presumed rare at the time, in which a woman's lawsuit against her therapist was based on actual therapist–patient sex. He described how those plaintiffs can prey on vulnerable therapists: Some "consumers recognize the vulnerability of the provider and are attempting to exploit that vulnerability for economic gain" (p. 114). He explained how women who are patients bear a responsibility to set limits on the male therapist's behavior. "The very strong probability that the real reason 'victim/patient' didn't set a limit for the provider . . . was the unwillingness of that same 'victim' to give up personal gratification [the consumer enjoyed in the relationship]" (p. 116; bracketed text appears in the original).

Although Wright attributed an economic motivation to female patients in cases of actual therapist–patient sex, Stone (1990), a former president of the American Psychiatric Association, focused on the economic interests of that professional association: "The point is that the American Psychiatric Association will continue to have an economic interest in defending victimizing doctors who have committed the most egregious sexual exploitation if only to limit the amount of damages awarded" (p. 26).

These views began to shift in the 1970s and 1980s, largely due to the impact of the women's movement and its focus on rape and other kinds of sexual assault of women and girls and to the books and surveys previously mentioned. Another factor was likely the rising number of women entering the profession. Unfortunately, many of them had experiences of sexual harassment or worse by professors in their academic departments, professional training programs, and institutes. The topic of sexual contact in graduate programs and psychotherapy began to open up. This book describes changes to the APA Ethics Code over this time period and into the present. The book also traces how therapist sexual boundary violations largely went underground again over the course of the past 2 decades with only the most egregious coming to light. That has changed in recent years, along with society's increased ability to acknowledge the scope of sexual abuse and assault across society, even in the most private and intimate of settings, such as the family and psychotherapy.

In this Foreword, I've tried to highlight and document a few key aspects of the history in this area. Readers will decide for themselves—based on their own experience, study, discussions, and independent judgment—the degree to which this history lives only in the past or the willful blindness, moral disengagement, institutional betrayal, passive bystanding, active resistance, views of women, and the use of DARVO recounted here live on to some degree. If they live on, how does this influence training, policies, organizations, institutions, the handling of ethics, licensing, or malpractice complaints, and each of us as individuals? And what are we going to do about it?

Regardless of how each of us answers those questions, this history underscores what a remarkable achievement this book is and the potential impact it can have on the field and on each of us.

However, much remains to be done. The writings in this volume make clear that indiscretions, transgressions, misconduct, and criminal behavior continue. This volume provides practical recommendations for prevention, training, and policy development. It allows us to hear the voices of survivors and their stories. It also allows us to hear the voices of researchers, educators, clinical training program directors, treatment center staff, and therapists of different professions and theoretical orientations. Many of these writers have been involved with the topic of sexual boundary violations for decades. Those contributing to this volume focus on topics as varied as ethics, electronic and remote contact, cultural context, and violations outside cisgender–heterosexual dyads.

The fields owes a debt of gratitude to Drs. Steinberg, Alpert, and Courtois for this impressive achievement, and to every author in this book, for moving our field forward.

—*Kenneth S. Pope, PhD*

REFERENCES

American Psychological Association. (2017). *Ethical principles of psychologists and code of conduct* (2002, amended effective June 1, 2010, and January 1, 2017). https://www.apa.org/ethics/code/index.aspx

Bass, A. (1989, April 3). Sexual abuse of patients—Why? High incidence may be due to therapists sense of impunity, inaction by professional groups. *Boston Globe*, pp. 27–28.

Bates, C. M., & Brodsky, A. M. (1989). *Sex in the therapy hour: A case of professional incest*. Guilford Press.

Brodsky, A. M. (1989). Sex between patient and therapist: Psychology's data and response. In G. O. Gabbard (Ed.), *Sexual exploitation in professional relationships* (pp. 15–25). American Psychiatric Press.

Brownfain, J. J. (1971). The APA professional liability insurance program. *American Psychologist, 26*(7), 648–652. https://doi.org/10.1037/h0032052

Cantalupo, N. C. (2020). Title IX & the civil rights approach to sexual harassment in education. *Roger Williams University Law Review, 25*(2), 225–241.

Chen, W. R., & Chen, L. M. (2019). Self-blame tendency of bullied victims in elementary and secondary schools. *Educational Studies, 45*(4), 480–496. https://doi.org/10.1080/03055698.2018.1509772

Davidson, V. (1977). Psychiatry's problem with no name: Therapist–patient sex. *American Journal of Psychoanalysis, 37*, 43–50. https://doi.org/10.1007/BF01252822

de Moraes, L. (2017, October 26). Ashley Judd describes Harvey Weinstein campaign to "Deny, Attack, Reverse Order of Offender and Victim." *Deadline*. https://deadline.com/2017/10/ashley-judd-harvey-weinstein-diane-sawyer-sexual-harassment-attack-deny-abc-video-1202195085/

Forer, B. (1980, February). *The psychotherapeutic relationship: 1968* [Paper presentation]. Annual meeting of the California State Psychological Association, Pasadena, CA.

Frankfurter, F. (1963). John Henry Wigmore: A centennial tribute. *Northwestern University Law Review, 58*, 443.

Freeman, L., & Roy, J. (1976). *Betrayal*. Stein & Day.

Freyd, J. J. (1997). Violations of power, adaptive blindness, and betrayal trauma theory. *Feminism & Psychology, 7*(1), 22–32. https://doi.org/10.1177/0959353597071004

Freyd, J. J., & Birrell, P. J. (2013). *Blind to betrayal*. John Wiley & Sons.

Gould, R. (2019). Working psychodynamically and psychosocially with women who have been raped. *Psychodynamic Practice: Individuals. Groups and Organisations, 25*(3), 208–222.

Hare-Mustin, R. T. (1974). Ethical considerations in the use of sexual contact in psychotherapy. *Psychotherapy: Theory, Research, & Practice, 11*(4), 308–310. https://doi.org/10.1037/h0086370

Harsey, S. J., Zurbriggen, E. L., & Freyd, J. J. (2017). Perpetrator responses to victim confrontation: DARVO and victim self-blame. *Journal of Aggression, Maltreatment & Trauma, 26*(6), 644–663. https://doi.org/10.1080/10926771.2017.1320777

In the matter of the accusation against: Myron E. Howland. (1980). Before the Psychology Examining Committee, Board of Medical Quality Assurance, State of California, No. D-2212. Reporters' transcript. Vol. 3.

Javed, N. S., & Gerrard, N. (1998). Border crossing and living our contradictions. *Women & Therapy, 21*(2), 89–100. https://doi.org/10.1300/J015v21n02_07

Lubit, R. (2016). A child's perspective on the role of therapists in custody battles. *Journal of Psychology & Clinical Psychiatry, 6*(4), 364–368. https://doi.org/10.15406/jpcpy.2016.06.00364

Melville-Wiseman, J. (2016). The sexual abuse of vulnerable people by registered social workers in England: An analysis of the Health and Care Professions Council Fitness to Practise cases. *British Journal of Social Work, 46*(8), 2190–2207. https://doi.org/10.1093/bjsw/bcw150

Noel, B., & Watterson, K. (1992). *You must be dreaming.* Poseidon.

Parker, T., & Stone, M. (Executive Producers). (2019, November 8). It's called DARVO [Season finale]. *South Park* [TV series]. https://www.youtube.com/watch?v=4Jd3Ml7YsDk

Plaisil, E. (1985). *Therapist.* St. Martin's/Marek.

Shepard, M. (1971). *The love treatment: Sexual intimacy between patients and psychotherapists.* Wyden.

Shepp, V., O'Callaghan, E., & Ullman, S. E. (2020). Interactions with offenders post-assault and their impacts on recovery: A qualitative study of sexual assault survivors and support providers. *Journal of Aggression, Maltreatment & Trauma, 29*(6), 725–747. https://doi.org/10.1080/10926771.2019.1660443

Stone, A. A. (1990, March). No good deed goes unpunished. *The Psychiatric Times,* 24–27.

Walker, E., & Young, T. D. (1986). *A killing cure.* Holt, Rinehart & Winston.

Wigmore, J. H. (1970). *Evidence in trials at common law.* Little, Brown. (Original work published 1934)

Wright, R. H. (1985). The Wright way: Who needs enemies? *Psychotherapy in Private Practice, 3,* 111–118. https://doi.org/10.1300/J294v03n02_15

Acknowledgments

In editing this book, our focus is on those who have been violated in the course of psychotherapy. We want to acknowledge what they have been through and the impact such transgressions have had. We also wish to provide psychotherapists information and resources to facilitate the seeking of support and consultation and for these to be more accessible and less shame-laden. Each of us has either had personal experiences of sexual harassment and other inappropriate behavior as supervisees or have dealt with the transgressions of colleagues, supervisees, consultees, and employees and treated numerous victimized clients. These experiences have spurred our interest in addressing this important topic. It is our fervent hope that this volume contributes to making it less likely that others experience the betrayal of sexual boundary violation in psychotherapy. We thank those who have bravely come forward to attest to their experiences, and we particularly acknowledge those who shared their stories in this volume.

We are grateful to all the authors who contributed chapters to this volume. All of the chapter authors had to "meet" with and respond to all three of us at various points. This degree of intensive communication can be difficult, and we are most appreciative of their telling these important stories, as well as their exploring the history of and grappling with this difficult subject.

Lu and Judie wish to acknowledge and express particular appreciation to Elliot Jurist, as past editor of *Psychoanalytic Psychology*, the journal of the Society for Psychoanalysis and Psychoanalytic Psychology (American Psychological Association Division 39), who supported our first foray into addressing sexual boundary violations by editing a special issue (April 2017) on this important topic. The journal was dedicated to Muriel Dimen, a renowned psychoanalyst who died too early and at a time when she had so much more to say. Muriel was a pioneer sharing her own early experience of being violated (Dimen, 2011), making it easier for others to tell their story. We also thank Division 39 as well as Division 56 (Division of Trauma Psychology) for providing support in myriad ways and for giving us professional homes. We are especially thankful to Division 39 for being active and supportive in establishing the Division of Trauma Psychology.

All three of us also wish to acknowledge Susan Reynolds, our initial editor at APA Books, who encouraged and shepherded us along as this book developed. We also acknowledge the contributions of and support of Emily Ekle and Beth Hatch at APA Books, as well as others on the staff who buoyed us at various stages of this process.

I, Lu, thank my family, inspired by my Holocaust-survivor parents who withstood adversity; stressed the importance of ethics, integrity, and generosity; and worked to ameliorate the suffering of others. I thank my husband (Dr. Michael Schulder) for his encouragement and belief in me; his tireless commitment, hard work, and dedication to the healing of others has inspired me. I thank my children, Talia and Ilana (and Daniel Ross, who recently joined our family), for their kindness, sensitivity, integrity, and creativity. I am grateful for their endless inspiration. I thank Judie Alpert for being such a wonderful mentor and friend, for always encouraging the trauma story to be told, and for introducing me to Chris Courtois, whom I hope to meet in person one day. It has been an honor to work with you both.

I, Judie, thank my three grandchildren (Jake, Ben, and Sia Laddis), who, despite their youth, demonstrate integrity, decency, kindness, and honesty that I find inspiring; they make me even more committed to doing what I can to make the world a better place. Also I thank their parents, my daughter and son-in-law, Dr. Ivanya Alpert and Dr. Dimitri Laddis, for all that they do professionally and personally (and they do so much) to create a better world. I also thank Herb, Ronda, Michael, Noah, Meg, and Navah (who will be very excited to see her name in print). And Dan—just because! Editing a book with three editors can present challenges; I am delighted to say that I learned so much working with my coeditors and grew even fonder of both.

And I, Chris, wish to express my heartfelt thanks to Judie and Lu for the invitation to join them in this endeavor after they had started it and for the warm and productive working relationship that developed among us. I also express gratitude to those who have been there for me, foremost, my husband, Tom; my late and highly devoted parents; my sister Claire Riley;

my cousin Gail Sirois; my dear friend and former business partner, Dr. Joan Turkus; devoted friends and consultants Drs. Leslie Jadin and Cathi Sitzman; Drs. Ellen Baker, Bethany Brand, Laura Brown, Jean Carter, Marilene Cloitre, Julian Ford, Jeffrey Jay, Philip Kinsler, Sylvia Marotta-Walters, Laurie Anne Pearlman, Steven Stein, Philip Silverman, Kathy Steele, Deb Stokes, and colleagues in Division 56 of the American Psychological Association, the International Society for Traumatic Stress Studies, and the International Society for the Study of Trauma and Dissociation; as well and many others who have both supported and spurred me on over the years. A special outreach to and appreciation of the dedicated staff of The CENTER: Posttraumatic Disorders Program, who withstood both the impact and the turmoil of colleague betrayal and remained dedicated to the work.

All three of us also thank Talia Schulder for her help with this book. Talia's keen writing and editing ability were very helpful, as was her perspective on the contents of this volume. We also want to express appreciation to our friend/colleague/psychoanalyst Dr. Donna Bassin, who conveys in her photographs what can't be readily captured in words, and who agreed to let us use one for this book's cover. We also thank the #MeToo movement for bringing this topic to public attention. Let's hope societal awareness of the possibility for the abuse of power in so many professions and contexts will not again recede from memory.

We also wish to acknowledge those luminaries in the field who paved the way for this book, particularly Glen Gabbard, Andrea Celenza, Ken Pope, Peter Rutter, Gary Schoener, Nanette Gartrell, Annette Brodsky, Thomas Gutheil, Robert Simon, their colleagues, and Jan Wolberg and the responders at TELL, The Therapy Exploitation Link Line, who have never shied away from confronting the occupational danger of sexual boundary violations and who, while sharing sobering predictions, have never averted their gaze from this crucial topic.

—*Lu Steinberg, Judie Alpert, and Christine Courtois*

REFERENCE

Dimen, M. (2011). *Lapsus linguae*, or a slip of the tongue? A sexual violation in an analytic treatment and its personal and theoretical aftermath. *Contemporary Psychoanalysis, 47*(1), 35–79.

SEXUAL BOUNDARY VIOLATIONS IN PSYCHOTHERAPY

1 SEXUAL BOUNDARY VIOLATIONS IN THE PSYCHOTHERAPY SETTING

An Overview

ARLENE (LU) STEINBERG, JUDITH L. ALPERT, AND CHRISTINE A. COURTOIS

The recent #MeToo movement has placed a spotlight on various types of sexual intrusions and violations across many professions and occupations. The psychotherapy setting is not an exception, and in fact, the nature of psychotherapeutic work may contribute to particular vulnerabilities, given the powerful and intimate emotions and issues addressed in this dyadic process. Indiscretions, transgressions, and misconduct in all these settings may range from behaviors that are somewhat subtle and uncomfortable to those that are blatant, coerced, physically intrusive, and highly traumatic. They can range from comments and looks, increasingly intimate and invasive touching, sexual comments and conversation, and sexual contact and behaviors, up to and including rape. They can involve grooming, that is, deliberate manipulation, emotional abuse and pressure that can have profound and life-changing effects on the victimized client and others both at the time and later. Due to their occurrence within an ongoing relationship of significance, these violations have now also been identified as involving betrayal trauma. The perpetrators of such abuses may range from those with the intent to harm and manipulate; to those who begin a path of grooming

https://doi.org/10.1037/0000247-001
Sexual Boundary Violations in Psychotherapy: Facing Therapist Indiscretions, Transgressions, and Misconduct, A. Steinberg, J. L. Alpert, and C. A. Courtois (Editors)

and manipulation without awareness; to those who, in forming strong therapeutic bonds with their patients, develop unhealthy, and even harmful, dynamics. No matter the intent, all abusive behaviors must be addressed, understood, and, through greater analysis, thwarted.

Sexual boundary violations (SBVs), like other forms of sexual assault and harassment, have devastating consequences for victim-patients, including their subsequent mental and physical health, their intimate and parenting relationships, and their overall well-being. Furthermore, SBVs often have damaging, if not devastating, consequences for offending psychotherapists as well, and they can have profoundly detrimental effects (collateral damage) on third parties, such as spouses and children, and on colleagues, friends, or other patients of the transgressive therapist who often suffer directly or vicariously. For both victimized patient and perpetrating therapist, developmental trajectories can become skewed or derailed, with marriages and families shattered—and lives, careers, and reputations ruined. Suicide (and at times, homicide) might also be a risk for the victim, the perpetrator, and third parties, as intense emotions are evoked in all parties. In addition, institutions and organizations where misconduct occurs can be affected detrimentally, especially if its leaders or clinical supervisors have been sexually inappropriate and the organization has historically tolerated a sexualized atmosphere or "turned a blind eye" toward sexual misconduct. Organizations, their agents, and their members may resist developing ways to prevent boundary violations from recurring or to adequately process the impact of these transgressions on other members and patients. Lawsuits and negative publicity may also derail an organization, even to the point of causing its demise, as has happened in at least one psychoanalytic institute and several inpatient programs.

Psychotherapists therefore need to understand the vulnerabilities involved in committing such violations, their personal and professional impact and the number and seriousness of possible consequences. Because most violations rarely occur in a vacuum but may be part of a progression from boundary crossing to transgression to violation, training on means of identifying therapist vulnerability and risk factors (such as personal and relational crises, isolation, life changes and losses, inattention to one's self-care and emotional health, substance and behavioral addictions, or other impairment and personality dynamics) are crucial. Although some psychotherapists have been found to be serial perpetrators who carefully and systematically groom their patients into participation in sexual activities through manipulation and misinformation, many others may be in the throes of situational problems.

The term *slippery slope* refers to a process in which minor boundary *crossings* occur, accumulate, and lead to other, more serious boundary *violations*, such as progressive seduction, romantic entanglements, and sexual activities. Although this term connotes a therapist not being able to stop once in the process and on the downward slope, throughout this book, it is noted that there are many points along the way where the therapist could and should seek outside consultation rather than simply and passively continuing the slide (Wohlberg, 2019). Often therapists do not do so due to shame and fear of judgment and their resistance to addressing transference and countertransference or to their lack of understanding of posttraumatic enactments. Rather than being acted out, acted upon, enacted, or reenacted, these noted patterns of behavior leading to greater vulnerability need to be understood by the psychotherapist through training, self-reflection or with the help of peers, consultants, and supervisors and used to better understand their own and their patient's dynamics. Therapists who treat patients who have previously been relationally victimized (especially through incest and other forms of child sexual abuse and thus suffered significant betrayal trauma) must understand their patient's particular vulnerability to all forms of revictimization, especially sexual. They must understand that traumatic transference and enactments may instead be misunderstood as erotic transference and, rather than acting on it and retraumatizing the patient, use this differentiation to assist them in learning to stay safe and avoid further abuse.

To move toward prevention, we recommend detailed education about sexuality, appropriate boundaries, SBVs, and the typical dynamics of their occurrence, encouraging open discussion in mandatory and ongoing training, consultation, and supervisory settings that is repeated periodically over the course of the therapist's career. This book can provide a critical piece of that education by exploring the boundary challenges therapists confront, including discussion of the erotic transference and countertransference that can arise; considering SBVs among different orientations and within different settings, including the more recent risks confronted in digital and virtual communication; and addressing particular risks arising within racial and cultural contexts as well as outside of cisgender/heterosexual dyads. This volume also explores grooming as viewed through the eyes of victim-peer advocates as well as explored by clinicians. It includes the voices of both the survivor and the clinician. The reverberating traumatic impact of SBVs within organizations, institutes, and professional communities is also discussed, even as it might contribute to their occurrence. In addition, the subsequent treatment of the SBV survivor, as well as the supervision and treatment of the offending therapist, are discussed. In addition, because clergy are frequently in a pastoral counseling role, a chapter is devoted to clergy abuse. The book intends to provide a framework for understanding and discussing these issues in training and supervision. As we emphasize, there is no substitute for education as well as quality clinical supervision and consultation.

This volume pays careful attention to the complex dynamics expressed in different transference–countertransference constellations and those associated with the patient's traumatic history. Although situations involving psychopathic predatory therapists are the most negative scenarios, viewing SBVs as binary occurrences (situational or slippery slope vs. psychopathic predator) is limiting and can be thought of as reductionist. Each therapeutic dyad has unique aspects and challenges. Therapeutic work takes place in terrain that at times can feel treacherous, as the most intimate aspects of patients' lives are expressed, enacted, and shared with another—namely, the therapist. Besides the personal characteristics of either therapist or patient that may contribute to vulnerability, there are likely to be particular characteristics of the dyad that create greater vulnerability.

Training programs and practice organizations or agencies should provide training and policies for all members on issues such as the following:

- What are warning signs?

- Are patients offered sufficient information regarding the impropriety and illegality of sexual contact between therapists and patients and means of reporting concerns and transgressions?

- How and when do supervisors or peers intervene if they notice something awry?

- When do they report their suspicions and to whom? What happens then?

- How are the victim-patient who report and disclose abuse and others who are impacted responded to and taken care of?

- When abuse is founded, how does the violation impact the agents and other members of the institution, whether patients or colleagues and the general public, and how is its impact dealt with?

- When and how should a therapist be removed, and how and when is rehabilitation and reinstatement possible?

- Was the institution somehow complicit due to lack of attention to reports of sexual and other boundary crossings and violations? Did it condone, whether implicitly or explicitly, various types of misbehavior on the part of staff?

- What about therapist–wrongdoers? Should they lose their job or be suspended or put on administrative leave?

- When a report is made to the licensing board or to police authorities, should their license be suspended immediately or revoked? How is that determined?

- If they are permitted to continue in practice during adjudication of the complaint, should they do so only under close supervision or monitoring? Should they be mandated into treatment and supervision, and if so, how should these be conducted?

- Can some offending therapists be rehabilitated and allowed to return to practice? Should they be? On what basis is that determined?

- What about criminal charges and civil lawsuits that often occur in parallel with reports of sexual misconduct? Should some offending therapists be jailed or made to register as sex offenders, as is called for in some states? Should they be barred from being able reestablish their credentials and return to practice by moving to another state, or should there be an effective national database available to all licensing boards that would prevent them from doing so?

These are some of the complex and often compounding issues that command attention and that we address in this specialized text.

The remainder of this chapter presents a broad cultural context for understanding SBVs in psychotherapy, followed by an overview of the book's content and organization.

SEXUAL BOUNDARY VIOLATIONS IN CONTEXT

The problem of SBVs in psychotherapy is not new. The history of #Me too–like movements runs parallel to the mental health field's ongoing difficulty confronting sexual abuse and boundary violations. Approximately 40 years ago, the women's liberation movement began to address sexual and physical harassment and assaults of women in the family, the workplace, and in the larger community, topics that had previously been taboo. During that time period, women met in a new format known as consciousness-raising groups, disclosing their secrets, emotions, and life stories. Among other topics, some divulged being violated in their own homes by fathers, other relatives, trusted friends or acquaintances, within professional relationships, and in their communities by total strangers. Inappropriate and sexualized relationships with and manipulative ploys by psychotherapists were also disclosed, as was sex between medical professionals and patients and educators and students or supervisees in clinical as well as other training settings across virtually all professions. In addition, sexual abuse by clergy members, pastoral counselors, coaches, bosses, colleagues, senior officers and peers in the military, and in virtually any setting was disclosed. It became depressingly clear that virtually nowhere was safe from such pressure or predation.

There was limited legal attention to these issues at the time. Although rape and incest had criminal statutes in most states, other forms of sexual assault and child abuse less so. The ongoing study of all forms of child abuse led to the tightening of some laws and reporting statutes in most states. Much changed when the U.S. Supreme Court held that sexual harassment is sex discrimination and is subject to prosecution. MacKinnon (1979) had previously identified that sexual harassment should be subject to equal protection laws as sex discrimination had been.

Nevertheless, between these two periods of time (roughly the early 1970s to the present), despite having been so widely publicized and acknowledged (Kilberg et al., 1986; Rutter, 1991; Schoener et al., 1989), issues of the sexual violation of women and children again began to fade into the background. During that middle period, several myths regarding such abuse developed. Among the most pervasive was that such transgressions are rare, not serious, and cause little harm. Stated simply but conclusively, these myths are just that—myths. Moreover, they are a form of denial, of whitewashing or gaslighting the problem to make it go away. Because these topics are uncomfortable, controversial, and continue to be taboo, they tend to be avoided, denied, or downplayed, with reports and complaints often delayed as well as disbelieved, especially if the alleged perpetrator is powerful, famous, rich, violent, or vindictive. Victims who complained were (and are) frequently discredited and disbelieved—and at worst, attacked, shamed, and shunned. The pushback and backlash could be brutal as many survivors, advocates, and psychotherapists learned when they were singled out for "suggesting memories of abuse that had not occurred" by "false memory" critics (Alpert, 1995) or were accused of consenting to the sexual contact and seeking financial gain in civil lawsuits by aggressive attorneys. Rape and sexual abuse deniers jumped on this bandwagon, in the process setting back the burgeoning movement and once again placing the blame on the victims and their supporters.

Feminist activist and clinical researcher Dr. Judith Herman (1992) wrote that the topic of trauma in general—and various types of interpersonal and gender-based trauma in particular—has had a strange intellectual and cultural history. Trauma tends to be identified and studied extensively during periods of societal upheaval, such as during wartime and afterward, only to fade from view when the social surround is less urgent and vocal. She argued that emotionally aversive issues such as child abuse and the sexual assault of children and adults can only receive ongoing attention if a large enough segment of society is willing to believe in their occurrence and to consistently take up the causes of identification, intervention, and prevention (Herman, 1992). *Collective shrouding* seems to have also happened between the two "MeToo moments," when not only sexual harassment and assault of women but also issues of incest and child sexual abuse again began to recede into the shadows. In clinical and other professional circles, accurate descriptive language became muted (i.e., incest was referred to as child sexual abuse or child maltreatment, obscuring that the perpetrator was a relative or that the abuse was sexual).

Research at the time substantiated that most victims of sexual violations were female. Another common yet hidden form of sexual victimization, that of boys and men, came to light in 2002, when the clergy abuse scandal in the Catholic Church could no longer be contained or concealed. It exploded into public awareness due to the dogged investigation conducted by the investigative staff of the *Boston Globe* (2002) and the determination of victims, both alone and in groups, to bring the abuse and its coverup to public scrutiny. Consequently, more men overcame their shame and their gender training to disclose that they had been sexually abused. More abuses were disclosed including those perpetrated not only by members of the Catholic clergy but by those in other denominations, as well as by others in positions of authority over young boys, including family members; teachers and staff in public, private, and residential schools; in the Boy Scouts; in sports; and in the military. Significant coverups by organization leadership and bystander members demonstrated "organizational betrayal" (Smith & Freyd, 2014).

Increasingly, other organizations where abuse occurred and had been covered up are being held accountable. In addition, the issue of sexual harassment in the workplace is being addressed in Hollywood, with celebrities disclosing their experiences of sexual pressure, harassment, exploitation, abuse, assault, and rape at the hands of famous producers, directors, and fellow actors. Extensive coverups by the perpetrators and others in the news and entertainment industry were also exposed, some of which involved settlements in the millions, paired with nondisclosure agreements to keep the abuses concealed (Farrow, 2019; Kantor & Twohey, 2019). Many women in Hollywood began using the #MeToo tag, originally started by Tarana Burke in 2006 as a social media tool to raise awareness of and show solidarity with victims of sexual violence (Ohlheiser, 2017). Victims are now more likely to be believed than at any time previously, although activists expect a backlash and fear that one is already underway, even as headway is being made. At the time of this writing, Harvey Weinstein had just been found guilty on two counts and sentenced to 23 years behind bars. He purports not to understand why this has happened *now* because that's essentially how things happened *then*. That says it all. Despite this, it is a hopeful sign that millions are now more attuned to the problem of sexual misconduct and predation and their broad scope; activists are working hard to educate the public to the nuances associated with the trauma of sexual assault. They are also working to intervene and curb it by pressing state legislatures to change archaic laws such as statutes of limitations.

In this milieu, it is only fitting that sexual harassment, violations, and misconduct in all professional settings should emerge for greater public scrutiny. Psychotherapy is one such setting. It is an unfortunate truth that SBVs were known to occur in psychotherapy virtually from its inception (Gabbard & Lester, 1995; Celenza, 2007), involving many of the pioneers of the early fields of psychoanalysis and the human potential movement. Some early feminist therapists also developed sexual relationships with clients under the aegis of empowerment and equality, and sexual contact between religious leaders—some of them in their pastoral role and others serving as pastoral counselors—and their congregant clients have long been an open secret in some congregations and settings. Historically, sexual contact between a therapist and patient has even been the subject of some debate as to its morality, ethicality, propriety, and legitimacy, with the pendulum swinging widely between the two extremes from the few advocates who considered its occurrence therapeutic to those critics, in much greater number, who damned it as extremely damaging to all parties but especially the victim-patient (Pope, 1990; Pope et al., 2006).

Today, sexual contact between a psychotherapist and a patient is regarded as unethical and as morally and ethically wrong in all major mental health and medical professions. In many states, it is against the law. Therapists owe a fiduciary duty of protection and safety as part of their professional obligation to the patient (Pope & Keith-Spiegel, 2008; Reamer, 2012). However, despite these ethical and legal prohibitions, such SBVs unfortunately have not gone away. In fact, they may have increased (Gabbard, 2017). Clearly, not every psychotherapist or other mental health professional becomes sexually involved with patients. Yet data derived from a national pool of mental health professionals representing various disciplines indicate that in the United States, between 7% and 12% of therapists have sexual contact with their patients (Borys & Pope, 1989; Jackson & Nuttal, 2001; Pope et al., 1987), although these prevalence studies are in need of updating. Because sexual misconduct is a difficult topic to research due to secrecy, conceal-ment, shame, nondisclosure, and other attachment-based trauma dynamics (e.g., attachment and loyalty to the abuser) and because most of the studies involve self-report by abusive therapists and victims, it is reasonable to suggest that the problem might be more pervasive than has been believed or previously reported. Whatever the true prevalence, a conservative rate of 10% is both shocking and totally unacceptable.

Therapist SBVs merit ongoing and increased investigation and more sophisticated attempts at education, prevention, and intervention for both offender and victim. At present, services for victims who formally report their experiences of abuse are lacking. It is ironic that licensing boards offer intervention to accused therapists but do not offer the same to reporting victims, a disparity that has largely gone unrecognized until recently. The result is that many victims remain isolated and left to cope on their own. In addition, many organizations and training facilities have few mechanisms or clear policies for prevention or addressing reported violations.

PURPOSE OF THIS BOOK

This book is designed as a core resource for clinical and counseling psychology, other mental health and behavioral health training and service programs, and practicing psychotherapists. It should be of value to trainers, super-visors, students and supervisees, employers, and practitioners who seek a real-world practical resource on the topic of SBVs in psychotherapy and other professional relationships. It will also be of interest to members of allied professions; members of state licensing boards, state lawmakers, and their staff; attorneys involved in criminal and civil litigation of cases of sexual transgression; and victims and their supporters.

The primary focus of the text is sexual misconduct in psychotherapy; however, such violations also occur in related contexts, such as clinical training programs, academic settings and institutes, and within teaching, supervisory, counseling, and employment relationships. The content of this text is suitable as a foundation for professional and training curricula and additionally for continuing education programs. The topics of boundaries, including the various dilemmas that occur in clinical relationships requiring careful navigation and the risks of SBVs, belong in all ethics courses and across the clinical training program; unfortunately, at present, it is usually squeezed into such training, often with the admonishment that because it is the major cause of malpractice lawsuits against therapists, it is to be avoided. Warnings of this sort primarily address monetary and status loss and not the other more personal damage to all parties that can accrue from such malpractice. Historically, some of the ethics training and the responses to reports by licensing boards and outside authorities have involved victim-blaming rather than holding the therapist responsible. This type of tepid ethical and risk management warning and associated victim-blaming rarely, if ever, includes attention to the characteristics of transgressive therapists, to risk factors and vulnerabilities, to difficulties addressing sexual feelings (Pope et al., 1993) and identifying and addressing erotic transference or countertransference (Celenza, 2014) in treatment relationships, or to the severe consequences of sexual enactment to these psychotherapists, their patients, and others.

When held responsible, transgressive therapists are frequently treated as "the other" and shunned by their colleagues, with the implication that such temptations or violations do not occur to the average practitioner, whether in private practice or institutional settings. However, according to research on the topic, this is far from the case. In addition to idiosyncratic factors in the treatment relationship, which might be contributory, research has identified other personal-subjective, contextual, or situational factors that can result in the loss of boundaries that result in sexual contact between therapist and patient. For example, some victims and therapists are particularly vulnerable due to their own histories of attachment trauma and child abuse. Whatever the circumstance, the ultimate responsibility for the maintenance of boundaries and a professional relationship and treatment rests exclusively with the professional. To a lesser extent, it rests with the training programs, institutions, employers, and supervisors (vicarious responsibility and liability), especially those who do not adequately prepare therapists for the challenges they might encounter treating a particular population of patients or who do not provide them with resources for support and consultation. Additionally, it might implicate colleagues and other third parties who turn a blind eye, minimize, or otherwise do not notice or who, in other ways, protect the therapist or do not intervene when something is obviously awry (the passive bystander phenomenon).

We have sought to include topics that have not received much attention in the extant professional literature, such as the narratives and voices of the abused; power dynamics outside of traditional cisgender-heterosexual (cishet) pairings; those related to race and ethnicity and exacerbated by racism; the special vulnerability of patients who are victims of incest; the grooming, reenactments, and other dynamics that result in "professional incest"; the matter of colleagues and institutions who stand by and do not intervene when abuse is suspected or reported or who actively cover up and attack the reporting victim or their supporters; the impact on the transgressor's other patients should the abuse become known; the dilemmas of the therapist treating patients abused in a previous psychotherapy (some of whom may still be in the relationship with that therapist or who are left with significant feelings of ambivalence and distress due to traumatic rupture); and the dilemmas associated with treating or providing remedial supervision to the perpetrator therapist (completely different roles and functions that need to be kept separate so as not to create another dual relationship).

Also included is a focus on the transgressions of pastoral counselors, a topic that has not yet received enough consideration in the psychotherapy literature. The possibility of remediation for the offending therapist or counselor and a return to the practice of psychotherapy and counseling are addressed, as are the circumstances where it is inadvisable, even with a supervisor in place. The roles of licensing boards and state laws as well as ethics codes and policies in professional organizations in making these determinations are also discussed. In addition, the unique challenges and the new "slippery slope" associated with the digital age and its various forms of communication are addressed. Despite the inclusion of these many topics, this text is not comprehensive. It does not include the voices of perpetrators. Nor does it address in any detail issues of public policy and legislation or the need for a comprehensive national reporting database that is effective in keeping therapists whose licenses were revoked from moving from state to state to start anew. We encourage our colleagues to take up the study of these topics to better understand them and their dynamics and to prevent and intervene.

Recent work by two of the coeditors supports the relevance of this effort and prospectus. Alpert and Steinberg coedited a special issue of *Psychoanalytic Psychology* (Volume 34, No. 2, April 2017) on SBVs. The journal was well received, attesting to the need for such material. In fact, Alpert's and Steinberg's (2017) article, "Sexual Boundary Violations: A Century of Violations and a Time to Analyze," was the top-downloaded article from *Psychoanalytic Psychology* on the PsycNet platform in 2017. The journal issue included exploration of historical, theoretical, and conceptual issues and the impact of sexual violations, including those that do not involve physical enactments but that are more verbal, emotionally coercive, or seductive. Also, there was consideration of why an SBV is, in fact, a collapse of the relationship and a betrayal to the commitment made to the patient, why SBVs occur, and why they result in such distressing consequences. Attention was also given to the issue of collective silence and shrouding and to the collateral damage or the impact of the violation on the professional community, the transgenerational aspect of SBVs, the perspective of the field of sex therapy and its firm stand against therapist sexual or romantical involvement with patients, and the ethics and other codes of conduct of various professional organizations.

Additionally, the third editor (Courtois) has written and edited a number of books on the treatment of adults with histories of incest (Courtois, 2010) and other forms of child abuse, adult rape, complex trauma, the spiritual impact of such abuses, and betrayal trauma (including colleague betrayal on the part of transgressive therapists and their supporters or passive bystanders) (Courtois, 2017). These writings also have been well received across the helping professions.

ORGANIZATION OF THIS BOOK

This text includes 20 chapters and an epilogue, divided into five parts. The majority of the chapter contributors are therapists, representing many treatment orientations and professions. They are also clinical researchers and educator/supervisors of clinical training programs and directors and staff of treatment clinics or private practices. The voices of survivors, including some who serve as peer advocates, are also included in this volume. Ken Pope, one of the pioneer researchers of therapist SBVs, whose writing focuses on education, intervention, and prevention of such abuses, provided the Foreword to the book.

Part I begins with a historical overview, including discussion of the ethics code as well as boundaries, as a context for discussion of SBVs and other misconduct. Chapter 2, by Linda Campbell, Linda Knauss, and Lauren Meaux, traces the development of the American Psychological Association (APA; 2017) *Ethical Principles of Psychologists and Code of Conduct*. Trends in APA disciplinary sanctions are discussed, along with legal statutes regarding sexual misconduct in psychotherapy and forensic trends and patterns within and across states. In Chapter 3, Stephen Levine and Christine Courtois focus on the need for integrity, morality, and appropriate limitations and boundaries in the psychotherapeutic relationship, all intended to protect the patient and the treatment.

The text's Part II addresses how SBVs have been understood and discussed within several different treatment orientations and approaches. Many of the authors note the dearth of literature on this topic—despite indications that SBVs occur across all orientations—and discuss the difficult histories of boundary violations in their own. In Chapter 4, Andrea Celenza, a psychoanalyst and a pioneer in the field, discusses the history of her work with both transgressors and victims in an interview conducted by Alpert and Steinberg. She shares a variety of perspectives derived from her experience working with a range of individuals, the fallout for all involved, her views and beliefs about possibilities for rehabilitation, and her stance on prevention. She also discusses her thoughts regarding erotic transferences.

In Chapter 5, Elizabeth Goren and Sue Grand discuss erotic idealization within a psychodynamic/psychoanalytic treatment. In Chapter 6, Amy Wenzel presents a cognitive-behavioral approach to understanding SBVs. Monique Rodriguez, in Chapter 7, discusses going beyond the contact boundary in gestalt therapy, noting a difficult history within the humanistic tradition. In Chapter 8, Elizabeth Goren presents an analytic sex therapy perspective, and Laura Brown and Christine Courtois discuss sexual misconduct in the feminist therapy realm in Chapter 9.

Part III focuses on unique settings and populations. In Chapter 10, Courtois and Steinberg address violations by clergy in their roles as spiritual authorities and pastoral counselors and the unique issues and vulnerabilities involved in these settings. Frederick Reamer confronts the unique challenges and novel boundary crossings of the digital age in Chapter 11, reflecting on both the risks and benefits of clients and therapists using various forms of electronic and remote contact as well as social media. Given the recent impact of the pandemic, and the increase in virtual psychotherapy, his writing is particularly timely. He discusses emerging ethical standards and risk management guidelines to protect therapist and client. Pratyusha Tummala-Narra, in Chapter 12, explores the way diversity and cultural context can pose unique risks to therapeutic dyads—namely, the ways power dynamics of cultural and ethnic difference related to race and racism can influence SBVs. Elizabeth Clark and Kori Bennett (Chapter 13) follow with a look at SBVs and power dynamics outside of cishet dyads. These include dyads in which one or both parties are nonheterosexual or are trans/gender expansive, as well as dyads consisting of two cishet women or men.

Part IV focuses on the dynamics and effects of abuse. In Chapter 14, Christine Courtois and Judie Alpert elaborate on the dynamics of grooming, including "gaslighting," attachment and betrayal trauma, trauma reenactment and trauma bonding, and the narcissism that fuels the control and sub-jugation needs of some transgressors. They note that adults who were sexually abused as children are particularly vulnerable to being multiply sexually revictimized later in life, including by psychotherapists and other professionals, and that posttraumatic and dissociative enactments can be misconstrued as erotic transference. In Chapter 15, a companion chapter to Chapter 14, Jan Wohlberg, a cofounder of the Therapist Exploitation Link Line (TELL), a grassroots peer advocacy organization, along with several of the organization's peer responders, discuss the grooming process, includ-ing first-person accounts, by which some therapists manipulate and coerce their patients into sexual relationships. Christine Courtois, Judith Alpert, and Goldie Eder (Chapter 16) gained firsthand information from interviews conducted with three individuals who were sexually abused in treatment, each at a different age and life stage. In Chapter 17, Jennifer Gomez, Laura Knoll, Alexis Adams-Clark, and Christine Courtois examine the relevance of different types of betrayal trauma in understanding SBVs, including the way organizations may enable them and additionally contribute to the trauma-tization of victims and colleague betrayal.

Part IV addresses the aftermath of SBVs in psychotherapy. Tyson Bailey and Laura Brown (Chapter 18) address the unique challenges of being the subsequent treating therapist of clients who have been sexually abused and suffered psychological damage in their prior treatment. In Chapter 19, Gary Schoener, another pioneer in the field, discusses issues in mandated super-vision with those who have engaged in sexual misconduct. In Chapter 20, Philip Hemphill, Christine Courtois, Mark Gold, Alexis Pollis, and Drew Edwards discuss the demands of treating offending therapists and criteria used to assess their possible rehabilitation.

In the epilogue, "Where Can We Go From Here?," Judie Alpert, Lu Steinberg, and Christine Courtois summarize many of the issues discussed in this volume, include clinical material that could help well-intentioned therapists avoid becoming transgressors, and point to the need for ongoing research and education. They make a case for offering more comprehen-sive and sophisticated information on the topic of SBVs on an ongoing and mandatory basis in professional training and license renewal programs. They call for more understanding of erotic transferences and countertransferences and their mismanagement that commonly precede the occurrence of SBVs. Ongoing supervision or expert consultation opportunities at all levels of experience—where therapists can receive assistance in disclosing and assess-ing their feelings without shame or fear of judgment to develop a plan of safe boundary management for all involved—is stressed throughout this volume. Patients seeking psychological assistance deserve nothing less than a treatment that fulfills its mandate of healing.

REFERENCES

Alpert, J. L. (Ed.). (1995). *Sexual abuse recalled: Treating trauma in the era of the recovered memory debate*. Jason Aaronson.

Alpert, J. L., & Steinberg, A. (2017). Sexual boundary violations: A century of violations and a time to analyze. *Psychoanalytic Psychology, 34*(2), 144–150. https://doi.org/10.1037/pap0000094

American Psychological Association. (2017). *Ethical principles of psychologists and code of conduct* (2002, Amended June 1, 2010, and January 1, 2017). http://www.apa.org/ethics/code/ethics-code-2017.pdf

Borys, D. S., & Pope, K. S. (1989). Dual relationships between therapist and client: A national study of psychologist, psychiatrists, and social workers. *Professional Psychology: Research and Practice, 20*(5), 283–293. https://doi.org/10.1037/0735-7028.20.5.283

Boston Globe Investigative Staff. (2002). *Betrayal: The crisis in the Catholic Church*. Back Bay Books.

Celenza, A. (2007). *Sexual boundary violations: Therapeutic, supervisory and academic contexts*. Jason Aronson.

Celenza, A. (2014). *Erotic revelations: Clinical applications and perverse scenarios*. Routledge. https://doi.org/10.4324/9781315773056

Courtois, C. A. (2010). *Healing the incest wound: Adult survivors in therapy* (2nd ed.). W. W. Norton.

Courtois, C. A. (2017). Colleague betrayal: Countertrauma manifestation? In R. B. Gartner (Ed.), *Trauma and countertrauma, resilience and counterresilience: Insight from psychoanalysts and trauma experts* (pp. 251–281). Routledge, Taylor & Francis.

Farrow, R. (2019). *Catch and kill: Lies, spies, and a conspiracy to protect predators*. Little, Brown & Co.

Gabbard, G. O. (2017). Sexual boundary violations in psychoanalysis: A 30-year retrospective. In J. L. Alpert & A. Steinberg (Eds.). (2017). *Psychoanalytic Psychology, 34*(2), 1–24.

Gabbard, G. O., & Lester, E. (1995). *Boundaries and boundary violations in psychoanalysis*. American Psychiatric Press.

Herman, J. (1992). *Trauma and recovery: The aftermath of violence—from domestic abuse to political terror*. Basic Books.

Jackson, H., & Nuttal, R. L. (2001). A relationship between childhood sexual abuse and professional sexual misconduct. *Professional Psychology: Research and Practice, 32*(2), 200–204. https://doi.org/10.1037/0735-7028.32.2.200

Kantor, J., & Twohey, M. (2019). *She said: Breaking the sexual harassment story that helped ignite a movement*. Penguin Books.

Kilberg, R., Nathan, P., & Thoresen, R. (Eds.). (1986). *Professionals in distress: Issues, syndromes, and solutions in psychology*. American Psychological Association. https://doi.org/10.1037/10056-000

MacKinnon, C. (1979). *Sexual harassment of working women: A case of sex discrimination*. Yale University Press.

Ohlheiser, A. (2017, October 19). The woman behind "Me Too" knew the power of the phrase when she created it—10 years ago. *Washington Post.* https://www.washingtonpost.com/news/the-intersect/wp/2017/10/19/the-woman-behind-me-too-knew-the-power-of-the-phrase-when-she-created-it-10-years-ago/

Pope, K. S. (1990). Therapist–patient sexual involvement: A review of the research. *Clinical Psychology Review, 10,* 477–490. https://doi.org/10.1016/0272-7358(90)90049-G

Pope, K. S., & Keith-Spiegel, P. (2008). A practical approach to boundaries in psychotherapy: Making decisions, bypassing blunders, and mending fences. *Journal of Clinical Psychology, 64*(5), 638–652. https://doi.org/10.1002/jclp.20477

Pope, K. S., Sonne, J. L., & Greene, B. (2006). *What therapists don't talk about and why: Understanding taboos that hurt us and our clients.* American Psychological Association. https://doi.org/10.1037/11413-000

Pope, K. S., Sonne, J. L., & Holroyd, J. (1993). *Sexual feelings in psychotherapy: Exploration for therapists and therapists-in-training.* American Psychological Association. https://doi.org/10.1037/10124-000

Pope, K. S., Tabachnick, B. G., & Keith-Spiegel, P. (1987). Ethics of practice: The beliefs and behaviors of psychologists as therapists. *American Psychologist, 42,* 993–1006. https://doi.org/10.1037/0003-066X.42.11.993

Reamer, F. (2012). *Boundary issues and dual relationships in the human services.* Columbia University Press.

Rutter, P. (1991). *Sex in the forbidden zone: When men in power—therapists, doctors, clergy, teachers and others—betray women's trust.* Fawcett.

Schoener, G. R., Milgrom, J. H., Gonsiorek, J. C., Luepker, E. T., & Conroe, R. M. (Eds.). (1989). *Psychotherapists' sexual involvement with clients: Intervention and prevention.* Walk-In Counseling Center.

Smith, C. P., & Freyd, J. J. (2014). Institutional betrayal. *American Psychologist, 69*(6), 575–587. https://doi.org/10.1037/a0037564

Wohlberg, J. (2019). What you should know first: A history of TELL. In Therapy Exploitation Link Line (Ed.), *TELLing it like it is: When therapists abuse and exploit.* https://www.therapyabuse.org/ebook-TELLing-It-Like-It-Is.pdf

PART I ETHICAL AND LEGAL ISSUES

ETHICAL AND
LEGAL ISSUE
Part
1

THE AMERICAN PSYCHOLOGICAL ASSOCIATION ETHICS CODE AND LEGAL STATUTES REGARDING SEXUAL BOUNDARY VIOLATIONS

2

History and Current Status

LINDA CAMPBELL, LINDA KNAUSS, LAUREN MEAUX

The treatment of therapists' sexual behavior in the American Psychological Association's (APA's; 2017) *Ethical Principles of Psychologists and Code of Conduct* (hereinafter, APA Ethics Code) and various state statutes reflects the values and priorities of the profession at the time and represents some of the association's most labored and conflicted decisions. Ambiguity often characterizes the development of APA Ethics Code revisions, particularly on sexual behavior. All psychologists do not share the definition of ethical behavior, the purpose of an ethics code, or acceptance of public accountability. Components of ethics include (a) virtue ethics referencing character, morality, integrity, respect for others, and values; (b) principle ethics in the form of a code of conduct that guides professional behavior; and (c) an educational tool to facilitate decision making. Psychologists may adopt one or more or none of these aspects of ethics, resulting in the ambiguity with which the inclusion of sexual misconduct has evolved in the APA Ethics Code and in legal statutes.

This chapter presents the development of the topic of sexual misconduct in the APA Ethics Code from its inception to the present. The current status

https://doi.org/10.1037/0000247-002
Sexual Boundary Violations in Psychotherapy: Facing Therapist Indiscretions, Transgressions, and Misconduct, A. Steinberg, J. L. Alpert, and C. A. Courtois (Editors)

of state statutes, the APA Ethics Committee reports on sexual misconduct, and licensure regulatory data on sexual misconduct are described. Although the APA Ethics Code does not specify a statement on sexual misconduct until 1977, a brief review of the earlier development of the code in this chapter provides a context.

1953 *ETHICAL STANDARDS OF PSYCHOLOGISTS*

In 1938, APA created the Committee on Scientific and Professional Ethics (the 1938 Committee) and, for the first time in the association's history, developed a procedure to investigate ethics complaints. The 1938 Committee carried out its responsibility through informal and private dispensation of complaints, citing that "it would be never be practical or desirable to devise a complete or rigid code" (Hobbs, 1948, p.80). By 1947, this same committee realized that the association was outgrowing the a priori method and reversed its recommendation in saying that the unwritten code was tenuous, elusive, and unsatisfactory (APA, 1952). Strong positions were taken on the proposal to develop a written code. Calvin Hall declared, "Decent mature people do not need to be told how to conduct themselves" (APA, 1952, p. 430). Contrastingly, James Miller wrote, "In recent decades, major American professional and trade organizations have realized the democratic importance of recording the common will, so should the APA" (APA, 1952, p. 438). By 1947, the new Committee on Ethical Standards decided to adopt the critical incident model of identifying the type and frequency of ethical dilemmas experienced by member psychologists. This critical incident model became the reliable method by which future codes would be developed; however, only in 1952 was the entire membership of 7,500 psychologists surveyed. More than 1,000 responses were submitted and compiled, resulting in the first six sections of the 1953 Code (i.e., public responsibility, client relationships, teaching, research, writing and publishing, and professional relationships).

Among these sections, client relationships laid the foundation for the development of ethical thinking about relationships between psychologists and clients/patients. This section addressed matters such as the prohibition of exaggerating credentials to clients, awareness of one's inadequacies which may bias observations of others (i.e., current terminology of loss of objectivity), the prohibition against misleading clients, use of untrained personnel, and the prohibition against offering psychological services through means of newspaper, magazines, radio, or television. These statements are noted inasmuch as descriptions of client relationships did not broach personal, dual relationships, or sexual relationships.

The 1953 Code did, however, establish the foundation of the continued and current-day standard regarding provision of dual role services: "A psychologist normally should not enter into a clinical relationship with members of his own family, with intimate friends, or with persons so close that their welfare might be jeopardized by the dual relationship" (APA, 1953, p. 4). This 1953 statement became more expansive in subsequent codes but was a core element of the first code. The framers demonstrated a sound perspective also on the inclusion of the initial informed consent statement: "The psychologist is obligated to inform his client of all aspects of the clinical relationship . . . that might reasonably be considered important factors in the client's decision to enter the relationship" (APA, 1953, p. 6). Both dual relationships and informed consent are pillars of the code today and conceptually support the contemporary sexual misconduct standards.

1959 *ETHICAL STANDARDS OF PSYCHOLOGISTS*

The first ethics code, *Ethical Standards of Psychologists*, was adopted in 1953; however, dissatisfaction with the code was immediate. The 1953 Code was viewed as too long (171 pages) and replete with courtesies and moral stances, many of which were not related to ethical conduct. Despite cries of reductionism, a revision of the 1953 code, approved by the APA Council in 1959, included only 18 principles compared with the 1953 Code of 162 principles. All 18 principles have remained in every revision of the code, including the current one, as either principles or standards. A 19th principle was added in 1964 concluding that industrial psychologists were ethically bound to protect the public. As noted earlier, sexual misconduct does not appear in the code per se until 1977; however, an early hint of relational conduct is introduced in Principle 3 of the 1959 Ethics Code. That principle, titled, Moral and Legal Standards, stated,

> The psychologist in the practice of his profession shows sensible regard for the social codes and moral expectations of the community in which he works, recognizing that violations of accepted moral and legal standards on his part may involve his clients, students, or colleagues in damaging personal conflicts, and impugn his own name and the reputation of his profession. (APA, 1959, p. 268)

Additionally, Principle 8(c), Client Relationships, states, "Psychologists do not normally enter into a clinical relationship with members of their own family, intimate friends, close associates, students, or others whose welfare might be jeopardized by such a dual relationship" (APA, 1959, p. 270). This statement is derived from the 1953 Code and expands the principle to include close associates and students.

Between 1959 and 1977, three minor revisions were conducted, in 1963, 1968, and 1972. The only revision made with relevance to the current topic is the change made from *clinical* to *professional* relationships in the principle regarding dual relationships (APA, 1963). Although a small change, this descriptor significantly expanded the clinical range of cautionary dual relationships to include advisor, supervisor, researcher, and others.

1977 *ETHICAL STANDARDS OF PSYCHOLOGISTS*

The 1977 *Ethical Standards of Psychologists* explicitly prohibited, for the first time, sexual intimacies with clients, shifting the focus from dual relationships to the more highly specific relationship with clients. Furthermore, for the first time, the concepts of *loss of objectivity* and *exploitation* were introduced in this same principle (i.e., Principle 6[aa]; APA, 1977, p. 23). These two constructs are the measures used today to determine appropriateness of multiple relationships. Reference materials describing the decision-making process, the conflicts, and the controversies of each code development did not reflect any discussion of sexual contact with clients. The appearance of the prohibition in the 1977 Ethics Code was not a topic of explanation in reference materials on this code either. A curiosity is whether the framers and the subsequent developers did not perceive sexual interaction as likely or conceivable or whether the subject was avoided. A likely deduction is that given the critical incident model, the feedback and scenarios from the membership identified this relationship as a problem.

The power differential between psychologist and clients was recognized in the 1977 Ethics Code: "Psychologists are continually cognizant of their own needs and of their inherently powerful position *vis a vis* client in order to avoid exploiting their trust and dependency" (APA, 1977, p. 23). In other words, the recognition of the potential for loss of objectivity or exploitation and the attention to the power differential in therapy should be significant guiding principles in psychologists' decision making about the boundaries of interaction with clients (Koocher & Campbell, 2016).

1981 *ETHICAL PRINCIPLES OF PSYCHOLOGISTS*

The 1981 *Ethical Principles of Psychologists* (1981 Ethics Code) refined two of the principles introduced in prior codes. The category of dual relationships to be avoided was expanded to include students. Further, a Professional Relationship standard was introduced that echoed other principles in moving toward specificity of sexual conduct boundaries: "Psychologists do not exploit their professional relationships with clients, supervisees, students, employees, or research participants sexually or otherwise. Psychologists do not condone or engage in sexual harassment" (APA, 1981, p. 636).

1992 *ETHICAL PRINCIPLES OF PSYCHOLOGISTS AND CODE OF CONDUCT*

The 1992 *Ethical Principles of Psychologists and Code of Conduct* (1992 Ethics Code; APA, 1992) introduced an entirely new structure for the document. Significant restructuring differentiated between aspirational principles and enforceable standards. The *aspirational principles* were moral ideals to which all psychologists should aspire, and the *enforceable standards* were intended to be used as rules potentially resulting in sanctions if they are broken. The only reference to sexual intimacies with clients/patients in the 1981 Ethics Code was incorporated into the 1992 Ethics Code as Standard 4.05, Sexual Intimacies with Current Patients or Clients. This standard, which specifies, "Psychologists do not engage in sexual intimacies with current patients or clients" (APA, 1992), was conceptually the same as in the 1977 and 1981 Ethics Codes but was incorporated into the revised structure of the 1992 Ethics Code.

Several new standards with regard to sexual intimacies were introduced in the 1992 Ethics Code. The most controversial of these was Standard 4.07, Sexual Intimacies with Former Therapy Patients. How controversial this change was is reflected in the fact that the first 15 drafts of the 1992 Ethics Code banned all posttermination sex with clients (Gabbard, 1994). Before 1992, the APA Ethics Code was silent on the question of posttermination sex with clients, as were most state licensing boards and ethics committees (Sell et al., 1986).

After a lengthy debate about the issue of posttermination sex with clients, the members of the 1992 Ethics Code Revision Task Force created a 2-year prohibition on posttermination sexual intimacies, but they did not impose a complete ban. According to Fisher (2017), a 2-year moratorium period was chosen rather than a permanent prohibition against sex with former clients/patients because most complaints involving sexual intimacies with former clients/patients were about relationships that began during the first year posttermination. Standard 4.07 of the 1992 Ethics Code states, "(a) Psychologists do not engage in sexual intimacies with a former therapy patient or client for at least two years after cessation or termination of professional services" (APA, 1992). The 1992 Ethics Code also included a rationale for this moratorium:

> Because sexual intimacies with a former therapy patient or client are so frequently harmful to the patient or client, and because such intimacies undermine public confidence in the psychology profession and thereby deter the public's use of needed services, psychologists do not engage in sexual intimacies with former therapy patients and clients even after a two-year interval except in the most unusual circumstances. (APA, 1992)

The rationale, and especially the last sentence, make it clear that posttermination sexual intimacies should seldom occur.

This is followed by a list of considerations demonstrating that sexual intimacies with former therapy clients/patients is not unconditionally acceptable even after 2 years because exploitation and harm could occur after that period. This list includes:

> (1) the amount of time that has passed since therapy terminated, (2) the nature and duration of the therapy, (3) the circumstances of termination, (4) the patient's or client's personal history, (5) the patient's or client's current mental status, (6) the likelihood of adverse impact on the patient or client and others, and (7) any statements or actions made by the therapist during the course of therapy suggesting or inviting the possibility of a post-termination sexual or romantic relationship with the patient or client. (APA, 1992)

Thus, although there are numerous restrictions on and considerations regarding sex with former clients/patients, the Ethics Code Revision Task Force stopped short of prohibiting sexual intimacies with former clients/patients. However, the 1992 Task Force made it clear that if an ethics complaint is made against a psychologist 2 or more years after termination, the burden is on the psychologist to demonstrate that the sexual relationship is or was not exploitative (Fisher, 2017).

There are numerous arguments both for and against the possibility of posttermination sexual intimacies. Arguments against posttermination sexual relationships include issues of transference and the power differential between therapists and clients/patients, which do not necessarily end when therapy ends and for some clients continue for a very long time. Although "transference" is a psychoanalytic term, the concept it represents is a part of most other theoretical orientations (Koocher & Keith-Spiegel, 1998). Other arguments for the perpetuity of a ban include the fact that even the possibility of posttermination sex could alter the therapy relationship from the beginning (Gabbard, 1994; Gabbard & Pope, 1989). Therefore, clients/patients who are attracted to their therapist may not want to discuss certain things in therapy if they think doing so would interfere with a possible future romantic relationship with the therapist. In addition, therapists may not be able to be objective toward a client/patient to whom they are attracted (Koocher & Keith-Spiegel, 1998).

Gabbard (1994) drew a parallel between the prohibition of consensual sexual activity between parents and adult children, which supports the structure and meaning of family and society, and the prohibition of consensual sexual activity between psychologists and clients/patients, which preserves the structure and meaning of therapy. He also stressed that the professional responsibilities of psychologists persist long after termination. Sexual relationships create role confusion and conflicts of interest in carrying out these responsibilities. Therapists may be required not only to maintain treatment records for a specified amount of time after termination (which is always longer than 2 years) but also to provide those records to a third party or to testify in court regarding the former client's/patient's mental status. A sexual relationship between a psychologist and a former client/patient also compromises the psychologist's ability to provide or appear to provide objective information to the court, information that may be crucial, for example, for the former client/patient to receive disability insurance (Fisher, 2017).

Confidentiality, privacy, and privilege also endure in perpetuity and are compromised by a sexual relationship. Also, many clients/patients request services from a former therapist even many years after termination, which would not be possible if the former therapist had become a romantic or sexual partner. Furthermore, if a former client/patient makes a complaint of harm to a licensing board or an ethics committee, even if all of the provisions of the Ethics Code are met, and even if they are married, a former therapist will have a difficult time defending themselves because of the many factors that could contribute to a charge of exploitation (Koocher & Keith-Spiegel, 1998).

In contrast, consider an argument for allowing posttermination sexual relationships between therapists and clients/patients. Perhaps, following a chance meeting at a barbeque several years after a three-session group smoking cessation treatment program, a therapist and former client/patient develop a romantic/sexual relationship. It is unlikely that concerns of transference, power differential, and a need for future treatment would prohibit this relationship. Also, a prohibition against posttermination sexual relationships would mean that former clients/patients would never be able to give informed consent to a sexual relationship with a former therapist. While proponents of this position agree with this hypothesis, Bersoff (1994) believed more data were needed before the position is converted into an ethical rule relegating clients (usually female clients) to the role of passive victims rather than reinforcing that they are autonomous, self-determining, consenting adults.

Many questions remain unanswered. For example, under what circumstances do posttermination sexual relationships result in harm, and are individuals able to make an autonomous choice to enter into a sexual relationship with a former therapist (Behnke, 2004)? Just as the APA Ethics Code has not successfully eliminated sexual involvement with current clients/patients, it has not completely eliminated sexual involvement with former clients/patients. Some have used this as a justification for permitting posttermination sexual relationships. However, no one suggests it is a justification for sex with current clients/patients. Most therapists are likely to experience sexual attraction to at least one client/patient. The problem is not the presence of sexual feelings but the way psychologists handle those feelings. Unfortunately, the topic of sexual involvement with current or former clients/patients causes such discomfort that careful consideration of the relevant issues is difficult (Gabbard, 1994).

Another standard related to sexual intimacies that was new in the 1992 Ethics Code was Standard 4.06, Therapy with Former Sexual Partners. This standard succinctly says, "Psychologists do not accept as therapy patients or clients, persons with whom they have engaged in sexual intimacies" (APA, 1992). There has not been much, if any, research or literature on the topic of accepting former sexual partners as therapy clients/patients. However, doing so signals poor professional judgment: It is difficult to see how anyone could remain objective while treating a person with whom they have had a sexual relationship (Koocher & Keith-Spiegel, 1998). This lack of objectivity is likely to compromise the effectiveness of therapy. Not only could romantic and sexual feelings reemerge during therapy on the part of both the therapist and the client/patient, but the knowledge that the latter has about the psychologist could interfere with their ability to benefit from the psychologist's professional communications (Fisher, 2017).

Standard 1.19 of the 1992 Ethics Code (APA, 1992) was also the first time that sexual intimacies between professors and students and supervisors and supervisees were explicitly prohibited parallel to the prohibition of sexual intimacies between psychologists and current clients/patients. This standard, which is still current, states,

> (a) Psychologists do not exploit persons over whom they have supervisory, evaluative, or other authority such as students, supervisees, employees, research participants, and clients or patients. (b) Psychologists do not engage in sexual relationships with students or supervisees in training over whom the psychologist has evaluative or direct authority, because such relationships are so likely to impair judgment or be exploitative. (APA, 1992)

Educators and supervisors do not have as much influence over supervisees and students as psychologists have over clients/patients; however, they cannot be objective if they are having a sexual relationship with their students or supervisees (L. Sullivan & Ogloff, 1998). Teachers and supervisors can influence students and supervisees through grades, research and professional opportunities, letters of recommendation, work on dissertation projects, and reputation among other faculty members and professionals. Thus, these dual relationships can become exploitative and harmful. In addition, when other students or supervisees learn about such relationships, this knowledge can jeopardize the psychologist's ability to be effective as a teacher or supervisor, as well as to appear professional and impartial (Fisher, 2017). The prohibition of sexual relationships in this standard also applies to graduate students serving as teaching or research assistants who are evaluating undergraduate students or other graduate students.

Can students and supervisees or clients/patients give true consent to sexual relationships with persons who have authority or evaluative power over them? In general, the power differential and the potential for negative consequences suggest that completely voluntary consent is not possible (Quatrella & Wentworth, 1995) and that clearly coerced sexual activity would not be acceptable in any situation.

The 1992 Ethics Code is silent on whether professors in the same department can have romantic or sexual relationships with students or supervisees they will likely never teach or evaluate. The standard seems to imply that relationships outside of authority or evaluation could be acceptable. The extent of authority and evaluation is not clear in the 1992 Ethics Code (Koocher & Keith-Spiegel, 1998). This is made more explicit in the 2002 Ethics Code, but not without creating further ambiguities. In contrast to the controversial standard regarding sexual intimacies with former therapy clients/patients, both the 1992 and the 2002 Ethics Codes are silent about sexual relationships between psychologists and former students or supervisees. In fact, some students and faculty members or supervisees and supervisors do become involved romantically and sexually and sometimes marry.

However, "the dynamics of the therapy and the student-supervisory relationship are somewhat different, with the latter typically being less intense and, when concluded, ushering the absolute closing of an era" (Koocher & Keith-Spiegel, 1998, p. 228).

2002 ETHICAL PRINCIPLES OF PSYCHOLOGISTS AND CODE OF CONDUCT

The current version of the *Ethical Principles of Psychologists and Code of Conduct* (APA, 2017) was adopted in its entirety in 2002. Although amendments were adopted in 2010 and 2016, they did not change Standards 10.05, Sexual Intimacies with Current Therapy Clients/Patients; 10.06, Sexual Intimacies with Relatives or Significant Others of Current Therapy Clients/Patients; 10.07, Therapy with Former Sexual Partners; or 10.08, Sexual Intimacies with Former Therapy Clients/Patients. Standard 7.07, Sexual Relationships with Students and Supervisees, has also remained unchanged since 2002.

In general, the 2002 Ethics Code was a conservative revision of the 1992 Ethics Code (APA, 1992). Although there was no less protection of the public, some of the changes were designed to prevent the Ethics Code from being unnecessarily punitive for psychologists (Knapp & VandeCreek, 2003). Also unchanged is the language in Standard 10.05 (formerly Standard 4.05): "Psychologists do not engage in sexual intimacies with current therapy/patients." According to Knapp et al. (2017), "This is one of the few absolute statements in the APA Ethics Code" (p. 115). Thus, there is no room and no need for psychologists to use clinical judgment in deciding whether or not to have a sexual relationship with a client/patient.

In the area of sexual relationships, a 2002 change was the addition of Standard 10.06, which states, "Psychologists do not engage in sexual intimacies with individuals they know to be close relatives, guardians, or significant others of current clients/patients" (APA, 2017). There is scant literature on this topic, although it was the subject of the movie *The Prince of Tides* (Streisand, 1991). These relationships have the potential to impair the psychologist's objectivity and risk exploitation. Relationships included in this definition include clients'/patients' parents, siblings, children, legal guardians, and significant others, and other relatives who may be emotionally close to the client/patient. The phrase "they know to be" is included in case a psychologist does not know that someone they are involved with romantically is a close relative or significant other of a client/patient (Fisher, 2017). This standard also states that "psychologists do not terminate therapy to circumvent this standard" (APA, 2017).

This standard is especially important when the client is a child. A romantic relationship with the parent of a child client might be harmful to the child and possibly betray the child's trust in the psychologist. In addition, in most jurisdictions, when working with a child, the parent(s) are the identified client; therefore, the psychologist has an ethical obligation to the parent(s) as well as to the child. The importance of this standard also becomes clear in the situation in which a psychologist has a sexual or romantic relationship with the adult child of a therapy client/patient. The therapist may learn information about the client/patient that causes them to lose objectivity, or the client/patient may worry that the psychologist will not maintain confidentiality about what was shared in therapy (Koocher & Keith-Spiegel, 2008).

Another change to the 2002 Ethics Code was that it eliminated the rationale related to the prohibition against sexual relationships with former clients/patients ("because sexual intimacies with a former therapy patient or client are so frequently harmful to the patient or client, and because such intimacies undermine public confidence in the psychology profession and thereby deter the public's use of needed services"; APA, 1992). The 2002 Ethics Code Task Force deleted the rationale because it appeared to be beyond the scope of the Ethics Code to explain the rationale for each of the standards (Knapp & VandeCreek, 2003) and because not every standard had a rationale. Standard 1.19 of the 1992 Ethics Code regarding exploitative relationships with students and supervisees also included a rationale ("because such relationships are so likely to impair judgment or be exploitative"; APA, 1992), but this rationale was eliminated in the 2002 Ethics Code for the same reason.

Other possible changes to the 2002 Ethics Code were discussed but not made. A controversial change that was made in 1992 permitted sexual intimacies with former therapy clients/patients after 2 years in certain limited circumstances. In discussing the 2002 Ethics Code, there were those who wanted to prohibit all sexual contact between therapists and both current and former clients/patients. However, the 2-year rule appeared to eliminate the most egregious examples of exploitation, and there was concern that an in-perpetuity standard would not stand up to legal challenges (Knapp & VandeCreek, 2003).

Whereas Standard 1.19 in the 1992 Ethics Code said, "Psychologists do not engage in sexual relationships with students or supervisees in training over whom the psychologist has evaluative or direct authority," the 2002 standard (7.07) says, "Psychologists do not engage in sexual relationships with students or supervisees *who are in their department, agency, or training center or* over whom psychologists have or are likely to have evaluative authority" (APA, 2017; italics added). According to Knapp and VandeCreek (2003), this new wording could lead to unintended consequences beyond the desirable outcome of protecting students and supervisees from sexual exploitation. It is not clear what is meant by "in their department, agency, or training center." Would this include situations in which a psychologist is teaching a course as an adjunct faculty member, supervising a practicum student at an external site, or serving as a member of a dissertation committee? If this is what is meant by this standard, psychologists would violate the Ethics Code if their spouse or life partner is a student or supervisee in the department or agency where they have a very limited role with no evaluative authority over the person with whom they have a relationship. It was much clearer in the 1992 Ethics Code, when the standard restricted sexual relationships only with students or supervisees in training over whom the psychologist had evaluative or direct authority (Knapp & VandeCreek, 2003). Standard 10.07, Therapy with Former Sexual Partners, did not change between the 1992 Ethics Code and the 2002 Ethics Code other than the number of the standard, which was 4.06 in 1992.

FUTURE DIRECTIONS

Although sexual intimacies between psychologists and current clients, students, and supervisees have been prohibited in the APA Ethics Code for decades, they still occur. In addition, every state prohibits sexual intimacies through state licensing laws that either incorporate the Ethics Code or include this prohibition separately. Some states have also criminalized sexual contact with clients, and others have mandated reporting requirements that psychologists must inform the licensing board when they learn that a client/ patient has had sexual contact with a former therapist. What can be done about this problem, and how can the Ethics Code help? The increased visibility of movements such as #NoMore, #TimesUp, and #MeToo, and the public showcase of accused perpetrators in highly visible national positions, including elected officials, suggest that more needs to be done both within the field of psychology and nationally.

All psychologists know that sexual intimacies with clients, students, and supervisees are unethical and in many jurisdictions illegal. This is also the most common reason for disciplinary action against psychologists. Thus, most psychologists believe that they would never have a sexual relationship with a patient. Unfortunately, sexual intimacies are the extreme manifestation of sexual attraction to clients, which is more common. Too often these feelings are not acknowledged, and there are few opportunities to discuss them. Focusing only on eliminating sexual exploitation may suggest that it is desirable to suppress or minimize sexual feelings. It is important for psychologists to have a safe setting in which to process these feelings so they may handle them productively. According to Knapp et al. (2013),

> Sexual exploitation can be reduced if individual psychologists focus on technical skills in maintaining boundaries; embed themselves in a system of protection; and recognize that strong feelings, including sexual feelings, will arise with certain patients during the course of therapy. Continuing education programs, graduate training, supervision, consultation, and other venues can be used to help psychologists learn how to control, modify, or channel those emotions to productive ends. (p. 94)

The most significant part of this recommendation is the need to shift the culture of psychology to include a profession-wide atmosphere to eliminate sexual misconduct. This could be accomplished through the APA Ethics Code.

An additional suggestion is to strengthen the self-care standard in the Ethics Code. Psychologists are at increased risk for sexual intimacies with clients/patients when they have had a recent stressor in their private lives, such as divorce, death in the family, severe financial problems, or too much stress in their practice. Standard 2.06, Personal Problems and Conflicts, now states,

> (a) Psychologists refrain from initiating an activity when they know or should know that there is a substantial likelihood that their personal problems will prevent them from performing their work-related activities in a competent manner. (b) When psychologists become aware of personal problems that may interfere with their performing work-related duties adequately, they take appropriate measures, such as obtaining professional consultation or assistance, and determine whether they should limit, suspend, or terminate their work-related duties. (APA, 2017)

Psychologists could be educated at every stage of their training and career about the effects of sexual intimacies on clients/patients, how to avoid this behavior, and where to seek help if they are struggling with challenges to their professional boundaries with clients/patients. This area could be made a part of mandatory continuing education for psychologists in every jurisdiction to renew their licenses. Educating the public about how to prevent, recognize, and report sexually inappropriate behavior in therapy could also be an ethical requirement. Language that encourages client/patient reporting of sexual intimacies between psychologists and clients/patients could be added to the Ethics Code. Finally, the Ethics Code could mandate that psychologists must inform the licensing board when they learn that a client/patient has had sexual contact with a former therapist, and additional states could criminalize sexual contact between psychologists and clients/patients (AbuDagga et al., 2019).

STATE STATUTES, RULES, AND REGULATIONS

State licensing boards, which are responsible for the licensure and certification of psychologists in their respective state, are also responsible for investigating and, if applicable, penalizing psychologists for unethical conduct (e.g., revoking or suspending a license). For this reason, state licensing boards designate which behaviors constitute unethical conduct via their rules and regulations. An analysis of each state's rules and regulations written by licensing boards for psychologists revealed that all but two state licensing boards clearly name sexual misconduct by psychologists as unethical behavior and grounds for discipline (see Table 2.1 for a summary of data or findings).

Of the state licensing boards that forbid sexual misconduct by psychologists, 58.3% address sexual misconduct by psychologists in their official rules and regulations, whereas 48% simply make reference to APA's (2017) *Ethical Principles of Psychologists and Code of Conduct,* and some licensing boards do both (see Table 2.1).

An advantage of those licensing boards that rely on the APA Ethics Code is that of a more expansive definition of potential victims. The present APA Ethics Code expressly forbids psychologists from engaging in sexual relations with current clients, individuals closely associated with current clients, students, supervisees, and former clients for at least 2 years; it also forbids psychologists from accepting as clients any individuals with whom they have had sexual relations (APA, 2017). When licensing boards define sexual misconduct in their rules and regulations, they often do not include these prohibitions.

One potential problem associated with licensing boards' reliance on the APA Ethics Code is that most references to the document do not specify a particular version (30.4%) or list an old version (52.2%; see Table 2.1). For example, even in their most recent rules and regulations, most licensing boards specified the 2002 version of the APA Ethics Code with the 2010 amendment but not the 2017 amendment. Indeed, some rules and regulations went so

TABLE 2.1. Descriptive Information of Rules and Regulations Specific to State Boards of Psychology

Source of state sexual misconduct rules	States
None	CT, MS
APA Ethics Code	AL, AK, AZ, AR, DE, GA, ID, IL, IA, LA, ME, MA, NE, NH, NC, ND, OK, OR, RI, TN, UT, VT, WY
Individual State Board Rules and Regulations	CA, CO, FL, HI, IN, IL, IA, KS, KY, MD, MI, MN, MO, MT, NV, NJ, NM, NY, OH, PA, SC, SD, TX, UT, VA, WA, WV, WI

Version of APA Ethics Code (if applicable)	States
Unspecified	DE, ID, ME, MA, NE, RI, VT
Earlier	AL, AK, AZ, GA, IL, IA, LA, NH, ND, TN, UT, WY
Latest	AR, NC, OK, OR

Prohibited relationships by state	States
Current clients	AL, AK, AZ, AR, CA, CO, DE, FL, GA, HI, ID, IL, IN, IA, KS, KY, LA, ME, MD, MA, MI, MN, MO, MT, NE, NV, NH, NJ, NM, NY, NC, ND, OH, OK, OR, PA, RI, SC, SD, TN, TX, UT, VT, VA, WA, WV, WI, WY
Former clients	AL, AK, AZ, AR, CA, DE, FL, GA, ID, IL, IN, IA, KY, LA, ME, MD, MA, MI, MN, MO, MT, NE, NV, NH, NJ, NM, NC, ND, OH, OK, OR, RI, SD, TN, TX, UT, VT, VA, WA, WV, WI, WY
Close relations of clients	AL, AK, AZ, AR, CO, DE, GA, ID, IL, IA, KS, LA, ME, MD, MA, MI, NE, NV, NH, NM, NC, ND, OH, OK, OR, RI, SD, TN, TX, UT, VT, VA, WA, WV, WY
Students/supervisees	AL, AK, AZ, AR, DE, GA, ID, IL, IA, LA, ME, MD, MA, MI, MO, NE, NH, NJ, NC, ND, OH, OK, OR, PA, RI, SC, TN, TX, UT, VT, VA, WI, WY
Former partners as clients	AL, AK, AZ, AR, DE, GA, ID, IL, IN, IA, LA, ME, MA, MT, NE, NH, NJ, NC, ND, OH, OK, OR, RI, SD, TN, TX, UT, VT, WA, WV, WI, WY

far as to exclude more recent versions; for example, Arizona's rules and regulations for psychologists states, "the incorporated materials do not include any later amendments or editions" (Ariz. Rev. Stat. Ann. § R4-26-301, 2019). However, these omissions do not likely affect the board's ability to sanction sexual misconduct given that the 2017 amendment to Standard 3.04, Avoiding Harm, was specific to psychologists assisting or engaging in torture (APA, 2017).

An advantage of expanding beyond the APA Ethics Code to define unethical sexual behavior is that licensing boards may also prohibit other harmful behaviors that are not explicitly addressed in that document. For example, some state licensing boards (e.g., Florida, Kentucky) forbid a psychologist from making statements of a sexual nature to a client, with an exception for professionally accepted treatment (e.g., in the course of treating a psychosexual disorder). Additionally, some state licensing boards (e.g., Washington, New Jersey) expressly prohibit psychologists from accepting sexual activities as payment for psychological services; however, this behavior, although not explicitly stated, can reasonably be assumed to be covered by the APA Ethics Code Standard 6.05, Barter with Clients/Patients.

Overall, of those state licensing board rules and regulations that address sexual misconduct, all (100%) prohibit psychologists from having sexual relations with current clients (see Table 2.1). Most (87.5%) forbid sexual relations with former clients for at least 2 years, with some (e.g., Virginia, Washington) increasing the required length of time since last therapeutic service to 5 years. In most cases, a sexual relationship with former clients is prohibited indefinitely if the client is emotionally dependent on the therapist or is otherwise mentally vulnerable. The burden of proof is on the therapist to show there was no exploitation of the former client. Many state licensing boards also forbid psychologists from engaging in sexual relationships with individuals closely related to current clients (72.9%) and students and supervisees (68.8%). Many (66.7%) also prohibit psychologists from providing therapeutic services for individuals with whom the psychologist has previously had sexual intimacies. Additionally, most licensing boards stipulate psychologists cannot terminate therapeutic services in order to circumvent these rules.

CRIMINAL STATUTES

An analysis of criminal statutes for each state revealed significant variation between states regarding laws specific to sexual abuse and boundary violations in psychotherapy (see Table 2.2 for a summary). Over half (54%) of the states do not have statutes specifically criminalizing sexual relations between a psychologist and a current or former client. The remainder of the states have laws that explicitly reference psychologists (36%) or that may apply to psychologists (10%; these statutes use terms such as "mandated reporter" and "health care provider"). Notably, the only mention

TABLE 2.2. Descriptive Information of State Criminal Statutes

Degree of statute's relevance to psychologists	States
None	AL, DE, HI, ID, IL, IN, KY, LA, MA, MS, MO, MT, NE, NV, NJ, NM, NC, OK, OR, PA, RI, SC, TN, VT, VA, WV, WY
Peripherally relevant	AR, KS, MI, NH, WA
Explicit mention	AK, AZ, CA, CO, CT, FL, GA, IA, ME, MD, MN, NY, ND, OH, SD, TX, UT, WI

Crime classification of offense	States
Felony	AK, AZ, AR, CO, FL, GA, IA, KS, ME, MI, MN, NH, NY, ND, OH, SD, TX, UT, WA, WI
Misdemeanor	CA, CO, CT, IA, MD, NY, OH

Patient factors outlined by state law	States
Current client	AK, AZ, CA, CO, CT, FL, GA, IA, ME, MD, MN, NH, NY, ND, OH, SD, TX, UT, WA, WI
Former client	CA, CT, FL, IA, MD, MN, NH, TX
Consent is null	AR, CO, FL, GA, MN, SD, WI
Emotional dependence	CT, IA, MN, SD, TX
Therapeutic deception	CO, CT, FL, KS, MN, OH, UT

Note: The criminal statutes described above are only those pertinent to victims who have reached the age of majority.

of psychotherapist sexual misconduct in the New Mexico Criminal Code is to specify that

> criminal sexual contact does not include touching by a psychotherapist on his patient that is inadvertent, casual social contact not intended to be sexual in nature, or generally recognized by mental health professionals as being a legitimate element of psychotherapy. (N.M. Stat. Ann. § 30-9-12[B], 2019)

Of those statutes that do explicitly criminalize sexual contact between therapists and clients, there is again variation in the terms used to describe such an offense. While most states refer to these offenses as "criminal sexual conduct" (e.g., Minnesota, Michigan) or "sexual assault" (e.g., Texas, New Hampshire), some use terms such as "sexual battery" (e.g., Ohio), and "rape" (e.g., New York, Kansas). Furthermore, there is disagreement regarding the severity of such infractions; some states (40%) consider sexual misconduct by a psychologist a felony, and fewer (14%) consider it a misdemeanor, and some states have relevant statutes that contain both felony and misdemeanor offenses (see Table 2.2).

Regardless of the severity of the offense, of those states with criminal statutes outlawing sexual boundary crossings in a therapeutic relationship, most (82.6%) specifically forbid sexual intimacies with a current client, and a significant number (30.4%) explicitly state that consent on the part of the client does not constitute a defense. Far fewer states (34.8%) include former patients, and a handful of those specifically prohibit sexual relationships if the former client is emotionally dependent on the psychologist. A representative definition of *emotional dependency* states,

> The nature of the patient's or former patient's emotional condition and the nature of the treatment provided by the psychotherapist are such that the psychotherapist knows or has reason to believe that the patient or former patient is unable to withhold consent to sexual contact by the psychotherapist. (Minn. Stat. § 604.20.2-8 [2019])

Furthermore, some states (30.4%) solely or more harshly criminalize therapeutic deception. Therapeutic deception includes any "representation by a psychotherapist that sexual contact with the psychotherapist is consistent with or part of the patient's or former patient's treatment" (Minn. Stat.§ 604.20.2-8 [2019]). For example, a recent case in California involved a psychologist using therapeutic deception on patients who were seeking treatment for sexual abuse. The psychologist purported to be using exposure therapy when he forced his patients to have sex with him. These actions resulted in a conviction and a possible 11-year prison sentence (J. Sullivan, 2018).

SEXUAL BOUNDARY VIOLATIONS ACROSS LICENSING BOARDS

Although almost all state licensing boards that govern psychologists have prohibitions against sexual boundary crossings, there is still a fair amount of variation across states that results in inconsistent coverage of specific victims and actions. Referencing the APA Ethics Code may be one of the most comprehensive methods for addressing unethical sexual contact, although boards might consider updating their rules and regulations to reflect the most current version. More worrisome is the lack of state criminal statutes specific to sexual misconduct by a psychologist. Even those states that do criminalize sexual misconduct by a psychologist typically do so only when the psychologist engages in sexual activity with a current or former client and make no protections for close relations of clients, students, and supervisees. Indeed, organizations such as the Citizens Commission on Human Rights International have called for every state to adopt comprehensive and uniform statutes criminalizing sexual misconduct by psychotherapists

("When Your Psychiatrist or Therapist is a Sexual Predator #MeToo in the Mental Health Industry," 2018).

Given that sexual boundary violations by psychologists are frequently harmful to the victim and undermine public confidence in the profession of psychology, it is paramount that any such violations by psychologists with current clients be explicitly prohibited by licensing boards and criminalized in state criminal codes. Given the powerful and subtle effects of the relationship between a psychologist and client/former client and student/supervisee in which the victim may be influenced by the unequal distribution of power, these rules and statutes should consider the victim's inability to provide consent and the psychologist's possible exploitation of emotional dependence or use of therapeutic deception.

APA DISCIPLINARY TRENDS

The APA Ethics Committee publishes a report of APA Ethics Office activities for each year. Among the data offered in the reports are the number of cases opened, activated, closed, ongoing, and other summaries of the committee's productivity from the Office. The reported types of cases opened include inappropriate professional practice, child custody, competence, confidentiality, inappropriate public statements, loss of license, and response to the Ethics Committee. Among these types of cases are dual relationships: Sexual misconduct with adults, sexual misconduct with minors, sexual harassment, and nonsexual dual role relationships. Table 2.3 shows the number and percentage of cases opened across the years from 2005 through 2015. The reports subsequent to these dates have not been published in *American Psychologist*. The occurrence of sexual misconduct and subsequent adjudication between jurisdictional ethics committees, state boards of examiners, and the APA Ethics Committee are difficult to discern inasmuch as ethics committees and the APA Ethics Office have focused on ethics education in recent years and have adjudicated selectively in light of jurisdictional decision making in that adjudication is primarily conducted under the auspices of state licensing boards. The data do indicate, however, regardless of number of cases, that sexual misconduct cases with adults between 2005 and 2015 have been between 25% and 38% of all cases opened. In more recent years between 2011 and 2015, the occurrence of sexual misconduct with adults has trended toward 50%. A reasonable hypothesis is that other types of cases are decreasing in occurrence, but sexual misconduct occurrences are remaining stable. After 2010, APA did not report sexual misconduct with minors or sexual harassment.

TABLE 2.3. Reports of the APA Ethics Committee 2005-2015

Cases Opened	2005 No. (%)	2006 No. (%)	2007 No. (%)	2008 No. (%)	2009 No. (%)	2010 No. (%)
Dual Relationship						
Sexual misconduct (with adults)	12-38	6-21	9-28	4-25	4-33	6-30
Sexual misconduct (with minors)	4-13	1-3	5-16	0-0	1-8	2-10
Sexual harassment	0-0	0-0	0-0	1-16	0-0	1-5
Nonsexual dual relationships	4-13	4-4	5-16	2-13	0-0	5-25

	2011 No. (%)	2012 No. (%)	2013 No. (%)	2014 No. (%)	2015 No. (%)
Sexual misconduct (with adults)	5-55	5-38	4-57	4-40	4-50
Nonsexual dual relationships	2-22	2-15	1-14	1-10	0-0

In comparison with data from 1983 (Sell et al., 1986) that capture the inclusion of the 1977 prohibition against sexual misconduct with clients, a significant reduction in reporting is noted. In the 1983 study, 41 reports were made to ethics committees or state licensing boards. Among those, 19 led to disciplinary action. Noteworthy is a related finding that upon being asked, "Would a policy on minimum length of time which must elapse before a social/sexual relationship between psychologist and client be helpful?" the overwhelming answer was "yes" (78%). The 1992 Ethics Code did include definitive new standards after much debate and disagreement. Studies have shown that sexual misconduct with current clients is primarily between older male therapists and younger female clients (Zelen, 1985). The two references just cited span 31 years—and the power imbalance appears not to have changed. Given that the sheer number of cases have decreased, as noted in Table 2.3, one might speculate that the empowerment of women resulting from broader employment and career opportunities, self-earned wages, social policies, and regulation has provided an environment in which women can exercise self-determination. Important, however, must be the recognition that personality, family of origin history, self-perception, maladapted schemas, and diagnostic classification can remove options for self-determination. Regardless of a client's cognitive or emotional capability, the responsibility for appropriate conduct remains with the psychologist.

CONCLUSION

Movement across the ethics codes from 1952 to the present reflects the ecological environment in which psychology resides. That is, the societal mores, political climate, and the profession's domains of education and training, research, and practice have been shifting across decades. The late 1977 entry of sexual misconduct in the code and the opposition in 1992 and 2002 to specificity in sexual-conduct-related standards alert us to the continued influence of power, privilege, and other dynamics that need to be addressed through definitive means (e.g., licensing boards, ethics committees) in order to promote the respect and welfare of others, autonomy, self-determination, and transparent informed consent. "Sexual boundaries" is not a term typically used in ethics code vernacular nor in regulatory parlance. The meaning, however, is captured in the development of sexual conduct standards in the APA Ethics Code across time and in the movement evidenced in the data describing regulatory rules and statutes. Ethics codes and regulation are both responsive to the public and to their constituencies. The critical incident method of attaining information from the APA membership is a strong force against those who would opt for no road maps and no blueprints. Licensing boards are commissioned to protect the rights of the public and most often prioritize the protection of those rights. Sexual boundaries between therapist and client remain a topic of high energy, strong opinions, and provide a litmus test of our professional values and commitment to our professed values of justice, truth, benevolence, and the welfare of others.

REFERENCES

AbuDagga, A., Carome, M., & Wolfe, S.M. (2019). *Time to end physician sexual abuse of patients: Calling the U.S. medical community to action.* https://doi.org/10.1007/s11606-019-05014-6

American Psychological Association. (1952). Discussion on ethics. *American Psychologist, 7*(8), 425–455. https://doi.org/10.1037/h0057724

American Psychological Association. (1953). *Ethical standards of psychologists.* https://doi.org/10.1037/e485172008-001

American Psychological Association. (1959). Ethical standards of psychologists. *American Psychologist, 14*(6), 279–282. https://doi.org/10.1037/h0048469

American Psychological Association. (1963). Ethical standards of psychologists. *American Psychologist, 18*(1), 56–60. https://doi.org/10.1037/h0041847

American Psychological Association. (1977, March). Revised ethical standards of psychologists. *APA Monitor*, 22–23. https://doi.org/10.1037/e388842004-024

American Psychological Association. (1981). Ethical principles of psychologists. *American Psychologist, 36*(6), 633–638. https://doi.org/10.1037/0003-066X.36.6.633

American Psychological Association. (1992). Ethical principles of psychologists and code of conduct. *American Psychologist, 47*(12), 1597–1611. https://doi.org/10.1037/0003-066X.47.12.1597

American Psychological Association. (2017). *Ethical principles of psychologists and code of conduct* (2002, Amended June 1, 2010, and January 1, 2017). http://www.apa.org/ethics/code/index.aspx

Ariz. Rev. Stat. Ann. § R4-26-301 (2019).

Behnke, S. (2004, December). Sexual involvements with former clients: A delicate balance of core values. *Monitor on Psychology, 35*(11), 76–77. https://doi.org/10.1037/e312342005-054

Bersoff, D. N. (1994). Explicit ambiguity: The 1992 ethics code as an oxymoron. *Professional Psychology: Research and Practice, 25*(4), 382–387. https://doi.org/10.1037/0735-7028.25.4.382

Fisher, C. B. (2017). *Decoding the ethics code: A practical guide for psychologists* (4th ed.). Sage.

Gabbard, G. O. (1994). Reconsidering the American Psychological Association's policy on sex with former patients: Is it justifiable? *Professional Psychology: Research and Practice, 25*(4), 329–335. https://doi.org/10.1037/0735-7028.25.4.329

Gabbard, G. O., & Pope, K. S. (1989). Sexual intimacies after termination: Clinical, ethical, and legal aspects. In G. O. Gabbbard (Ed.), *Sexual exploitation in professional relationships* (pp. 116–127). American Psychiatric Press.

Hobbs, N. (1948). The development of a code of ethical standards for psychology. *American Psychologist, 3*(3), 80–84. https://doi.org/10.1037/h0060281

Knapp, S., & VandeCreek, L. (2003). An overview of the major changes in the 2002 APA Ethics Code. *Professional Psychology: Research and Practice, 34*(3), 301–308. https://doi.org/10.1037/0735-7028.34.3.301

Knapp, S. J., VandeCreek, L. D., & Fingerhut, R. (2017). *Practical ethics for psychologists: A positive approach* (3rd ed.). American Psychological Association. https://doi.org/10.1037/0000036-000

Knapp, S. J., Younggren, J. N., VandeCreek, L., Harris, E., & Martin, J. N. (2013). *Assessing and managing risk in psychological practice: An individualized approach* (2nd ed.). The Trust.

Koocher, G. P., & Campbell, L. F. (2016). Professional ethics in the United States. In J. C. Norcross, G. R. VandenBos, D. K. Freedheim, & L. F. Campbell (Eds.), *APA handbook of clinical psychology: Vol. 5. Education and profession* (pp. 301–337). American Psychological Association. https://doi.org/10.1037/14774-020

Koocher, G. P., & Keith-Spiegel, P. (1998). *Ethics in psychology: Professional standards and cases* (2nd ed.). Oxford University Press.

Koocher, G. P., & Keith-Spiegel, P. (2008). *Ethics is psychology and the mental health profession: Standards and cases* (3rd ed.). Oxford University Press.

Minn. Stat. §604.20.2-8 (2019).

N. M. Stat. §30-9-12(B) (2019).

Quatrella, L. A., & Wentworth, K. (1995). Student's perception of unequal status dating relationships in academia. *Ethics & Behavior, 5*(3), 249–259. https://doi.org/10.1207/s15327019eb0503_4

Sell, J. M., Gottlieb, M. C., & Schoenfeld, L. (1986). Ethical considerations of social/romantic relationships with present and former clients. *Professional Psychology: Research and Practice, 17*(6), 504–508. https://doi.org/10.1037/0735-7028.17.6.504

Streisand, B. (Director). (1991). *The prince of tides* [Film]. Columbia Pictures.

Sullivan, J. (2018, December 1). *Jury finds former Travis psychologist guilty in sexual abuse case*. https://www.dailyrepublic.com/all-dr-news/solano-news/crime-solano-county-courts/jury-finds-former-travis-psychologist-guilty-in-sexual-abuse-case/

Sullivan, L., & Ogloff, J. (1998). Appropriate supervisor–graduate student relationships. *Ethics & Behavior, 8*(3), 229–248. https://doi.org/10.1207/s15327019eb0803_4

When your psychiatrist or therapist is a sexual predator #MeToo in the mental health industry. (2018, February 8). CCHR International. https://www.cchrint.org/2018/02/07/when-your-psychiatrist-or-therapist-is-a-sexual-predator-metoo-in-the-mental-health-industry/#_edn1

Zelen, S. L. (1985). Sexualization of therapeutic relationships: The dual vulnerability of patient and therapist. *Psychotherapy: Theory, Research, Practice, & Training, 22*(2), 178–185. https://doi.org/10.1037/h0085491

3 BOUNDARIES AND ETHICS OF PROFESSIONAL CONDUCT

STEPHEN B. LEVINE AND CHRISTINE A. COURTOIS

Discussions about the importance of maintaining sexual and other boundaries between professionals and their clients began in earnest in the early 1990s. State licensing boards had registered a dramatic increase in the number of health professionals being accused of having sexual relationships with their patients (d'Oronzio, 2015). For example, the rate of recognized violations doubled between 1989 and 1996 to 4.4% of those disciplined by state medical boards. It has been estimated that 1.6% or less of physicians have had sex with their patients (Sansone & Sansone, 2009), yet in some anonymous surveys as many as 9.2% have admitted to at least one instance (Gartrell et al., 1992). Relevant studies have estimated sexual contact in psychotherapy in the range of 10% across different professions (Borys & Pope, 1989). These survey studies were first undertaken after increased societal awareness of the prevalence of sexual abuse during childhood. Data first emerged in the 1960s and 1970s on the sexual abuse of girls, then boys, between adults and children, health care professionals and patients, psychotherapists and clients, teachers and students, clergy and congregants, and, more recently, by those (the vast majority of them men and

https://doi.org/10.1037/0000247-003
Sexual Boundary Violations in Psychotherapy: Facing Therapist Indiscretions, Transgressions, and Misconduct, A. Steinberg, J. L. Alpert, and C. A. Courtois (Editors)

some women) in positions of power in all fields. Since then, there continues to be ever-increasing societal acknowledgment of sexual harassment and other sexual violations in a wide range of fiduciary relationships and workplace settings.

The question of frequency is still not definitively answered; however, it is a fair assumption that a far lesser number are ever reported or disclosed, causing many to speculate that the 10% number is low. Significant questions remain: Are these incidents more common in any one mental health discipline? If so, why? Are there personality and characterological features about these professionals and their clients that predispose to this behavior? Are there other factors, such as stereotypes and discrimination at work? Are professionals adequately trained regarding the damage that can be caused by sexual boundary violations? The reader can refer to various chapters of the present text for currently available information about these and other issues of professionals who violate sexual boundaries with their clients. Although significant advances have been made, much more remains to be studied and implemented going forward.

Although sex with those seeking care has been known to be a temptation since the beginning of recorded medical history, it has also been a prohibited behavior for physicians since that time. Today, this prohibition has been extended to all health care providers, including mental health caregivers and allied professionals with differing educational degrees. Those who defy this widely shared cultural expectation for professional conduct and relationships free from exploitation do so at considerable risk to the client or patient, to themselves and their loved ones, and to the entire profession.

BEING A PROFESSIONAL

Professionals, of course, were once laypersons. From their early days in graduate and medical schools, they are expected to internalize the values of their profession with increasing clarity as their early years of experience accumulate.

The Moral Responsibilities of Professionals

Mental health providers have a moral responsibility, with obligations incumbent upon them by virtue of their training and expertise in a healing profession and the needs and vulnerabilities of those who seek their help. The professional may understand these obligations in various ways depending on their individual values system. For example, some sense it as an allegiance to conscience, God, society, the patient, or the law (Markel, 2004). How one thinks of it matters less than the fundamental need to grasp the obligation to conduct one's professional life under the time-honored "moral umbrella." Professionals who fail to intuitively grasp this universal expectation that the therapist works for the client's benefit may be surprised to learn that their professions, colleagues, and the courts do.

Although morality is generally thought of as the rules for civilized human behavior regardless of era or culture, separating moral guidance from ethical guidance can at times be difficult to achieve. Ethics involves the rules for conduct within a profession. It is a narrower concept than morality, although some refer to professionals' exploitation of their clients as immoral. Psychologists, physicians, counselors, and nurses draw up their own guidelines for the conduct of their peers within their profession.

It is a compliment to be thought of at the end of one's professional life as having lived with integrity. A person with integrity has a set of stable, coherent, and well-regarded values and behaves in a manner that integrates personal and historical rules of conduct. Professionals are a part of a historical chain of countless previous others. Mental health professionals with integrity can articulate their professional values, know their origins, and conduct their lives governed by them. The attribution of integrity means that another person perceives that the individual professional understands, can articulate, and lives by the ethics of the profession. Therapists not only talk about professional values, they apply them in their work.

Principles and Standards of Professionalism

The following are five principles that characterize respectable professional behaviors: (a) altruism, where welfare of the patient is foremost; (b) accountability to those served and to others in the profession; (c) excellence, with interventions based on knowledge and expertise; (d) felt duty to help others and to serve the patient; and (e) respect for patients, colleagues, students and trainees, assistants, and employees. Other descriptions pertaining to professionalism include respect for human life, absence of prejudice in care provision, confidentiality, attending to one's own physical and mental health, and not using knowledge to violate human rights or civil liberties (World Medical Association, 2017).

Even before graduate students, psychiatric residents, or medical students are provided with a lecture on professionalism, they are expected to understand its key elements. Theoretically, the internalization of values and virtues of the profession is part of the professional identity process from the first day of training. Recognizing that a reliance on such expectations may not be wise or adequate, most schools today explicitly discuss the principles and standards of professionalism in lectures, seminars, assigned readings, or innovative programming (Khandelwal et al., 2015). Trainees' learning is also expected to derive from outside their coursework in the environment created by their teachers in their schools and programs. When this includes sexual harassment or other sexual misconduct on the part of educator or supervisor, it sends the message that such sexual behavior is condoned rather than condemned or prohibited. This was such a problem in some programs that they developed the reputation of professor–graduate student sexual relationships, and certain professors were known for these advantage-taking sexual relationships. This is now understood to be a destructive process, as well as an ethical and legal violation by the faculty person. If an errant professional's development was characterized by or modeled on such relationships, it raises the question of whether it became a template for the professional to later violate the sexual boundaries of patients or trainees (McNulty et al., 2013).

Defining Sex in a Professional Relationship: Ethics Codes and Laws

Pertaining to professionals, state licensing boards define sex far more broadly than intimate touching; oral–genital stimulation; or acts of vaginal, anal, or oral intercourse. Sex is the use of the client's body or mind for the professional's pleasure or for other needs, such as control, sadism, and dependence. The behaviors do not have to involve intercourse or culminate in orgasm. The Ohio Medical Board of Medicine, for example, defines sex as the expression of thoughts, feelings, or gestures that are sexual or that reasonably may be construed by a patient as sexual. Verbal examples are as follows: "I'm attracted to you," "You have lovely legs," "Have you ever had sexual fantasies about me?" Other examples involve intrusive behaviors and comments that might be rationalized as part of the treatment or a therapist's sexual response, such as an obvious erection or sexualized touches, behaviors, or gestures. It is likely that far more "sex" and sexual contact occurs between professionals and clients/patients than ever gets perceived or, if perceived, ever gets reported.

The American Psychiatric Association and the American Psychological Association (APA), as well as other mental health organizations, have debated the issue of the contraindication of sexual contact between clinician and patient. When the American Psychiatric Association questioned the length of time after termination when it would be ethical to have a romantic relationship with a former patient, several suggestions were made (Shavit & Bucky, 2004), but the most prudent idea put forth was "never" (Appelbaum & Jorgenson, 1991; Lazarus, 1992).

The history of the APA's development and periodic revision of its *Ethical Principles of Psychologists and Code of Conduct* (APA, 2017; hereinafter, APA Ethics Code), including its standards regarding sexual contact between therapist and client, is detailed in Chapter 2. Considerable debate existed within the organization about whether a lifelong ban on any sexual or romantic contact between a therapist and patient was necessary. Proponents of allowing such a relationship after a set period of prohibition argued that former clients, as responsible adults, have the right and the ability to consent. Opponents cautioned that the ongoing power differential and transference–countertransference dynamics between the parties despite the end of treatment created potential for exploitation or other misadventure. After considering both positions, the developers of the psychological code decided on mandating a 2-year window posttermination—a seemingly random choice without any clear rationale or research substantiation—before any personal romantic or sexual contact could take place. Cautionary language was included in the Ethics Code indicating that such a relationship should be the exception rather than the norm and that the onus always rests with the therapist for evaluating the potential for harm before engaging in such a relationship. This 2-year posttermination stance has remained controversial within the organization and is at odds with those of other mental health professions, all of which have determined that "never" is the most responsible course of action (Snyder, 2012). Lifelong prohibitions are warranted for many reasons, but the primary one is the damage that can be done to the ex-client/patient, even long after the treatment has ended. The following example is illustrative:

A patient told the first author that her psychoanalyst of 20 years earlier called her to ask if he could visit her briefly when he returned to town. Pleased, curious, and a bit concerned, she agreed. When she opened the door, the older man greeted her with a long, close hug. Their hour-long chat in her living room left her with unanticipated emotional upheaval. When she had a session a week later, she spoke of again having to recall her unpleasant feelings about her father's familiarity with her and many of her transient erotic feelings about her analyst, then and now. She was uncertain what his intentions really were when he said, "I just wanted to know how you were getting on in life." She told the first author, "He told me too much about his life. I could not begin to tell him the actual answers. I have not slept well since. I wish I had never agreed to the meeting."

Appreciating Eroticism and Its Many Meanings

Psychotherapy training used to emphasize transference and countertransference as universal phenomena that privately occurred during long-term therapy. Patients were expected to have some degree of love, dependence, and other intense feelings about their therapists. Therapists were expected to interpret these subjective states into feelings, conflicts, and motivations that were being displaced from parents or former spouses to the therapist. Therapists in training were alerted to appreciate that every person may have a dramatic eroticism within their private conscious subjectivity. Within this privacy, affection, sexual fantasies, and hostility to loved ones were played out. As these are discussed, the client was to learn about the conflicted nature of love (Kernberg, 2012). Erotic transferences are more likely to be discussed in depth in psychoanalytic and psychodynamic training programs. Client eroticism can occur in any type of therapy, however. See the chapters on various therapeutic orientations in Part II of this text.

Therapist–client sex typically occurs without revealing the eroticism that motivated it. Young professionals were taught to consider that their clients' sexual desires for them were resistances to uncovering its developmental meanings. As such, sexual behavior with a client was the result of inadequate or incompetent dealing with the erotic transferences that preceded the behaviors (Levine, 1992, Chapter 15). Such incompetence is expected among nonpsychiatric physicians, but all mental health professionals are expected to understand these phenomena, even though their training may not have included discussing the conscious subjective process of being a client.

When the erotic is dealt with in psychotherapy, sexual impulses and fantasies lose their power to overwhelm. Clients gain confidence in regulating their impulses, wishes, and imagery; they learn about themselves in love; and they realize that if this subjective drama is occurring in them, it must also be occurring in others. Such learning precludes acting out. At the beginning of such discussions of attractions or fantasies, some clients subtly or directly suggest or joke about changing the therapy to a sexual relationship. This probe of the therapist's professionalism is not to be ignored. Calmly, without anger, evident temptation, or harsh censure, the therapist can reply, "You must understand that there is no way that is actually going to happen," "You can ask many things of me, but not to make me a bad doctor in my and my profession's eyes," or "I see we have a lot of important work to do." When the first author was a resident, his supervisor told him that when a young woman at her first session looked at him and said that she wanted to have sex with him, he replied, "That is a hell of a way to say hello!" and went on to establish a clear boundary against such an interaction between them.

Defining Boundaries in Professional Relationships

Boundaries can be articulated with a variety of synonyms—among them, edge, frame, rule, guideline, and line. Each of these is indicative of the same concept, namely, that a boundary is the edge or the line of demarcation and distinction between one thing and another. A boundary can refer to the differentiation between self and other, what is regarded as therapeutic rather than intrusive or exploitive, what is and what is not contained within the invisible social contract and fiduciary duty between the professional and the client, behavior that is appropriate and inappropriate, moral and immoral, and what may be freely consented to and what may not be.

In terms of boundaries and their maintenance, the issue of consent is critical. How consent has been defined has changed over time. Whereas it was once seen as the client's prerogative to give consent in all matters, freely given consent in most, if not all professional relationships is now seen as an impossibility due mainly to the power and authority differential between a professional and a client. That power and status discrepancy, as well as trauma-based and transference reenactments, create a relationship in which clients are unable to offer true consent to sexual involvement with their therapist. For that matter, this also applies to any other dual relationship. The power inequality is too great: Clients' conditions may cause high susceptibility to influence and dependence. They may be pressured or coerced to meet the needs of their therapists in ways that they may or may not be able to perceive.

Purposes of Boundaries in Psychotherapy and Other Professional Relationships

Boundaries are designed to attain four important goals:

1. To maximize the potential of the therapist–client relationship to overcome the problems for which the client seeks assistance. It is understood that well-intentioned and well-conducted therapies can fail; however, they are far more likely to fail when boundaries are violated because they are not safe, are coercive, and trap the client.

2. To minimize the risk of harm to the client. Research has documented the harm that may be caused to clients psychologically and interpersonally with their families.

3. To minimize the risk of social, psychological, economic, and reputational harm and loss to the therapist.

4. To maintain the public trust in the profession and its integrity. Reports of sexually abusive professionals and their various methods of patient engagement are thought to inhibit some clients from seeking needed mental health services. These clinicians tarnish the profession to such a degree that it is a Hollywood cliché that psychotherapists routinely engage in sexual relationships with their patients. It is only recently that professions, legislatures, licensing boards, and criminal justice organizations are making efforts to clarify that sex with patients is unethical and illegal and not a Hollywood romance. Over several decades, understanding has shifted from patient blame and protection of the abuser to holding the professional responsible.

The need to maintain suitable boundaries over an entire career, regardless of the vicissitudes of the professional's personal life, can be understood by using two analogies. Professional–client boundaries are like a suit of armor to be worn daily as a safeguard against external or internal dangers. Boundaries can also be comparable to vaccinations used to inoculate the individual and reduce the risk of a serious disease. Some therapists directly educate patients verbally and in writing at the start of treatment to make the demarcation clear and a point of mutual effort to maintain boundaries. This education is in line with other limitations, such as telling patients, "You may and are encouraged to say whatever you feel during the session, but you may not do whatever you feel like doing. For instance, you may tell me of your anger at me, but you may not throw anything at me." The therapist must be clear that he or she is solely responsible for the maintenance of boundaries and not the patient. It must be understood that this is the case even when the patient behaves badly and in ways to provoke or tempt the therapist. Professionals are ethically, legally, and even criminally responsible, whether they or the patient invites or initiates sexual contact as illustrated by this case:

> The husband of a psychiatrist's patient found a note she had written to her doctor referring to their recent sexual behavior. The enraged and outraged husband called the doctor to tell him what he thought of him and sent a copy of the note along with a formal complaint to the licensing board. His wife, the patient, was greatly upset by her husband's responses. She violated his demand that she no longer have anything to do with her psychiatrist by approaching the doctor in his parking lot to apologize for her carelessness. "I would never have reported you!" The doctor's response was to plan his suicide, for which his wife immediately and luckily got him into psychiatric care.

When the board learned that the doctor had tolerated the woman's stimulation of her clothed genitalia during a long series of sessions, it charged him with that number of sexual violations. The fact that she repeatedly begged him to have intercourse and refused to stop masturbating in front of him as he instructed and then implored her did not sway the board. On the two occasions that he succumbed to her entreaties, he immediately stopped the sexual contact saying it was wrong. Despite this, the psychiatrist permanently lost his license and his professional standing.

When a client breaks a rule of therapy or violates an established boundary, the therapist generally has five primary options, not mutually exclusive:

1. To firmly remind the client of boundaries and of the limits of expression while working with them to understand the affects, conflicts, or memories that lay behind the sexual or other acting out.

2. To seek a consultation with a colleague about the situation with or without the client's knowledge. This can sometimes be done with the client.

3. To seek supervision for the case with or without the client's knowledge to directly focus on the therapist's vulnerabilities and the dynamics of the situation. The ideal goal is to get the treatment back on track or to end it in a nonharmful manner.

4. To seek personal psychotherapy to better understand needs and vulnerabilities and to support the therapists' clarification and enforcement of boundaries.

5. To terminate the treatment and transfer the client to another therapist. Of course, such termination is not done to begin a sexual relationship.

The therapist should include a description of the issue in the patient's chart from all perspectives: the perceived problem, both patient and the professional's reactions and responses, and how the course of action was determined. Many therapists are reluctant to describe such circumstances due to shame or the fear of negative repercussions. Actually, such documentation is self-protective. It describes a conscientious effort to maintain appropriate boundaries. It alerts future readers of the record of the client's responses and the therapist's struggle to use these responses in a therapeutic way.

In the preceding example, the psychiatrist did not realize that his patient had been sexually abused. He had not asked about such a history, and none had been disclosed to him. He did not understand her traumatic reenactments. He was only aware that the patient was an emotionally unstable "borderline" and that he was uncertain what to do with her. He was too embarrassed to seek help.

HOW BOUNDARIES ERODE AND RESULT IN CROSSINGS AND VIOLATIONS

The suit of armor, vaccinated status, and patient education are sometimes not enough to prevent boundary crossings and violations. Throughout their career, psychotherapists have responsibilities to maintain their overall health and emotional resilience enough to handle the challenges of the work and other life issues and must allow themselves to seek personal and professional assistance when needed. Life difficulties and transitions happen to everyone and can drain even the most resilient individual. Professionals must overcome arrogance about their perceived psychological hardiness and sophistication and their seeming invulnerability to weakness, life stress, temptation, and misconduct. It is hubris and denial that generate the notion that "this could not happen to me." When professionals' or their loved ones' health fails, career becomes stymied, finances get stressed, intimate relationship becomes asexual or is lost, children leave home or don't meet expectations, or another tragedy occurs, they can become susceptible to sexualization of a therapy. The resultant need for personal nurturance may lead them to throw caution to the wind and seek support from their clients.

Lovelorn therapists find many reasons to rationalize their behavior, sometimes railing at the restrictions that are placed on them as professionals. Loving or being in love with the client is not a free pass, even though it is both tempting and powerful. Rationalizations are proffered: "All my life, I have been waiting to meet such a person and now here she (he) is in my office. This is not about sex, this is about finding my missing half and filling the void that I have never until this moment fully understood." As moving as this explanation may be, it does not constitute an excuse or an exception to the ethics code or the law.

It is the case that clients may become overly dependent on and aggrandizing of their therapists, and some may have a different intent of breaking rules and boundaries and exploiting the therapist in some way (e.g., for financial gain or to get prescription medications, to get revenge for prior professional misconduct, or to prove all men are the same and the therapist's venality and lack of trustworthiness). They may inflate their therapist's ego by flattery (e.g., "You are the best therapist I have ever had," "You understand me in ways that no one ever has," "I don't know what I would do without you"). They may attempt to tempt or seduce by behaving in suggestive ways that may create an obsessive interest on the part of the therapist. Whether on a conscious or unconscious basis, they may engage in a reenactment of prior abuse dynamics. A psychotic version of the seduction scenario is seen in clients with erotomania.

Far less intense versions of clients' love for their therapists, however, can be disruptive to the therapists' mental health. Some version of falling in love with the therapist or with the client can undermine the therapist's assumption that "I will always act properly." Acting properly in the face of a client's eroticized transference can be considerable challenge (Levine, 1992, Chapter 15). Therapists are not immune from psychiatric conditions that may create sexual risk. Most therapists do not consider situations such as these until they happen to them.

Assume There Are No Exceptions

Boundary maintenance and the expectation of integrity apply at all times to all mental health professionals in all settings: to psychiatrists, psychologists, social workers, nurses, counselors, family and marital therapists, nurses, clergy, and allied professionals. They apply to students, residents, young adult, middle-aged, and older professionals. They apply to heterosexual, bisexual, lesbian, and gay and gender fluid therapists and those of all races and cultures.

In a practical sense, physicians, PhDs, and master's-prepared professionals who conduct psychotherapies are held to higher standards than those without the same degree of responsibility for the clients' welfare. The most highly educated or experienced mental health professionals are expected, regardless of their ideology or training, to understand and effectively manage erotic transferences and countertransferences (Levine, 2007, Chapter 3). Although a dermatologist may be excused for not initially appreciating a patient's seductive behaviors, mental health professionals are expected to better understand the contents of their clients' mind and what is behind seductive behaviors. It may be surprising to some therapists that the motivation for seduction of the therapist may include anger, contempt, financial gain, or a desire to seduce, toy with, or destroy.

Mental health professionals work in a vast array of settings, care for a wide range of individuals and problems, and use a variety of therapy techniques. Therefore, it should not be expected that the means of dealing with one type of situation applies equally to all. Boundary and ethical questions can abound. For example, is it wise or even ethical for a therapist to take a socially phobic person alone out for dinner to create an in vivo desensitization process? The therapist must balance what is known about the patient's condition, the behavioral therapy strategy being used, and what is unknown about having a therapeutic dinner out with one's therapist. No therapist should believe that he or she knows exactly how a client feels about what is occurring.

Moreover, other than the absolutes of boundary violations, there is no fixed line between what is appropriate and what is not, and what is therapeutic or not. It varies with the patient's age, presenting problem, the therapist's schema for conducting therapy, stage in the relationship, and perhaps other factors, such as illness and life threat. For example, a therapist's personal revelation is generally discouraged, but there are some circumstances where personal disclosure enhances the therapeutic alliance due to a greater sense of the therapist's empathy. There are also times when making a disclosure of an illness or other limitation in the therapist is necessary, although it might be uncomfortable and sad for both parties. Therapists who overdisclose can ruin the therapeutic frame by making the patient a friend and confidante, thereby creating a dual relationship. Over time, this can put the client in the role of helper while their needs for assistance and their therapy are ignored or derailed.

Boundary Crossings

Boundary crossings are different from boundary violations and can have both positive and negative effects. And they may be inevitable and virtually impossible to avoid. Additionally, modes of engagement, rules of conduct, and types of activities or exercises included in various treatment orientations may vary widely, and these need to be considered as well (Glass, 2003). Boundary crossings may involve unplanned contact outside of sessions, impulsive behaviors or mistakes on the part of the therapist, or more deliberate behaviors that are thought through ahead of time. The possible consequences of crossing a boundary, however it occurred, should be carefully ascertained and discussed ahead of time or afterward. Therapists are sometimes faced with the challenge or dilemma of doing something that is outside their usual way of practicing or the procedures of their preferred treatment orientation. For example, the second author treated a sexual abuse survivor who, despite having bouts of uterine hemorrhaging that was becoming increasingly dangerous, refused to be examined because she had had a highly negative prior gynecological experience and was now phobic. Due to the urgency, after the client asked and despite her reservations, Dr. Courtois did accompany her at her examination. They discussed ahead of time what this action would mean for the treatment relationship and how they would approach the appointment. After receiving the gynecologist's permission, Dr. Courtois sat behind her patient with her hand on her shoulder during the procedure. She remained uncertain about the wisdom of her decision until her client told her that she had never in her life felt such a sense of safety. With ongoing coaching, the client felt triumphant that she was able to attend subsequent appointments on her own.

When therapists do something out of the ordinary, make a mistake, or break a rule, it should be brought to the client's attention and labeled as such. The feelings of the client about the behavior are elicited and appreciated. If the situation warrants it, the therapist apologizes. Such a sequence of relational repair can advance trust and understanding, enhancing the relationship in the process. Some boundary crossings are relatively harmless deviations from traditional practice, behavior, or demeanor, and some can be quite helpful. For example, one generally does not touch the client except for a handshake, but when a client trips or falls, the therapist may help the client up without much discussion about the touch unless the patient brings it up in the next session. The reason therapists avoid touching is that even simple contact may be misinterpreted and elaborated into something it is not, something that usually goes undiscussed. Another example is the patient who unexpectedly hugs the therapist at the end of a session. This, and anything out of the ordinary, needs to be discussed at the next session.

The first author once paid for a patient's cab fare home, fed another who had not eaten in two days, and attended a wedding of a chronically mentally ill patient. A far more serious crossing occurred when, early in the treatment of a well-to-do married man for repeated episodes of infidelity, the same author ran into a problem with his department chair who wanted to terminate staff to save money, leaving Dr. Levine agitated, uncertain, and depressed. Soon afterward when his patient said, "How are you?" Dr. Levine found himself telling him the details of his academic political woes for 15 minutes, in the hopes of getting some sage advice. The patient listened until Dr. Levine stopped himself and apologized for his lack of restraint and misuse of their time. Embarrassed, he asked the patient if they could stop the session and resume the next day, and he did not charge for the session. The next day, Dr. Levine again apologized. The patient responded, "Listen, it is okay. I understand. I always knew you were a human being. We all have bad days. Good luck with your situation." Treatment continued to a successful outcome several months later.

Boundaries become an issue when therapists encounter their patients in social situations such as in church, synagogue, or mosque; when their children attend the same school; or when their spouses come to know each other in some community activity. Therapists may attend the same institutional meetings or social activities as their clients. Some of these crossovers are unavoidable, especially in small and isolated communities and social groups. It can be helpful to anticipate them with a client and discuss how to handle them. Such situations call for politeness and discretion, minimizing interaction without ignoring the client. The therapist has the obligation of maintaining the client's confidentiality, and it is solely the client's prerogative to make a self-introduction outside of the treatment setting. Informing a spouse as to who is a client before or during such an encounter is a breach of patient confidentiality. When any social encounter between therapist and client occurs, especially if unexpected, it is best if both parties at least briefly discuss it in the following session, if only to acknowledge its occurrence and any mutual awkwardness. It may be particularly uncomfortable for the therapist whose client may now know about aspects of the therapist's life that would not have been revealed otherwise.

Therapists know when their boundary crossings have gone too far when they don't document in the chart, they resist discussing their actions with a colleague, or they feel the need but fail to obtain a consultation (Martinez, 2000). They don't want to discuss the feelings of the client about the behavior at the next contact and are embarrassed to apologize. These are warning signs.

Dual Relationships

Dual relationships in which the parties have a relationship of some sort apart from and often simultaneously with the treatment, usually constitute boundary violations rather than crossings. They are to be avoided because they create dual loyalties and confound relationships that can compromise and permanently disrupt the treatment, harming both parties. Some therapists and clients enter into business relationships, buy and sell things to one another, or give expensive gifts and favors to each other. Some inappropriately offer to become supervisors, academic advisors, and mentors to their clients who are mental health trainees, hire clients as employees, use their services for office help or cleaning, or hire them as housekeepers and baby-sitters at home. Either party may end up feeling unappreciated or duped over the course of such an arrangement. For example, a patient may feel overcharged after purchasing a product, boat, car, or house from their therapist that they later perceive, rightly or wrongly, was too expensive.

Some idiosyncratic examples illustrate such scenarios: A numismatist therapist learned of his client's deceased father's extensive coin collection and made an offer to relieve her of the burden of having it catalogued and sold. Initially she was relieved, but a year after the transaction, she learned that the collection was worth five times what the therapist had paid her. She accused him of exploiting her due to his privileged knowledge from their sessions and terminated the treatment, threatening him with a lawsuit and a board complaint. By purchasing the coin collection at a highly discounted price, the doctor established a dual relationship between them, while exploiting his knowledge of her circumstance and the true value of the coin collection.

In another case, a psychologist's administrative assistant abruptly quit, posing her many logistical stresses. The next day, a client who had recently left college complained of financial need and uncertainty about her future. Quite impulsively, without any thought to problematic entanglements and intending to be helpful by creating a solution to their respective problems, the therapist offered her the job. Quickly, the new admin came to know much about the doctor's private life. The other clients in the practice lost their anonymity and confidentiality as they and their records became known to her. Within 2 weeks, the psychologist realized that her admin was disorganized and could not follow instructions to limit talking about herself and the doctor to clients. Mistakes were made several times each day. The psychologist wanted to terminate the young woman's employment but feared increasing her already high anxiety. Because they had not discussed ending the therapy when the job offer was extended or the issues that might arise in the dual relationship, their sessions became awkward, with feelings and issues left unstated. Before long, the young woman abruptly quit both roles, leaving the therapist in a worse office predicament than before and the therapy unfinished; her status worsened. The therapist had compromised herself as she had compromised her fiduciary duty to her client's welfare.

The lesson is clear: The potential of a treatment to be therapeutic is based on the doctor being devoted solely to the client's welfare and having no competing self-interest in the path to that goal. The therapist is expected to know better, but many therapists have never considered the dangers of dual relationships until they become trapped in them.

Boundary Violations

When boundary crossings become the norm and are repeated, some tend to get more conspicuous and serious, eventuating in one or more boundary violations. This tendency to escalate the breaking of ethical codes and standard professional conduct is referred to as the slippery slope of boundary crossings (Brooks et al., 2012) in the belief that the momentum may increase to the point where a violation is almost inevitable. Janet Wohlberg, who has studied sexual violations by psychotherapists for years (see Chapter 15), has argued against the wholesale use and acceptance of this concept and terminology, believing it suggests that therapists are helpless to stop their downward trajectory. Rather, she believes that there are many points along such a hypothetical slope when the therapist has choices and can take action that prevents a violation from occurring. We agree.

We elucidated some of the major choices earlier in this chapter. Yet once on the slippery slope, it is common for therapists to become paralyzed or to rationalize their inaction. They don't seek professional consultation or supervision due to being self-conscious and steeped in shame, because they have thoroughly rationalized their behavior and want it to continue (i.e., "this is true love"), or they don't care, in the case of serial predators, narcissists, and psychopaths. Moreover, they may express concern about taking time away from their practices, the expense of consultation, the breach of patient confidentiality, and what the consultant/supervisor will think of them. If the relationship has become sexual, they reassure themselves that the client has promised never to tell a soul and that no one suspects. The client is much happier now, and the professional tells himself that he can stop it later. It is simply too enjoyable to stop now.

Nor is it typical for the therapist to discuss the sexual involvement as a serious boundary violation with the client (although that does happen in some cases when therapists express their remorse, guilt, or shame in the aftermath and promise not to let it happen again) because the therapist is motivated to obscure his or her motives. This, despite the fact that such violations waste the opportunity for genuine therapy, ruin the possibility of effective future therapy and have high potential to traumatize the patient, immediately or later. The use of the client's body or mind for the therapist's pleasure is an egregious violation. The violation then has a life of its own. It may be a one-time occurrence, or it may escalate into a frequent years-long escalation within or outside of the regularly scheduled sessions. Some therapists have been known to bill for the sessions during which sex occurs, adding to the egregiousness of the violation when it becomes known. The second author evaluated a psychiatrist who initiated a sexual relationship with a patient whom he eventually married and had children with, then subsequently divorced. During the divorce, the psychiatrist's wife reported him to his licensing board for taking advantage of her while in therapy 17 years earlier. In a variation of this case, the second author interviewed a man who was in couples therapy with a therapist who "fired" him from the treatment, claiming that no progress was being made. Nevertheless, the therapist continued to treat the man's wife and then seduced her, then convinced her to divorce her husband and marry him. The husband sued for alienation of affection and mounted a board complaint. The therapist's license was permanently revoked.

Why Sexual Abuse Happens

There are many discernable reasons that sexual violations occur: For example, the therapist is lonely, depressed, sexually anxious or deprived, and unhappily married and encounters a client who is sensitive to the therapist's distress, expresses concern, and offers comfort. This begins a two-way psychological intimacy that can prove to be irresistible to the professional and involves increased self-disclosure and mutual dependency on the part of both individuals Eventually, talk may begin to move on to touch, nonsexual at first but increasingly suggestive and sexual. The client or therapist may express an interest in something social outside the office—meet for coffee, or direct encouragement of a hug or kiss in the office. Clients may love the therapist to varying degrees and instead of dealing with these appreciative feelings and fantasies of being loved in a full way by the therapist, their "confession" results in a change in the nature of their relationship from professional to personal.

In addition to those therapists who get caught up in sexualized contact due to situational issues, there are other who recognize the sexual opportunities inherent in practice or seek them out and periodically or serially take advantage of them, sometimes concurrently. When such a scenario comes to light, it shocks all of the involved clients who were led to believe that the therapist's love was exclusive to them and is shocking to others as well. These therapists are predators. They seek to identify clients who are particularly susceptible and naive and begin the process of engagement by complimenting them in a seemingly innocuous fashion. When these comments are met with gratitude, they escalate to indications of attraction and appreciation of the client's physical and sexual appeal and to increasingly sexually tinged comments. Therapists explain their comments as directed toward boosting the client's self-esteem, but as they continue, authorities refer to the process as one of grooming designed to disarm the patient and to satisfy the therapist's desires. The therapist cleverly finds additional ways to influence the client and to increase their dependency on the relationship. The client comes to misinterpret the process as one of love and desire rather than exploitation.

This type of therapist has a pattern of advantage-taking and a need for control, domination, and even sadism and can be quite dangerous. They have strong narcissistic and sociopathic features and recognize those clients whom they can influence to act out their erotic pleasures. Therapists who are serially accused of sexual misconduct by clients or patients tend to be dealt with by the judicial system rather than their state boards. Some of them end up in prison.

Many victimized patients describe experiencing great confusion during the period of grooming by a perpetrator of this type and feel as though their minds and their lives have been taken over and that they no longer know themselves or have control of their decisions and actions. In response, they paradoxically turn to the very person who is exploiting them. They develop an intense dependence on the therapist, including compulsive need for contact, approval, and explanation (Ishee, 2020). They believe what their therapists tell them because their own ability to judge the situation has been compromised. They often tell no one because they have been enjoined into secrecy and silence and due to their shame, confusion, and fear of being judged. For the therapist, the secrecy is necessary for protection from negative outcomes but is also a requirement for the relationship to continue uninterrupted and unabated (Ishee, 2020).

This situation, of course, is the opposite of what therapy is supposed to be and to provide. Most of these relationships end badly—often abruptly and in a deeply painful way. Only then do some clients "come to their senses," a process that may take months, years, or a lifetime. Many are deeply shamed and scarred by their "participation" and left with a host of other painful feelings as well. Although some react in ways that are vengeful, most want acknowledgment and apology and for the therapist to stop or be stopped from abusing others. To this end, some report the malfeasance to the licensing board, others to the police, still others to both. Others never tell, too ashamed to discuss their sexual relationship with their therapist with a subsequent therapist if they dare to see one.

Every Evaluated Professional Boundary Violator Has a Psychiatric Diagnosis

By the time boundary violators have been reported to a state licensing board and mandated to evaluation and treatment, most are usually emotionally frail and psychologically depleted. They have made a bad judgment or a series of them, which have had major consequences on their ability to work, as well as their financial resources, marriage, children, and colleagues, not to mention the patient(s) they took advantage of. The evaluation attempts to understand how and why the violation occurred and whether they can be rehabilitated with appropriate treatment and supervision (see Chapters 19 and 20). They may qualify for several diagnoses, the least of which is adjustment disorder with anxiety and depressed mood. Are they mentally or physically ill? Were they in a hypomanic state? Do they have a frontal lobe disease? Do they have a character trait that led to this, such as a manipulative, exploitative, advantage-taking tendencies, dysthymia, or naiveté?

Are they narcissists or sociopaths or do they have such tendencies? Do they have a major sexual disorder or conflict? Are they an addict? Are they a recently unhappy depressed person, or is their depression more charactero-logical? Has some childhood trauma or attachment issue been reactivated? Are they unable to assert themselves, or are they overly confident in a narcissistic manner? Do they make responsible clinical judgments, or is the client the one who has been in control of the treatment in some way, through threats of exposure, extortion, suicide? Is the therapist suicidal or homicidal? These possibilities are not mutually exclusive.

After a detailed inquiry when the evaluator does not know why this happened (this is not uncommon), it is reasonable to conclude that the frightened professional has not trusted the evaluation process because of shame, fear of the consequences of telling the truth, due to sociopathy, or for some other reason. This can make it incumbent on the evaluator to involve victims and hear from them what transpired. Victims' psychological status and the degree of damage done may be pertinent to a determination of whether a wayward and abusive therapist can be treated and rehabilitated or should be banned from the profession (see Chapters 19 and 20).

FINAL THOUGHTS

By virtue of the training, roles, and the right to practice sanctioned by their licenses, mental health professionals have the responsibility to maintain high standards and ethics of practice over the entire course of their career. To vaccinate oneself against these problems, to put on a suit of boundary armor each day of one's career, is to focus on the responsibilities inherent in the role of professional—namely, to restore mentally pained individuals to an improved state of internal and behavioral equilibrium.

Perfection in boundary maintenance, paradoxically, may not be ideal because an occasional crossing, when discussed as deviation from the usual rules of treatment or when undertaken for a particular therapeutic reason, can enhance the treatment. This includes the client's understanding of the therapist's struggle to do the right thing, which is not that different from the client's internal struggles. Like parents who occasionally misbehave in their roles with their children and who apologize, therapists attest to the dignity and rights of their clients by apologizing to them when appropriate and necessary. Boundary crossings can facilitate the therapy but must be dis-cussed openly, focusing on the client's feelings and conflicts.

Dual relationships are boundary crossings that manipulate the client or that allow the client to manipulate the therapist; these are far more destructive—often preludes to various forms of violation or abrupt, painful termination of treatment and the relationship. In this discussion, we have focused on how they can presage a collusion to act out sexually within the therapy, but they also can presage the conversion of the therapy to friendship or a business arrangement while billing for sessions, constituting fraudulent billing.

When egregious violations have occurred, the errant therapist should be recognized to be in an emotionally vulnerable state with periods of desperation. It is likely that most middle-aged and older professionals encounter colleagues in such a state who ask to become a client. They need the support of a caring professional who does not condemn but seeks to understand the steps taken that culminated in the violation. The treating professional will quickly become acquainted with the array of feelings of being a disgraced therapist.

Although it is, of course, far safer to resist the temptation, seek consultation, and spend time and money to understand the antecedent errors that enabled movement down the slippery slope than pay the profound career-changing price of a state board investigation and adjudication, we have far more experience with the latter group. In our experience those who have violated sexual or romantic boundaries seek care only when they feel in immediate danger of being reported and investigated. If this crisis passes, their participation in therapy quickly ends.

The ever-increasing social awareness of boundary violations by professionals has created a public health imperative of preventative actions and care, as well as aftercare, for all parties. Virtually all mental health disciplines now have courses on ethics or professionalism that cover many topics (Parran et al., 2013), yet some still omit sexual violations from the curriculum. Boundaries exist for the purpose of safety and protection. To ignore and violate boundaries is to defeat the cultural, moral, and ethical purposes of all the health professions and, in the process, to betray the client.

REFERENCES

American Psychological Association. (2017). *Ethical principles of psychologists and code of conduct* (2002, amended effective June 1, 2010, and January 1, 2017). https://www.apa.org/ethics/code/index.aspx

Appelbaum, P. S., & Jorgenson, L. (1991). Psychotherapist–patient sexual contact after termination of treatment: An analysis and a proposal. *American Journal of Psychiatry, 148*(11), 1466–1473.

Borys, D. S., & Pope, K. S. (1989). Dual relationships between therapist and client: A national study of psychologist, psychiatrists, and social workers. *Professional Psychology: Research and Practice, 20*(5), 283–293. https://doi.org/10.1037/0735-7028.20.5.283

Brooks, E., Gendel, M. H., Early, S. R., Gundersen, D. C., & Shore, J. H. (2012). Physician boundary violations in a physician's health program: A 19-year review. *The Journal of the American Academy of Psychiatry and the Law, 40*(1), 59–66.

d'Oronzio, J. C. (2015). Professional codes, public regulations, and the rebuilding of judgment following physicians' boundary violations. *American Medical Association Journal of Ethics, 17*(5), 448–455.

Gartrell, N. K., Milliken, N., Goodson, W. H., Thiemann, S., & Lo, B. (1992). Physician–patient sexual contact: Prevalence and problems. *The Western Journal of Medicine, 157*(2), 139–143.

Glass, L. L. (2003). The gray areas of boundary crossings and violations. *American Journal of Psychotherapy, 57*(4), 429–444. https://doi.org/10.1176/appi.psychotherapy.2003.57.4.429

Ishee, C. T. (2020). *Seduced into darkness: Transcending my psychiatrist's sexual abuse.* Terra Nova Books.

Kernberg, O. (2012). The psychology of sexual love. In O. Kernberg (Ed.), *The inseparable nature of love and aggression: Clinical and theoretical perspectives* (pp. 247–306). American Psychiatric Publishing.

Khandelwal, A., Nugus, P., Elkoushy, M. A., Cruess, R. L., Cruess, S. R., Smilovitch, M., & Andonian, S. (2015). How we made professionalism relevant to twenty-first century residents. *Medical Teacher, 37*(6), 538–542. https://doi.org/10.3109/0142159X.2014.990878

Lazarus, J. A. (1992). Sex with former patients almost always unethical. *The American Journal of Psychiatry, 149*(7), 855–857. https://doi.org/10.1176/ajp.149.7.855

Levine, S. B. (1992). *Sexual life: A clinician's guide.* Springer.

Levine, S. B. (2007). *Demystifying love: Plain talk for the mental health professional.* Routledge.

Markel, H. (2004). "I swear by Apollo"—On taking the Hippocratic oath. *The New England Journal of Medicine, 350*(20), 2026–2029. https://doi.org/10.1056/NEJMp048092

Martinez, R. (2000). A model for boundary dilemmas: Ethical decision-making in the patient-professional relationship. *Ethical Human Sciences and Services, 2*(1), 43–61.

McNulty, N., Ogden, J., & Warren, F. (2013). "Neutralizing the patient": Therapists' accounts of sexual boundary violations. *Clinical Psychology & Psychotherapy, 20*(3), 189–198. https://doi.org/10.1002/cpp.799

Parran, T. V., Pisman, A. R., Youngner, S. J., & Levine, S. B. (2013). Evolution of remedial CME course in professionalism: Addressing learner needs, developing content, and evaluating outcomes. *The Journal of Continuing Education in the Health Professions, 33*(3), 174–179.

Sansone, R. A., & Sansone, L. A. (2009). Crossing the line: Sexual boundary violations by physicians. *Psychiatry, 6*(6), 45–48.

Shavit, N., & Bucky, S. (2004). Sexual contact between psychologists and their former therapy patients: Psychoanalytic perspective and professional implications. *American Journal of Psychoanalysis, 64*(3), 229–248. https://doi.org/10.1023/B:TAJP.0000041259.60877.14

Snyder, L. (2012). American College of Physicians ethics manual (6th ed.). *Annals of Internal Medicine, 156*, 73–104. https://doi.org/10.7326/0003-4819-156-1-201201031-00001

World Medical Association. (2017). *Declaration of Geneva.* https://www.wma.net/policiespost/wma-declaration-of-geneva/

PART **II** PERSPECTIVES
FROM DIFFERENT
THEORETICAL
ORIENTATIONS

4

EROTIC TRANSFERENCES AND COUNTERTRANSFERENCES IN SEXUAL BOUNDARY VIOLATIONS

An Interview With Andrea Celenza

INTERVIEWERS: ARLENE (LU) STEINBERG AND JUDITH L. ALPERT

QUESTION: We chose to interview you for this book because you are a leading expert in the area of sexual boundary violations and have been working in this area for a long time. Tell us about your work in the area of sexual boundary violations.

ANSWER: I am a licensed psychologist (since 1985), training and supervising psychoanalyst at the Boston Psychoanalytic Society and Institute, and an assistant professor at Harvard Medical School. At this point, I have consulted on approximately 400 cases of boundary violations, including sexual boundary violations with a patient by a caregiver. I have been hired by boards of registration for all professional disciplines to consult on cases of boundary crossings, violations, and sexual misconduct. I have consulted to and served on ethics committees, peer review boards, task forces, and study groups on these subjects. I have also been involved in teaching and program development for a variety of institutions. I have published more than 30 articles in peer-reviewed journals and published a book, *Sexual Boundary Violations: Therapeutic,*

https://doi.org/10.1037/0000247-004
Sexual Boundary Violations in Psychotherapy: Facing Therapist Indiscretions,
Transgressions, and Misconduct, A. Steinberg, J. L. Alpert, and C. A. Courtois (Editors)

Supervisory and Academic Contexts, on these subjects. I have been an invited speaker locally, nationally, and internationally on the subject of boundary violations. I have served as an expert witness on many cases of all kinds of boundary violations.

QUESTION: How did you got involved in this field?

ANSWER: If you mean how I got involved in psychoanalysis, that's a big and deep question. Like so many of us, I came by it honestly, which is to say I came to our field because I wanted to think deeply, *needed* to think deeply about my life, and others around me. We all come to this work wounded and needing to be healed. Also to find ourselves, that synergistic process of finding oneself through finding others.

But if you mean, how did I get involved in the area of sexual boundary violations, that is also a question with many layers. I became interested in sexual boundary violations with the referral of a patient (the story of which I tell later in this interview). This led me to conduct research and perform more and more clinical work in this area. Like all psychoanalysts, I am a person who likes to look beyond the external, to the underlying motives. What particularly intrigued me was how well-intentioned most of the violators are—I was drawn to the paradox of this vexing problem And there is an amusing backstory. I had a colleague who was on the licensing board in another state and she had remembered—I should say *mis*remembered—the title of my dissertation, *The Capacity for Empathy, Regression and Ego Boundaries.* The only thing she seemed to have remembered was that the title had the word boundaries in it. It so happened that this licensing board was taking a very progressive step with one of their transgressing therapists—they wanted to rehabilitate him. Innocently, she announced to the board, "Andrea Celenza did her dissertation on sexual boundary violations." As you can see, this referral was based on a mistake.

When my colleague called and asked if I'd be interested in seeing a therapist who had had a sexual relationship with his patient for over a year, I naturally said to myself, "No!" I was thinking he'd be a psychopath, perhaps lying to me throughout the treatment, unremorseful, and maybe there would be other patients he'd exploited too. This was the stereotype in my mind and I would venture to say this is the stereotype we all had about these characters at that point in time. But then I looked at my appointment book. This was the first year of my private practice, and I only had a few patients. I knew there weren't others who had expertise in this area. I thought to myself, "Full fee, mandated treatment" (in other words, he can't leave), so I responded, "Yes, I would be happy to see this person."

Part of me dreaded meeting him. Little did I know how attached I would become and how sympathetic I would find him to be.

QUESTION: Have your writing and clinical work influenced each other, and if so, how?

ANSWER: At this point I guess it is fair to say that I have written a lot. Many years ago, my first job as a licensed psychologist entailed administering psychological testing, sometimes more than one test battery a week. It was not much fun, but I did get a lot of experience writing narratives suitable for my colleagues to read. That experience helped me get words on paper.

The other thing that helped me write is my enjoyment for presenting papers. To this day, I use conferences, clinical presentations, and teaching for the deadlines they require of me. I try not to prepare anything unless it might be suitable for publication at some point. I also try to write something new and enjoyable—not just for the audience I'm imagining in my head, but for me—something that I'm interested in learning more about, and something that I think might be a contribution to our field.

The nature of my clinical work is, of course, always psychoanalytic, even if a person is coming once weekly or never uses the couch. To be a psychoanalyst is to have that worldview. I always have a psychoanalytic lens that I view everything through, but I am not always functioning as a psychoanalyst—that entails the asymmetric role and that's only relevant in the office.

There are different kinds of psychoanalysis, as we know. I now consider myself a pluralist in terms of the kinds of theories I rely on and unconsciously embody. To be more specific, I would say I rely on a social constructivist epistemology (the assumption that we are always in relation, be they unconscious internalized self–other configurations or external relationships) and that everything we experience is influential. Beyond this epistemology, I incorporate everything I've been exposed to into my practice and thinking, whether psychoanalytic insights derive from drive, Kleinian, ego, self, object-relations theories, relational, or post-Bionian field theories—our platform is vast, and I find all the different orientations useful and intriguing.

Of course, my patients have led me to where I am. I began writing about sexual boundary violations through the patient I mentioned earlier. At that time, we didn't know much about the problem, what motivates violators, except to dismiss them as predators and that is not what I found in that first referral and in many others that followed. I felt a responsibility to get this information out, and that helped me write as well.

QUESTION: Within the area of sexual boundary violations, do you work with victims, clinicians who have been violated, bystanders, i.e., those who have suffered collateral damage such as family members, other patients, or members of the same professional community—or all of these?

ANSWER: I see the full range of people who have become involved in or are affected by sexual boundary violations in some way. This very much does include the therapists and analysts, the victim-patients, and others who suffer so-called collateral damage, such as spouses, colleagues, friends, and analytic siblings. Among the most damaging sequelae for those who are related to the victim-patient or therapist/analyst is the tremendous disillusionment in our field and industry. I often say that the most tragic consequence of sexual boundary violations is how it closes the door to subsequent, reparative treatment and this is true for all those involved, even if the involvement was not direct. The problem corrupts the core of our work upon which everything else depends, that being the trust in our character and in the setting. That is the only way our patients can reveal themselves to us.

As I have written elsewhere (Celenza, 2017, 2020), one of the most vexing, persistent, and painful sequelae of the particular posttraumatic stress syndrome associated with sexual boundary violations is directly derived from the corruption of the asymmetric structure of the treatment. The treatment contract consists of a promise by the analyst to maintain asymmetry (the asymmetric distribution of attention paid). When the asymmetry is corrupted, the betrayal comprises *a lie*—the use of the treatment (perversely) to convey some sense of love in an upended fashion. The problem is not the love—unhealthy, incestuous, and asymmetric as it is—but the broken promise upon which the relationship now rests. This, then, challenges the patient with an impossible task: *to believe in a love that rests upon a broken covenant.* The aftermath of sexual boundary violations revolves around this insecure foundation, where victim-patients are tortured by a lingering, persistent, and profound inner doubt of the verity and realness of this love and tragically, of love in general.

For those only indirectly related, there is an analogous disillusionment in the trustworthiness of the mental health professions. Some may never seek treatment for fear of being betrayed. To put an even finer point on this, I believe there is a type of profile of sexual boundary violations where the transgressor unconsciously targets the professional community, with a desire to pervert, corrupt, and bring down the profession through a grandiose, self-destructive act. Sometimes hostility toward the professional institute or training facility is part of the unconscious perverse scenario. Sometimes institutions play a part by mistreating their employees, prompting a desire to expose an exploitative environment or culture.

When I began this work, I oversaw the training of psychologists at Cambridge Hospital and was very interested in the gaps in training that failed to address the problem of sexual boundary violations. Prevention was the goal, but so too was how to address the problem once it came to light. At the individual level, I believe personal self-care is the most important problem to address. Mental health professionals are, by nature, "other directed" in the sense that we tend to focus on the other's needs. This can become an occupational hazard, leading to enormous self-neglect and overwork. These are also problems at the cultural and institutional level since we tend to cultivate a work environment that reinforces an omnipotent fantasy that we can heal anyone, as long as we work hard enough at it. I believe all the helping professions have this fallibility.

I have found this problem to be endlessly interesting in the ways it led me to examine other issues as well, such as self-disclosure, erotic aspects of the analytic encounter, how to understand the frame, and, of course, countertransference.

QUESTION: In your opinion, what motivates sexual boundary violators?

ANSWER: The question of what motivates sexual boundary violators differs depending on the kind of transgressor that you are studying. There are different profiles that, in reality, span the full range in the diagnostic spectrum. But I have come to believe that it is useful, in very broad strokes, to think about the violators in at least one of two categories, differentiating the psychopathic predator and the so-called one-time transgressor, whom I call "narcissistically needy" and Gabbard (1994) has called "lovesick." The psychopathic predator is not remorseful, usually blames the patient, has little sense of the harm that he has caused, and usually lies about the violation(s)—even feels entitled in some way. The shorthand for this profile is a multiple offender, and it is easy to see how the serial nature comes about, given the absence of superego functioning and lack of empathic concern. In contrast, there's the one-time offender, where there is an unhealthy love affair, a mutual idealization, and fantasies of rescue. But this profile is associated with genuine remorse, an abiding concern for the patient and how she may have been harmed, and a masochistic tendency give everything up for her in a misguided sense of healing.

It might be tempting to imagine a continuum between these two characters (the predator and the narcissistically needy/ lovesick profile), but they really are qualitatively different, and the distinctions are not difficult to make. The offender is either remorseful or not, he is concerned about the victim or he blames her, he violates once or multiple times, and she is meaningful to him or not. On the other hand, it does happen that I sometimes see a multiple offender who has only violated once; i.e., he got caught with his first.

Diagnostically, these categories might also be considered to fall along a continuum of narcissism . . . from narcissistically needy to malignant narcissism. Perhaps the differentiation between the two types of narcissistic personality is useful here—the one who is deficient in self-esteem and the other who is defensively grandiose, but this can miss the quality of psychopathy in the predator profile.

Also, within these two broad-stroke categories, there is a variety of differentiations to be made, but that is like anything. The better one knows a person, the more complicated it gets, and diagnostic categories lose their usefulness. Still, I believe this differentiation goes a long way to begin to understand what motivates different therapists to do this kind of thing. Once you make this distinction, there are implications for what is needed to address the problem as well, such as whether rehabilitation might be considered (one-time offenders, probably yes; predators, no, probably never). Of course, as you get to know them each individually, the picture becomes more complex, and then what is needed is very individualized.

QUESTION: In your opinion, can violators be rehabilitated?

ANSWER: First, I think that it would be very helpful to our professional community if rehabilitation were part of the culture, part of what is considered in every case. This does not mean all violators will be amenable or have the potential to be rehabilitated, but our culture should have a more humane attitude toward this occupational hazard. Paradoxically, I think a change in the culture is one of the factors that holds out some hope for preventing sexual boundary violations. One of the troubling aspects of trying to address this problem is how punitive and hostile we are toward the transgressors, regardless of their motivations, context, or personal dynamics. This hostility is antiintellectual, antipsychoanalytic, and antihumane. It is also not helpful in providing an atmosphere where practitioners can turn to each other when they get into trouble. There is so much shame and judgment; this hostile culture renders the problem unspeakable, leaving our colleagues dangerously alone, trying to deal with a problem when they may feel over their head, and soon it will be too late.

The resistance to rehabilitation, in my view, is highly defensive on our part, because openness to it entails the acceptance of a vulnerability we *all* must own. If a particular person has potential to be rehabilitated, then we all have that potential, and it's a short step to say the same about the good work we do. Don't we believe persons are capable of being healed? Of course, I'm not including everyone here, but the one-time offender is more like us than is comfortable to admit. In fact, sexual boundary violations occur in every treatment orientation, including gestalt, CBT, humanistic, behavioral modification, DBT . . . even family therapists where multiple family members are clients of the therapist. They occur in every helping profession as well.

The idea that we can get rid of bad actors, engaging an "us versus them" kind of polarization is a defensive fantasy. We know that even when a violator is exiled, the problem does not go away. Tragically—and this is not a fantasy—the transgressors risk ruining their career, ostracization, and expulsion from their professional community, rendering it too risky for them to reveal themselves, even when the boundary crossings are relatively mild and not yet sexual. This creates a necessity for secrecy and an inability to get consultation or any kind of help. (In a more general way, erotic countertransference is pathologized too, and our theories are desexualized overall. I address these questions in my second book [see Celenza, 2014]).

I don't want to be misunderstood as saying that everyone should be rehabilitated or that we should turn a blind eye in some way. I am saying that the most common kind of sexual boundary violation, the so-called one-time offender who falls into an unconsciously self-deceptive, idealized, and unhealthy (i.e., exploitative) love affair, is more like us than not. Indeed, I believe the vulnerability to this is universal. This is not a conclusion I arrived at through personal introspection but by observing changes in colleagues, especially as they age, facing mortality, and/or other major stresses. In our current state of mind, we can all say, "I would never do that." But it is omnipotent to think we will always be in our current state and that we can know or be in control of how we feel and what we desire for the rest of our lives.

QUESTION: Are there personal characteristics or other factors that are conducive to the rehabilitation of a violator?

ANSWER: Yes, there are specific factors that help to differentiate the one-time offender from the psychopathic predator. These factors are also associated with amenability to rehabilitation and are spelled out in my first book in a chapter entitled "Precursors to Sexual Boundary Violations" (Celenza, 2007). In that chapter, I delineated eight personal characteristics that I believe are vulnerabilities for the one-time offender.

Before going into more detail about these factors, I want to state a reminder. When I talk about rehabilitation, I am talking about the one-time offender. We don't really know much about the psychopathic predators because they usually refuse to be evaluated. I've seen some, but they are not well studied. They typically lie about the violation continuously, they are unremorseful, and they often blame the patient (which I find intolerable).

For those who have the potential for rehabilitation, the most important factor is the presence of genuine remorse. I carefully differentiate this from narcissistic mortification (which everyone has whenever there is a complaint, i.e., they are mortified *for themselves*, what they have done to their career, etc.—this is not genuine remorse). The kind of remorse I am referring to involves *concern for the patient*, the willingness to look at the *harm* that the offender has wrought, the feeling of *regret* about the violation and finally, the desire to understand his or her actions *from within*. The abiding concern is for the well-being of the victim-patient and there's a capacity to take responsibility for one's actions. These are the important factors. There are several others, but I'd like to leave it there, to keep this front and center.

QUESTION: Do you think that therapists who are sexual boundary violators should be charged as criminals? If so, under what circumstances?

ANSWER: The question of criminality, criminal charges, and criminalization of sexual boundary violations stands in stark contrast to the idea that this is a universal vulnerability. Criminalization also contradicts my belief that we, as a professional community, should take a less hostile and punitive stance toward the one-time offenders while trying to help them and, at the same time, recognize that the victim-patient has been wronged and harmed, that it wasn't her fault, and that she likely is suffering greatly. I do not believe criminalization is the way to respond to this problem (although for the psychopathic predators, there is an argument to be made in certain cases, especially if assault or force are involved). But for the one-time offender, I do not think criminalizing this very human problem is a helpful way to think about it or respond to it.

QUESTION: How has your involvement with lawsuits, expert witness testimony, and the court conflicted with your role as treating therapist?

ANSWER: If I am the treating therapist in a specific case, I do not become involved in any other role (consultation, evaluation, supervision, advocacy, or expert witness). I may write a letter sharing my clinical observations with the appropriate waiver of confidentiality, but this is not an agreement between me and an overseeing body; it is something I negotiate based on my patient's wishes. All of my treatments of violators are nonreporting to any overseeing body, otherwise the treatment is compromised.

If I am *not* the treating therapist, however, I do provide expert witness consultation, supervision, other advocacy, or expert opinion given my knowledge base in this area. I also conduct evaluations of violators, usually to address the question of amenability to rehabilitation and to outline such a program if I think they have the potential.

I have consulted and have been involved in adjudicatory processes associated with lawsuits and complaint processes. There are multiple ways to address the problem from many angles, and I have been involved from many different vantage points.

Lately I have been leaning toward the idea that monetary settlements can be a good response for the victim-patient(s), but often the victim-patient(s) will tell you that an apology or evidence of taking responsibility for the exploitation is really all they want from the violator. I respect this. Still, I believe monetary compensation is also warranted because the victim-patient(s) paid for a perverted treatment and have consequent harm that is costly to be addressed. She will need a subsequent treatment where the harm for the violation needs to be addressed and she should be compensated for that. Why should she be harmed again?

QUESTION: We welcome your thoughts about working with erotic transference and erotic countertransference, an area that you have written a great deal about.

ANSWER: I did not arrive at my study of erotic transferences and erotic countertransferences via my work with sexual boundary violations (although of course these are all related). Once again, my interest came from my work with a patient, one who was extremely challenging and also frightening for a period of time. This is a patient I wrote about in my second book (Celenza, 2014), where after pressuring me to have sex with him, then wanting me to leave my marriage for him, he shared a fantasy of killing me. I was petrified for 3 weeks—an eternity!

Early on, when the treatment was in its initial challenging phases, I noticed that there was very little literature—not only on the general subject of erotic transference but especially lacking were reports of cases where the analyst is a woman. Consultations were key for me during this time. I needed help sorting out the dynamics of this treatment in order to know how best to help him. This inevitably involved my counter-transference as I was attempting to understand this confusing picture and I was able to see his unconscious communications in my own internal fantasy life. Since erotic countertransfer-ences come in as many varieties as erotic transferences, they often carry much unconscious significance as to the nature of the erotic transference in a particular treatment. Yet, erotic countertransference has been rendered taboo, much like our theories have been desexualized—there's a constant tendency to bury sexuality!—and normalizing all of these very human experiences would be a great help to furthering our under-standing about how to intervene. I often say that the absence of erotic countertransference should be problematized (i.e., the absence of any erotic attraction toward a patient should signal that something is missing).

I'm often asked if this case might have gone awry had I not had expertise in sexual boundary violations. But here, I think it is important to note that not all cases of erotic transferences risk the possibility of sexual boundary violations. Sometimes the under-lying, unconscious issues are in a different realm. Plus, erotic transferences arise in many forms, many of which are defensive and are negative transferences (e.g., a defense against mourn-ing, hatred, or envy). But not all erotic transferences have this structure nor do they necessarily tempt the therapist to cross boundaries. The transference–countertransference dynamics vary by the particular analyst–analysand pair and their indi-vidual proclivities.

QUESTION: Can you say more about erotic transference and counter-transference and their relationship to the vulnerability of committing sexual boundary violations?

ANSWER: As I stated just now, not every case of erotic transference or erotic countertransference leads one to feel a vulnerability to sexually violating boundaries. Erotic transferences span the full spectrum of meaning because sexualization is a very common defense. In the end, the manifestation of an erotic transference is highly individualized.

However, there is a group of erotic transferences that are involved in sexual boundary violations. This is usually a defensive or erotized transference culminating in an urgent demand from the patient to have sex with the therapist or analyst. To begin thinking about this, it is useful to distinguish between a sexualized transference and an erotic transference (this distinction is derived from Christopher Bollas's, 1994, work). The sexual transference is actually quite simple, even concrete, in the sense that it is not variegated in meaning. It is a blatant and often pressured demand to have sex with the therapist/analyst. In contrast, an erotic transference is where the therapist's or analyst's role in the patient's erotic fantasy life is more fully developed and eventually revealed. So, the first step is to transform the sexual transference into an erotic transference so that the fantasy behind the sexual transference can be understood. A lot of sexual boundary violations are responses to a sexual transference because the therapist or analyst takes the patient's demands at face value. If the therapist/analyst is able to tolerate the sexualization, explore the patient's fantasies, thereby transforming the sexual transference into an erotic transference, and then work with that, a sexual boundary violation may be averted. But this all depends on the capabilities of the therapist/analyst at that point in time.

It would be a mistake to think that falling into a sexual boundary violation only happens with the less well-trained or unseasoned. I have been stunned to see many otherwise highly seasoned and well-trained analysts suddenly become unusually concrete in relation to a sexual transference, motivated by his or her need to see the patient in this unidimensional way, at least at this moment in time. Added to this is the false dichotomization in our literature between so-called real and unreal analytic love that can serve self-deceptions as well (see Celenza, 2017, 2020). Suddenly, it seems you are experiencing a different analyst, one who normally doesn't function simplistically but is doing so with this particular patient because of the unconscious meaning of the patient to him or her. I write a lot about this sort of *perfect storm* where the analyst–analysand pair, in the erotic transference–countertransference dynamic, is highly meaningful for each. Much of this is only revealed in a subsequent treatment where it is possible to see how the complexity of what was played out had been greatly reduced.

QUESTION: Since there are more women than men in the field, have you noticed an increase in female sexual boundary violators?

ANSWER: It is an inescapable fact that our field is becoming feminized, as are many of the health care professions. It stands to reason that these changing demographics will also change prevalence rates according to gender. In my clinical work, I have seen a disturbing increase in female sexual boundary violators, but I am unaware of any empirical or systematically controlled studies that bear this out. I know this is an inconvenient fact because we like to think of women as having a lesser tendency toward exploitation. I still think it is true that there are fewer female psychopathic predators, but as for the one-time offender category, indeed, there has been an apparent rise in prevalence among female practitioners.

As I reported in my first book, two thirds of female transgressors end up violating female patients, and these therapists/analysts are not necessarily self-identified as gay before their relationship with the victim-patient. They also do not necessarily identify as gay afterward, although sometimes you do have same-sex pairs (female–female and male–male dyads), and here, often the sexual boundary violation occurs in the process of coming out.

QUESTION: In your experience, is the nature of the violations different depending on the sex or gender of the violator?

ANSWER: Yes, I believe that the nature of the violation, the dynamic underpinnings, and the unconscious meanings for female therapists/analysts are different from the meanings associated with male transgressors. What I have found is that the dynamic underpinnings for male therapists/analysts relates to an attempt to control the erotic transference as the idealization fades and its defensive structure is unmasked. In other words, the negative transferential underpinnings begin to be revealed, which of course, is a positive step in the treatment but is experienced as an intolerable transformation for the fragile therapist/analyst.

For whatever reason in the male therapist/analyst's unconscious, he is unable to tolerate the patient's hostility and attempts to recapture the earlier erotic transference in its idealized form. This is when the seduction occurs and is its purpose.

For the female transgressors, in contrast, there is usually an overidentification with the patient. This is especially true if it is a female–female analyst–analysand pair. Perhaps a merger fantasy fuels the violation, but not always. Still, there is an almost total disregard for difference in the victim-patient, i.e., for ways in which the view of the patient might diverge from what the therapist–analyst understands about herself.

QUESTION: We explore diverse communities in this volume. Are there situations of greater vulnerability when either the patient or the violator is a member of a marginalized community?

ANSWER: There is some literature on this specific context for sexual boundary violations—the prevalence and meanings in marginalized communities. John Gonsiorek (1995) has some very good papers on his research in these communities, although at this point they may be dated. He likes to analogize minority communities as "psychological small towns" even when members reside in big cities. What he reveals is the higher prevalence of all kinds of boundary crossings that tend to be viewed as inevitable, given that social, political, occupational, and personal lives overlap in these small communities. Some see this as unavoidable, much like in small towns and rural communities.

A particular study that I find helpful as well was conducted by Lyn (1995) from within the Society for the Psychology of Sexual Orientation and Gender Diversity (Division 44 of the American Psychological Association). Through anonymous questionnaires, she examined members' attitudes, beliefs, and actions within these communities and found a higher prevalence of sexual boundary violations (15%) despite strong feelings against these ethical violations. There is also one aspect of her study that I think is especially revealing, and I appreciate it for its generalizability. She asked participants for their assessment of their own experience of sexual relationships with patients and whether or not they pose a dilemma for themselves. Only 2% reported experiencing sexual relationships with patients as a dilemma *for themselves*. In contrast, when asked about colleagues' vulnerabilities, participants reported that they thought *almost half* of their colleagues would experience such relationships as posing a dilemma. This is a wide divergence and can be interpreted as believing others' have greater difficulty with sexual boundaries than oneself. I think this is a generalizable and quite common self-deception.

There is also a tendency toward retrospective revisionism when a sexual boundary violation comes to light, especially by a formerly trusted colleague. A sudden mistrust of that person and a rewriting of history emerges, as if they mistrusted that person all along.

QUESTION: We know that you treat individuals whose boundaries have been violated. What disciplines do the practitioner/violators represent?

ANSWER: I have seen practitioners of all disciplines, including psychoanalysts, psychologists, psychiatrists, social workers, and licensed or unlicensed mental health caregivers. I've even seen an occupational therapist and a massage therapist. Also, as you may know, this is a particular problem among clergy (and I'm excluding the problems of the Catholic Church here). But mostly I've seen mental health caregivers, and I can tell you that no discipline is immune to this problem.

I am not aware of any recent empirical and controlled studies that compare the prevalence rates among different types of therapies within the mental health professions. Older studies show that psychiatrists and psychologists have equivalent prevalence rates with a lower incidence among psychodynamic therapists and therapists who provide long-term intensive psychotherapy (see, e.g., Borys & Pope, 1989). It is speculated that this derives from greater awareness of the importance of clear, nonexploitative, and therapeutically oriented roles, boundaries, and responsibilities, such as maintaining the frame, the holding environment, and appreciation for transference. These studies imply that the more loosely bounded maintenance of the therapeutic frame in some humanistic and eclectic approaches may predispose clinicians to boundary crossings. Other approaches can be similarly unclear about boundary maintenance, as in those that may involve nonerotic touch (e.g., hugs, pats on the back). In general, the longer term therapies are conducted by therapists or analysts who are sensitized to unconscious factors and transference pressures. Many cognitive-behavioral therapists and practitioners of other short-term treatments are ill-equipped to understand complex, emotionally intense pressures on the therapist. We would expect these therapists to have a higher prevalence rate of sexual boundary violations, and many of the therapists I have seen bear this out. Further, they often report that they had nowhere to turn for help since their supervisors had similarly limited training to their own.

QUESTION: Within psychoanalysis, what are some differences you have noticed based on different theoretical orientations?

ANSWER: The question about theoretical orientation is very interesting, and I'm glad you asked. I suspect that many psychoanalytic practitioners would guess that relational practitioners would have a higher incidence of sexual boundary violations, but this is not the case. I have not seen any systematic studies on this question, but I do *not* think there is a difference in prevalence among the various theoretical orientations. The fact is, *our theories fail us differently*, and there is no refuge for sexual boundary violations within theoretical orientation.

For example, consider the relationally oriented analyst. Here, the vulnerability usually resides in the idealization of love and its healing power. While of course, the emphasis on the mutuality and humanness of the analytic relationship is a much-needed corrective to the wooden, inaccessible classical caricature, the overemphasis (by some practitioners in this tradition) on mutuality to the exclusion of the disciplined restraint of asymmetry is a real problem, especially as this imbalance evokes omnipotent rescue fantasies. This is a certain profile of sexual boundary transgression where the subjectivity of the analyst can be stirred to a level of grandiosity that knows few limits.

On the other hand, the problem in the valorization of anonymity and abstinence (two parts of the classical analytic triad), fails to guide the more schizoid, narcissistically impaired analyst when emotional connection and needs are stirred up. Like a boat in a storm without a mooring, intense erotic transferences can overwhelm the more schizoid, inhibited analyst who has only classical theories with their one-person epistemology—a mandate to "act like you're not there"—to provide guidance.

Or, to overemphasize the asymmetry in the analytic relationship can be interpreted as permission to hide behind the analyst's authority. A masochistic surrendering to the patient's intensely driven demands is more likely to derail this kind of limited analyst, whose subjectivity finds safety in the hidden, mysterious shroud of anonymity.

There is a great fallibility among mental health caregivers of other orientations outside of psychoanalytic and psychodynamic orientations as well. Many of these caregivers lack an understanding of transference in general and take the client's pleas for love (and sex) at face value. They can fall into unconscious enactments where they have limited familiarity with their own vulnerabilities as well.

QUESTION: How might existing professional ethics codes be improved?

ANSWER: This goes back to the question of what we need in order to possibly prevent sexual boundary violations. I don't think more rules or regulations will help, especially as education about this problem has become more widespread (though is not at the level of a required part of ethics courses as of yet). Nor do I think more committees will be helpful. I have consulted with institutes where there was every committee one would hope for as part of their infrastructure—professional relations committees, ethics committees, and ombudspersons—yet no one used these resources when they needed them because the atmosphere in the institute was too hostile and punitive. In contrast, I have consulted with institutes who had very little in the way of infrastructure, yet members turned to each other for help when they needed it. That was because the atmosphere and the overall culture in these institutes was more accepting of their human fallibilities, a more humble attitude toward each other's humanity. So, I think the cultural change has to happen as opposed to a structural change.

QUESTION: In your opinion, what are some public policy needs that should be addressed with respect to sexual boundary violations?

ANSWER: Basically, I don't think you can legislate attitudes and beliefs. I think that to try to address this problem from a public policy perspective is top-down rather than by addressing the problems at a more local level. This is parallel to the question of where the institutes may have every resource, committee, and structure but members don't have the requisite trust in one another to take advantage of these structures. I prefer a bottom-up approach through education and also through processing one's experiences perhaps with members who have violated boundaries. This would bring with it a potential to empathize with all sides of the problem. It is only at the level of experiencing each other and oneself in relation to one another that we can grow and develop a more transcendent culture.

QUESTION: How can training be improved to minimize or prevent sexual boundary violations?

ANSWER: I do think training can be greatly augmented by teaching about this problem in general. It should be part of required curriculum. It is also one of the avenues that might change the culture within a particular professional community, especially in relation to the universal vulnerability to sexual boundary violations. But I don't think this is largely an educative process at the level of cognition. As we all know only too well, we have analysts (who arguably are among the best trained mental health practitioners), even those who know a lot about sexual boundary violations in particular, who have still fallen into these problems.

I think we need to teach at the level of experience, as I was saying in the previous question, where we engage affectively with those who have transgressed, talk to victim-patients, and feel with them the harm that is wrought. I also believe we should take a developmental view of personal challenges across the lifespan. This would be really helpful to add to any kind of training where we take a more humble approach to our own omnipotence. We need to recognize that we may not always have the personal strengths that we have at the moment. When I teach about sexual boundary violations, I always emphasize the universal vulnerability, and I know that some members in the audience will be saying to themselves, "Not me." Then I recite these words and tell them that it might be true in their current state of mind, but we don't know what the future holds, and I think it is omnipotent to think that you would know. Perhaps I should more rightly say it is omniscient.

QUESTION: What is your prognosis for the field of mental health with respect to sexual boundary violations?

ANSWER: To state it in very simple terms, I would say that my prognosis for the field is twofold. First, I think we are well on our way to eradicating psychopathic predation within our institutes. This is due to our zero tolerance for such acting out, at least in the United States. However, I don't think we will ever be rid of the one-time offender because I think this is part of the human condition, part of human frailty, and the existential fear of death. We don't do well addressing this very present aspect of life, especially in America. This is part of what I mean when I say that it is a universal vulnerability. All the more reason I think it is incumbent upon us to have avenues of redress in ways that are humane. Of course, we want to avoid all sexual boundary violations. The cost of offending is significant. There are many who suffer when there is a violation, and this includes the profession, the institution, the bystanders and, especially the victim-patient.

QUESTION: You treat victims and violators. What impact does this have on you? How do you manage your own countertransference?

ANSWER: I think treating both victims and violators has helped me to empathize with and understand the complexity of this problem from all different angles. The fact that I have treated so many violators has helped me with victim-patients as well, especially when they need to address (and admit to themselves) how much they loved the therapist, even beyond the exploitation and betrayal. At the same time, when victim-patients are very hostile toward their therapist, I understand that too because they are usually leading with the awareness of the exploitation. Many of these have been victimized by psychopathic predators, and they should be outraged. It often takes them longer to talk about and be able to hold onto the love that they had, for fear of letting the violators off the hook. I think the deeper you understand a problem from all sides, the more you are able to empathize with the complexity of the problem overall. This, of course, is what psychoanalysis is all about.

           In terms of countertransference, I think I only find myself over time having less tolerance toward the psychopathic predators who are unable to see the harm that they have caused. I think in general, we all have trouble with that as time goes on.

QUESTION: Have you been personally affected by what you hear? Do you turn to others for support and consultation?

ANSWER: I frequently use consultation in all of my treatments (of course, without identifying my patients). I meet monthly with a consultative peer group, and I meet biweekly with a close colleague. I often call on colleagues who have special expertise in some area I find myself struggling with. I couldn't possibly have done this work without the great help and support of Glen Gabbard and Gary Schoener, both of whom have been terrific colleagues and friends. I rely on Glen for all kinds of cases as well, but especially those with sexual boundary violations.

I have come to believe that it is helpful to inform all of my patients at the beginning of every treatment that I regularly consult with other colleagues. One reason I inform everyone of this practice is that it guards against the experience of the analysis or therapy as if it is in some insulated bubble, separated in time and space. This is one of the characteristics of dyads where sexual boundary violations can occur.

QUESTION: In your opinion, has the #MeToo movement influenced reporting of abusive therapists? Do you think there is now more social understanding of sexual boundary violations in treatment as a result of the visibility of the #MeToo movement?

ANSWER: I don't think anything within our professional community has influenced the reporting of abusive therapists for the #MeToo movement. I believe the public is fairly uninformed of what goes on in the psychoanalytic world, and the #MeToo movement has had its own impetus, largely motivated by feminism and the greater respect for women within our culture. This is all to the good. I think the #MeToo movement is on its way toward diminishing and hopefully abolishing psychopathic predation in Hollywood, corporate America, politics, and academia.

On the other hand, I am very concerned about the impact of the #MeToo movement *on us*. Within our industry, psychopathic predators were brought to light back in the 80s, and we are well on our way to eradicating psychopathic predation within our industry, as I mentioned. For me, I fear the #MeToo movement will oversimplify the challenges we face so that we see every flirtation as an assault or every sexual boundary violation as predation. We have worked hard to differentiate the trees from the forest, and I fear the #MeToo movement will drag us backward. While that movement is in its first wave, we are actually in our third wave. (I am writing a paper that addresses these very problems; see Celenza, 2021). I fear important insights on prevention and modes of redress are threatened to be lost if the history of what we have already accomplished is overlooked or forgotten.

REFERENCES

Bollas, C. (1994). Aspects of the erotic transference. *Psychoanalytic Inquiry, 14,* 572–590. https://doi.org/10.1080/07351699409534007

Borys, D. S., & Pope, K. S. (1989). Dual relationships between therapist and client: A national study of psychologists, psychiatrist, and social workers. *Professional Psychology: Research and Practice, 20*(5), 283–293. https://doi.org/10.1037/0735-7028.20.5.283

Celenza, A. (2007). *Sexual boundary violations: Therapeutic, supervisory and academic contexts.* Jason Aronson.

Celenza, A. (2014). *Erotic revelations: Clinical applications and perverse scenarios.* Routledge. https://doi.org/10.4324/9781315773056

Celenza, A. (2017). Lessons learned on or about the couch: What sexual boundary violations can teach us about everyday practice. *Psychoanalytic Psychology, 34*(2), 157–162. https://doi.org/10.1037/pap0000095

Celenza, A. (2020). Righting a wrong: A commentary on "The Poetics of Boundary Violations: Anne Sexton and Her Psychiatrist" by Charles Levin and Dawn Skorczewski. *Psychoanalytic Dialogues, 30*(2), 222–229.

Celenza, A. (2021). *Psychoanalysis and #MeToo: Where are we in this movement* [Manuscript in preparation]?

Gabbard, G. O. (1994). Psychotherapists who transgress sexual boundaries with patients. *Bulletin of Menninger Clinic, 58*(1), 124–135.

Gonsiorek, J. (1995). *A breach of trust: Sexual exploitation by health care professionals and clergy.* Sage Publications.

Lyn, L. (1995). Lesbian, gay, and bisexual therapists' social and sexual interactions with clients. In J. Gonsiorek (Ed.), *A breach of trust: Sexual exploitation by health care professionals and clergy* (pp. 193–212). Sage Publications.

5

PSYCHODYNAMIC PERSPECTIVES ON THE PROBLEM OF EROTIC IDEALIZATION

ELIZABETH GOREN AND SUE GRAND

Addressing sexual boundary violations, this volume speaks across therapeutic practices. This mission implicitly asks: How do we help each other with boundary trouble? As two psychoanalysts, we hope to contribute to this dialogue. In this chapter, we speak to nonanalysts who may be interested in how psychoanalysts anticipate, understand, and navigate this knotty predicament. What theories and techniques guide us? These questions recur in this chapter as we consider a specific form of erotic boundary trouble. This form, most commonly found with sexually or romantically addictive (or hungry) patients, can occur in any gendered dyad. Here there is no actual sex between patient and therapist. In this situation, the therapeutic exchange calcifies into an overstimulating, romantically idealizing dynamism. In its extreme form, the therapeutic relation becomes fixated in mutual fantasies of a perfect erotic partner. In more subtle cases, the therapist feels vitalized by the patient's idealization and desire, while the patient becomes "hooked" on the "perfect" therapist. At the outset, it must be stated that love, including moments of feelings of attraction, in and of itself, is not necessarily a problem. Indeed, it can be therapeutic, a sign of the patient's growth.

https://doi.org/10.1037/0000247-005
Sexual Boundary Violations in Psychotherapy: Facing Therapist Indiscretions, Transgressions, and Misconduct, A. Steinberg, J. L. Alpert, and C. A. Courtois (Editors)

The trouble we are describing occurs when patient and therapist become embroiled in a mutually reinforcing combination of erotized love infused with toxic, intractable idealization. In these cases, therapeutic progress stagnates as dependency on the therapist increases, and the patient's real-life relationships are marginalized or diminished. The patient's growth is actually undermined by the therapeutic relationship. To varying degrees, therapist and patient may be conscious of this problem and may make attempts to extricate themselves. These efforts are sabotaged by the therapist's unconscious need to remain "the one."

In what follows, we trace the nuances of this scenario, together with the theories and methods that can restore therapeutic process, and we provide a clinical illustration. Before proceeding, it is important to note that there are many ways that patients can overidealize their therapists and that therapists can overidealize their patients (see Slochower, 2011). These processes can pose many problems for patient growth and individuation. But when this idealization is imbued with erotic or romantic heat, mutual idealization can be gripping for both parties, often for years. Implicitly or explicitly seduced by the therapist, the patient has an intensified craving for what Charles (2017) referred to as the "promise of love" from the therapist. For this dyad, the therapy relationship becomes a fixation that repeats, rather than heals, the patient's presenting problem. The patient's presenting problems contribute to this predicament, but it is the therapist's need for erotic idealization that paralyzes or destroys the therapy.

At times, therapists may be aware of their overinvestment in this adoration. The therapist can make "good faith" therapeutic efforts, attempts to work through the patient's sexual and romantic fantasies and compulsions, to help them find stable, *real-life* intimacy outside the treatment. But in cases where patient and therapist have become locked into a negative therapeutic dynamic, the therapist may unwittingly keep injecting a subversive undercurrent into the treatment. Unspoken distress signals are usually emergent in the process if the therapist is listening. The patient may be increasingly isolated and disengaged from their interpersonal world. Their mood and self-esteem fluctuate in reaction to the therapist's regard. Their good-enough love relationships are destabilized or dissolve. Sexual compulsivity may increase, as the overstimulated patient seeks more external outlets for frustrated desire. The comparative perfection of the analyst can prevent new romantic relationships from developing. Lovers cycle through the patient's life and are discarded. Meanwhile, the therapeutic bond grows ever more insular, privileged, and exclusive. The treatment relationship is elevated, while an intensifying devaluation is directed at the self or others.

Distress signals can be displaced "out there" onto the patient's romantic partner (or close family). Patients may mention that their partner is complaining about the chronicity, expense, and lack of change produced by treatment. The partner may express jealousy of the therapist, and in mentioning this, the patient is disowning their own concerns about their excessive, romanticized involvement. When the therapist is narcissistically attached to being the "only one," the therapist often counters the partner's complaints through "clinical" observations that devalue the partner. This increases the "us against them" affiliation of therapist and patient against the outside world. In chronic, extreme cases, this can cause partners to develop real antipathy toward, and distrust of, the therapist. This understandable reaction will then get labeled as a partner's wish to "destroy the treatment." In these extreme scenarios, the therapist remains good and the patient remains innocent, while the life partner becomes increasingly marginalized or pathologized. These circumstances can dysregulate a good-enough life partner, heighten conflict, and have a disintegrative effect on the real-life relationship.

THE TRANSFERENCE-COUNTERTRANSFERENCE FIELD: RISKS AND REPAIR

How do psychoanalysts anticipate, and avert, the therapeutic scenario just described? How do we understand and repair it once it has begun? Of course, many psychoanalysts have drawn patients into this exploitative encounter (see Alpert & Steinberg, 2017; Goren, 2017; Slochower, 2017). Certainly, analytic methods and precepts have been used to rationalize this exploitation. As Grand (2017) noted, analytic seduction has often been rationalized as the necessary exploration of the patient's "erotic transference." Psychoanalytic training, however, does offer methods and theories that can protect the therapy. These methods are grounded in our theory of the therapeutic field.

Every psychotherapeutic approach recognizes the importance of the therapeutic alliance. The therapeutic alliance, when responsibly conducted with warmth, care, and compassion, allows the patient to reveal the self in a safe, nonshaming environment. Patients seek a figure of benign authority: someone with wisdom and experience, a good, nonjudgmental listener. Patients thrive in therapies with a good match; *we* do our best work when *we* have that good match. The therapeutic relationship can model healthy intimate relatedness, both in the therapist's way of being present and also through explicit relational interventions and observations. If therapists appreciate their patients as human beings—if they see and highlights patients' strengths—this enhances therapeutic potential. Patients are more likely to appreciate themselves and to recognize their own flaws with less shame and defensiveness. They can more readily examine their own role in their life troubles. Through verbal and nonverbal communications, the therapist demonstrates respect and care, strengthening the patient's self-image and self-esteem. At the same time, we convey appropriate expectations about real-life, imperfect relatedness.

All therapeutic orientations recognize that the patient's trouble may interfere with basic trust and therapeutic alliance. But psychoanalysis turns a more specific lens on the vicissitudes of this relationship. For us, the relationship between patient and therapist—that is, the transference–countertransference field—occurs at multiple levels and involves both implicit and explicit communications. This field is an important locus of therapeutic study, of lived and transformative experience. Although the treatment relationship moves *toward* basic trust, all too often it does not begin with such trust. Rather, we expect that patients will relive their difficulties in the therapeutic relationship. Patients will implicitly communicate much of whatever is not readily known to themselves. Therapists will have to thoughtfully decode these communications to further the patient's growth, all while maintaining ongoing self-questioning of how one's own feeling, needs, and history may be influencing the patient.

We recognize, of course, that analysts themselves have complex counter-transferential feelings and reactions to a patient's verbal and nonverbal communications. The therapist's preexisting vulnerabilities can collide with the psychic pressures of a patient. This can be a transient moment, informative and illuminating for the therapy and readily corrected. But if this collision is chronic, it can produce a destructive repetition of the patient's trouble. To catch these moments before they undermine treatment, the therapist must be aware that therapy is an ongoing psychic exchange. The process is characterized by continuous, contingent communications—explicit and implicit, verbal and nonverbal—that shape the therapeutic field, even when the treatment is thriving. Aron (1996) and Fiscalini (2004) are just two of many authors who have written on this topic. They, respectively, referred to this field as "a-symmetrical mutual influence" and "co-participant observation." It is our job to see and care for patients, but patients also see and sense and react to *us*, despite our best intentions. Their reactions to us are filtered through their own psychic experience and, as Slochower (2006) suggested, these reactions may or may not be directly revealed to a therapist upon whom they feel dependent. The therapist must bear sole responsibility for the constructive course of the treatment, regardless of the psychic pressures a patient brings to bear upon the therapist. This is the ethical premise embedded in "asymmetrical mutual influence."

If we think about the therapeutic relationship in this way, we can anticipate the relational conundrums that may occur in the treatment. If a patient arrives with a sex or romance addiction, or if the patient is in a state of romantic hunger, we can think ahead about the possibility that this idealizing hunger may surface with the therapist. We can think about how we might become vulnerable to this hunger, even as we have confidence that there will be no sexual acting out. If, during the treatment, the patient's real-life lovers keep being diminished and discarded, we can consider that our interventions might be undermining these relationships.

What if our own needs and feelings are being subtly picked up by our patients, and responded to, without the patients even being aware of what they feel the therapist wants from them? For example, we need to ask ourselves, are we overemphasizing the negative qualities of the patient's relationships? Does our patient think we will be hurt if they leave us "for someone else"? Are we enjoying the attachment a little too much? Are we afraid of our patients growing up and "leaving home"? Have we been communicating our own dissociated dread of loss, failure, imperfection, aging, and depression? Do we share their resistance to negative feelings, such as anger, loss of control? Do we experience conflict as disruptive to attachment? Self-reflectivity is essential in our work, and it is bolstered, here, by analytic theories about idealization.

ANALYTIC THEORY: THE DUAL EDGE OF IDEALIZATION

In the form of boundary trouble under discussion, both members of the dyad are participating in the underlying fantasy that often haunts our sex or romantically addictive patients. This is a fantasy of an elusive but ecstatic and perfect love. This erotic love will never become banal or misattuned. It will erase psychic wounds, vanquish existential anxieties, and eliminate all human loneliness, conflict, and frailty. In our imagination, it neutralizes separation, disappointment, loss, and death. This fantasy is one of fusion, in which there is a maladaptive form of idealization. To help the patient and avoid this therapeutic knot, we need to focus on the dual nature of idealization. In early development and in psychotherapy, idealization can take facilitating or maladaptive forms (or both). Ranging from the work of Kohut (1971, 1977) to that of Winnicott (1945) and Slochower (1996, 2006, 2011), our theory illuminates these two pathways as they exist in development and in therapeutic process.

Watching young children with loving parents, we have all witnessed the positive, mutual glow that builds a child's self-esteem. Maturation, exploration, autonomy—these develop within a healthy, joyous loop of being adored by those they adore (see Kohut, 1971, 1977). As children inevitably experience disappointment with, and anger at, their parents, the perfect parent gradually becomes de-idealized. As the parent goes on loving the child without retaliation or withdrawal, the child's capacity for love, autonomy, and attachment becomes ever more solid and ever more flexible. We become able to manage difference, conflict, disappointments, and mutual imperfections in love relationships. "Good-enough" development facilitates adult relationships that can include exciting affects and deep trust but also manage feelings of anger, sadness, loss, and grief. This is the bedrock for stable, real-life, imperfect, erotic love.

Many of our patients have significant deficits in this developmental experience. For these patients, the healthy developmental process of benign idealization and de-idealization never occurred in their childhood, or this phase was never resolved. These patients often have sex or love trouble. They crave developmentally reparative idealization but, instead of seeking its benign form, they keep recapitulating counterproductive, maladaptive forms of idealization that collapse into deprivation, fragmentation, alienation, and devaluation. In this context, *idealization* is always predicated on a compensatory *devaluation* of the self or the other. The sense of self is fragile; patients with this problem cannot tolerate negative emotions (in self or other) without the loss of narcissistic equilibrium. Maintaining this equilibrium through fantasies of perfect love takes primacy over sustaining imperfect loving bonds.

Therapists, too, can have these developmental deficits and vulnerabilities in their backgrounds. Our personal therapy may have gone a long way toward healing these developmental fissures, but they can resurface in response to a particular patient or in reaction to our life stressors. Sometimes we just happen to really "click" with a patient who is suffering from developmental predicaments in a way that reignites our old longings for reparative idealization. But with our understanding of therapy as a bidirectional transference–countertransference field, we are trained to query our reactions and to listen to those unspoken warning signs described earlier.

With romantically or sexually addicted patients, we can anticipate our own vulnerability to this maladaptive idealization. We know that this form of idealization is not reparative. We know it will have its dark side: the patient's self-devaluation or devaluation of those who might really be able to love her. Maladaptive idealization can ignite ecstatic self-experience in the patient, but this is not benign. Rather, these ecstatic states evoke rapid surrender of the self; oscillations in mood and self-esteem; excessive dependency; unrealistic relational fantasies; deference toward the all-knowing therapist; rage, depression, and self-attack when transformation fails; the disintegration of real-life relationships; and an underlying dread of emptiness and loss. Often, these are the presenting complaints that need to be worked through in the therapy.

For us, the bubble of transference idealization can be pleasurable, a vitalizing reprieve from stressful work and our own real-life relationships. After all, none of our loved ones seem to think we are perfect! We can allow ourselves to enjoy this, even as we know that we must query and relinquish unquestioning loyalty and exclusive adoration. In this way, most therapists are like good-enough parents (Winnicott, 1956/1984, Chapter 24); our commitment to our patient's growth is not upstaged by our own narcissistic gratifications. We must celebrate our patient's autonomy, mastery, and growth, knowing that one day, our patient will "leave home." In this type of therapeutic engagement, patients evolve an attachment to an important but imperfect therapist. The therapeutic relationship can offer bedrock support, but it does not divert the focus from the world "out there." Patients can have some experience of benign (mutual) idealization, even as they mourn the "perfect" intimacy they have pursued. There is opportunity for completing the necessary developmental achievement of mature individuation with its acceptance of limitations in oneself and others. While they learn that early wounds can never be fully repaired, they build a tolerance for disappointment and ambivalence in their relationships; flaws (in self and other) are not so dysregulating, and painful affects can be contained. When this works, this kind of patient is able to sustain real-life, imperfect intimacy. This capacity is scarred by grief and regret, as patients reflect on those they have hurt and those they have lost.

ROBERT: A CASE STUDY

Robert[1] entered treatment in his early 40s. He is charming, witty, lively, and intelligent. He enjoyed making his therapist laugh and became one of her favorite patients. Similar in background and temperament, they

---

[1]The authors asked Robert for permission to publish this material. After reading it, he emphasized that the boundaries of therapy had never been in doubt: "You made that perfectly clear." His comment implies that there might have been a more problematic outcome, if the therapist had not maintained professionalism and clear, realistic limits at all times in their interactions.

"get each other"; they are vitalized in each other's presence, they are a good match. Robert is romantic and passionate. He dates and pursues hot sex; the sex turns banal. He is always disappointed by the women he pursues and decides that his analyst is "the one." Of course, he knows they are prohibited from dating.

The therapist is a trained psychoanalyst, couples, and sex therapist. She knows that to help this patient, she will have to work on certain ways that her resonance with him may end up getting in the way of therapeutic progress. They share an expressive, passionate personality style, while the vitality of their relationship is overshadowed at times by their shared proclivity to avoid negative emotions along the line of depression and sadness. For the therapist, this manifests in continuous motion—a life of overwork and overgiving. For the patient, this manifests in compulsive sexuality, in a manic oscillation of romantic idealization and devaluation. For Robert, the flight from loss actually results in the recurrent undoing of real-life intimacy. The patient will not achieve stable, good-enough love until this pattern is disrupted and worked through in the therapy and their relationship. To unpack this, the analyst will have to touch upon her own grief and losses. Together, they will have to contend with the patient's lifetime of infirmity and his childhood grief, helplessness, and loss.

Presenting Problem

Robert came to therapy in a crisis about his 20-year marriage. His marriage had become dull. Intimacy had been lost to the mundane parallel lives of professionals more occupied with their careers than with each other. A vulnerable sexual life was deadened further by a lengthy process of trying to conceive. The failure to conceive was compounded by their failure to realize their creative aspirations. These issues evoked profound disappointment, loss of romance, and a sense of mutual deadness. Robert's life was marked by a series of unmourned losses. When he entered therapy, a wild affair was enlivening him and forestalling his grief over his deadened marriage. He was in an agitated, ecstatic state; high on illicit sex; infatuated with his lover; and unclear whether to end the affair, the marriage, or both. Passionate sexuality riveted his entire being. However, he loved his wife, felt loved by her and was afraid to lose her.

In response to the therapist's inquiries about his marriage and his life, Robert would be manifestly compliant and reflective but distracted by the manic heat of sex. This manic energy indirectly infused the sessions with vitality and humor. Over the course of a year, Robert tried to work through the marital difficulties, but he could never seriously engage in this effort. His ambivalence provoked first his lover and then his wife into leaving him. He might have plummeted into grief. Instead, he became involved with one woman after another. Excitement about these women would always fade into devaluation and disappointment. Aside from his erotic adventures he led an isolated life; his only steady bond was with his therapist. He claimed the therapist as the only woman "who understood him."

The patient's recitations of sexual and romantic adventures did provide the possibility of analytically studying Robert's compulsive pattern of idealization–devaluation. These observations gained some traction, but in general, the patient's sexual-romantic patterns were resistant to change. His erotic stories were the locus of therapeutic work, but they were also a transference performance intended to entertain, seduce, and divert his idealized analyst. In a light, charming, and flirtatious way, Robert would say that he and the analyst would make perfect lovers. Aside from this comment, there were never any inappropriate gestures, and there was never a risk that boundaries would be broken. There was certainly a mutual allure, however. Being erotically adored by this witty man—this was enlivening to this aging, married, female therapist.

Robert's History: Flight From Grief

Beginning in early childhood, Robert had suffered from a life-threatening disease, chronic pain, and recurrent medical interventions. His psychosocial development was marred by bodily awkwardness and social marginalization; his internal experience was of defectiveness, loneliness, and shame. His masculine confidence was fragile. Robert's father died when Robert was 13. This father had always been esteemed in the family as a "manly man," strong and courageous. He held a contradictory place in Robert's imagination: He was a good identificatory object, but his masculine perfection lit up Robert's masculine defects. At age 13, Robert was left with his grieving mother, a timid, withdrawn woman who had always been sheltered by her husband. As a "sickly" child, Robert was already entwined with a devoted mother who was always afraid that he would die. Now she had no one else. Her love for Robert was protective and sustaining, but it was also needy, dependent, and smothering. He could never be angry at her and never felt he could individuate from her.

In high school, Robert discovered a natural flirtatiousness and ease with women. Erotic seduction and engagement offered a joyous and enlivening exception to his physical challenges. In addition, sex offered him a secret space, hidden and separate from mother. In this secret place, he could forget his damaged body and morph into a manly man. His physical disabilities did not prevent him from becoming a skilled lover. Women wanted him; in bed with a woman, he felt liberated, potent, and desired. Hot sex allowed him an escape from grief and loss and mortification—until the breakdown of his sexual life in marriage.

Clinical Process

Robert could not tolerate the loss of either his wife or his lover. He denied the possibility of loss and yet he precipitated loss when they *both* left him. He then went from relationship to relationship, leaving them before they could leave him. Desirous of perfect intimacy, compelled by each new lover, he could not tolerate any waning of lust. Women's lust was the barometer of intimacy, vitality, and his masculine self-esteem. Closeness threatened him with the total fealty and fusion he thought these women would require. He could not imagine more autonomous relationships, and he could not imagine a love that could incorporate difference or conflict. He repeated the same questions in his therapy sessions: Was the sex frequent enough, adventurous enough, and always passionate? Did the woman really "get him"? In between girlfriends, Robert was alone, suffered from regrets, and was preoccupied with sexual fantasies.

Robert was not oblivious to his predicament. He worked on his desire for fusion and his dread of suffocation, and he linked these issues to his mother's dependency. He explored his longing for manly perfection. Sex and seduction were understood as an antidote to the idealization of father and to the diminishment of Robert's sense of self. Therapist and patient looked at the ways the living father had offered a partial buffer to the maternal symbiosis and the ways that this buffer had failed. They examined the mother's heroic idealization of father and the protective function of her mythology. Robert had lost the opportunity to know his real, flawed father, a loved but imperfect masculine figure, with whom Robert might identify. He had no male role model for managing anger, and no one to help him separate from his grieving, desperate, and self-sacrificing mother.

Seduction, Enactment, Analytic Reflectivity

Despite considerable work, Robert's love addiction continued. He began to voice the fantasy that his therapist would be his perfect partner. At first the therapist understood this as a repetition of his previous pattern and reminded Robert that he would find her as disappointing as he found other women to be in real life. One day he mused with a laugh, "Why don't you run away with me?" Although the boundaries always felt firm, this became a mantra that remained one of those truth-in-humor lines that recurred for a long time in the therapy. Then, a troubling incident occurred. The therapy was taking place in New York City, where there was a very large pool of women for Robert to date. Thanks to the uncanny coincidences of Match.com, Robert began dating a close woman friend of the therapist. The therapist found herself in an impossible situation: She knew she would be listening to Robert describe sexual details of his encounters with her friend; she also knew he would seduce and hurt her friend. Confidentiality prohibited the therapist from warning her friend. It would feel perverse and false to listen to Robert's affair as if the therapist didn't know the woman involved. The therapist also felt encroached upon in her private life. The affair had an incestuous "feel." Was it Robert's unconscious fantasy that this woman would serve as a sexual surrogate for the therapist?

The therapist informed the patient that this woman was a close friend and that therapy would have to stop if Robert continued dating her. In another geographic context, with a much smaller pool of women to date, this might have been a questionable therapeutic stance. But the options for dating in New York City seemed near infinite for Robert, and the women he dated seemed interchangeable for him. For a brief period before he stopped dating her friend, this ultimatum intensified Robert's arousal, and he imagined that all three (he, the friend, and the therapist) would share social occasions. When the therapist reiterated the ultimatum, Robert rapidly lost interest in the friend and stopped dating her. This intervention reestablished a workable therapeutic frame for the therapist, but it was double-edged. The therapist was concerned: What implicit communication might Robert be hearing? Did Robert hear this as a demand to "stay home with mother"? Did it seem like a disguised declaration that the therapist wanted him for herself? Could this feel seductive or smothering? Did this seem like a confirmation from the therapist that, as Robert imagined, they were "meant for each other"?

The therapist explored these issues with Robert. He had little response. His compulsive sexuality continued with other partners while, in his mind, his therapist remained the perfect, but unavailable, partner. She had no defects, and possessed the constancy of empathy, understanding, and acceptance that no other woman could ever provide. Robert could express feelings to her, like anger and aggression, that he felt he could not express to his mother, wife, or lovers.

But after the incident with the therapist's friend, the therapist reflected more seriously about the stasis in the therapy. Why wasn't more change occurring for Robert? She also reflected on her own countertransference. Perhaps her own pleasure in the flirtation really was interfering in moving the patient forward? Perhaps she was too attached to the patient's flattery, adoration, and desire? Robert was appealing and charming, and he injected vitality into her day. With their shared ethnicity and working-class backgrounds, she found herself laughing at his jokes. She found his commitment to self-reflection and honesty compelling; he could even laugh about himself and his neurotic tendencies. As she questioned herself, she revisited the treatment and realized this: Robert and she had talked about his losses, but he had never actually grieved them. He understood that sexuality was a flight from loss. But this reflection was all cerebral; he thought about those losses without ever feeling them. Emptiness, sadness and grief were occluded by the mutually compulsive vitalization stirred up in the therapy room as well as by the ongoing affairs. She was complicit in Robert's manic pursuit of vitality. He helped her vacate her own depression and grief. Her other patients were suffering; she was aging, some of her friends were already dying. If Robert touched his own losses, they would trigger her own.

After this period of reflection, the therapist could tolerate more quiet and stillness in the sessions; she wasn't so effervescent in her engagement with Robert. Instead, she began to locate, and mirror, the underlying sadness and loneliness that Robert had suppressed. The therapy proceeded with no diminution of affection between therapist and patient. There was still laughter, but Robert also wept. The sessions became more somber and contemplative. Erotic stories disappeared; lovers stopped cycling through the treatment. Robert was less manic and less flirtatious toward his therapist. He cried about the good women he had rejected and began to look outside the therapy for a real relationship in the real world.

This case raises questions about the benefits, risks, and limits of therapeutic love. How and when does idealization of the therapist contribute to an impasse in real-life love? How does meeting a patient's fantasy with resonance and safe, realistic boundaries help a patient move toward a greater capacity for good-enough love? And finally, every therapist must ask: What is the effect of countertransference on a patient's persistent fantasy about having a relationship with his or her therapist, even knowing that the patient's fantasy will never be fulfilled? We can as therapists work with the growth-enhancing function of therapeutic love but, like all good parents, recognize the needs of our patients to separate, individuate, and relinquish idealization to pave the way for realistic love in life.

REFERENCES

Alpert, J., & Steinberg, A. (2017). Sexual boundary violations: A century of violations and a time to analyze. *Psychoanalytic Psychology*, *34*(2), 144–150. https://doi.org/10.1037/pap0000094

Aron, L. (1996). *A meeting of minds: Mutuality in psychoanalysis*. The Analytic Press.

Charles, M. (2017). The promise of love revisited: Healing ruptures through recognition. *Psychoanalytic Psychology*, *34*(2), 186–194. https://doi.org/10.1037/pap0000090

Fiscalini, J. (2004). *Co-participant psychoanalysis*. Columbia University Press.

Goren, E. (2017). A call for more talk and less abuse in the consulting room: One psychoanalyst-sex therapist's perspective. *Psychoanalytic Psychology*, *34*(2), 215–220. https://doi.org/10.1037/pap0000092

Grand, S. (2017). Seductive excess: Erotic transformations, secret predations. *Psychoanalytic Psychology*, *34*(2), 208–214. https://doi.org/10.1037/pap0000106

Kohut, H. (1971). *The analysis of the self: A systematic approach to the psychoanalytic treatment of narcissistic personality disorders*. International Universities Press.

Kohut, H. (1977). *The restoration of the self*. International Universities Press.

Slochower, J. (1996). Holding and the fate of the analyst's subjectivity. *Psychoanalytic Dialogues*, *6*(3), 323–353.

Slochower, J. (2006). The psychoanalytic other: Commentary on paper by Helen K. Gediman. *Psychoanalytic Dialogues*, *16*(3), 263–272.

Slochower, J. (2011). Analytic idealizations and the disavowed: Winnicott, his patients, and us. *Psychoanalytic Dialogues*, *21*, 3–21. https://doi.org/10.1080/10481885.2011.545317

Slochower, J. (2017). Don't tell anyone. *Psychoanalytic Psychology*, *34*(2), 195–200. https://doi.org/10.1037/pap0000082

Winnicott, D. W. (1945). Primitive emotional development. *International Journal of Psycho-Analysis*, *26*, 137–143.

Winnicott, D. W. (1984). *Collected papers, through paediatrics to psychoanalysis*. Karnac. (Original work published 1956)

6 A COGNITIVE BEHAVIORAL APPROACH TO UNDERSTANDING SEXUAL BOUNDARY VIOLATIONS

AMY WENZEL

Sexual boundary violations (SBVs) are transgressions in therapy that are discussed routinely in graduate school ethics courses (e.g., Knapp, 2011). Moreover, cognitive behavioral therapists place great importance on a wide array of ethical issues that affect their clinical practice (Sookman, 2015). It is surprising and unclear why, then, that there is a paucity of scholarly and clinical discussion on understanding, addressing, and resolving SBVs in the context of cognitive behavioral therapy (CBT). In this chapter, I outline the cognitive behavioral model that underlies cognitive behavioral therapists' understanding of their clients' clinical presentations with an eye toward considering personal beliefs (in both the therapist and client) that serve as cognitive vulnerabilities and that could put therapists, clients, or both at risk for an SBV. In addition, cognitive behavioral interventions will be described for therapists who notice themselves in situations with their clients that are ripe for SBVs to occur and wish to prevent such an outcome. Finally, therapeutic interventions for clients who are currently participating in CBT after experiencing an SBV with a previous therapist are considered.

https://doi.org/10.1037/0000247-006
Sexual Boundary Violations in Psychotherapy: Facing Therapist Indiscretions, Transgressions, and Misconduct, A. Steinberg, J. L. Alpert, and C. A. Courtois (Editors)
Copyright © 2021 by the American Psychological Association. All rights reserved.

Before proceeding, a definition of CBT is in order. CBT refers to a family of many specific psychotherapy packages that have their basis in cognitive and/or behavioral theories. The quintessential example of CBT is Aaron T. Beck's cognitive therapy (Beck et al., 1979), but the CBTs also include (but are not limited to) rational emotive behavior therapy (Ellis, 1994); problem-solving therapy (PST; Nezu et al., 2013); schema therapy (Young et al., 2003); exposure-based therapies, such as prolonged exposure (Foa et al., 2007) and cognitive processing therapy (Resick et al., 2017); dialectical behavior therapy (DBT; Linehan, 1993); metacognitive therapy (Wells, 2009); cognitive behavioral analysis of systems (McCullough, 2000); and acceptance and commitment therapy (Hayes et al., 2012). Although there are specific strategic interventions and therapeutic tools associated with each of these CBT packages, they all are guided by a coherent theoretical framework that lends itself to a customized case formulation of the individual client's clinical presentation. Whatever a therapist's theoretical orientation may be, it is always the responsibility of therapists to conduct themselves ethically and to refrain from committing an SBV regardless of the client's behavior or wishes. Nevertheless, the therapist's theoretical framework, and in this case, the cognitive behavioral framework, can provide guidance for therapists and clients to address, in a preventive manner, cognitive and behavioral factors that put the dyad at risk for an SBV. They can also be applied in a treatment package to help a client work through an SBV that he or she might have experienced in the past. There is no reason to believe that any of the specific CBT approaches would be more or less associated with risk of an SBV occurring during the course of treatment.

THE CBT MODEL AND ITS APPLICATION TO SBVs

Although the nuances of the theoretical models underlying specific formats and applications vary, according to the general cognitive behavioral theory, the way in which people think about and make sense of their world plays a large role in determining their emotional states and behavioral responses. To illustrate, say a male therapist makes the comment to a female patient, "I was thinking about you this past week." One client might interpret that remark as "My therapist really cares about me; I'm fortunate to be working with him," which could be associated with a positive emotional experience (e.g., a sense of warmth) and behaviors that would further contribute to a healthy therapeutic relationship (e.g., active engagement in treatment, completion of "homework" in between sessions). Another client might interpret that remark as "This therapist is creepy," which could be associated with a negative emotional experience (e.g., alarm) and behaviors that might have the potential to interfere with a healthy therapeutic relationship (e.g., guardedness in session, missing sessions). A third client might interpret that remark as "I've finally found someone who cares about and values me," which could be associated with feelings of love or lust and behaviors that could provide context for the client to make advances toward her therapist (e.g., excessive contact between sessions, sexual advances), thereby increasing the likelihood of the occurrence of an SBV. Although all these examples illustrate the way in which cognition affects later emotional and behavioral responses, it should be acknowledged that research shows that cognition does not always precede emotion and that at times, emotional and behavioral responses precede cognition (e.g., Clore & Ortony, 2000). For example, a therapist might experience an unexpected sensation of arousal toward a client (or vice versa) and take that arousal as an indication that there are mutual romantic feelings.

The thoughts and interpretations that people have in specific situations are not random; according to cognitive behavioral theory, they are influenced by underlying beliefs that are shaped over time by formative life experiences. For example, a client who reports a history of her parents' anger, volatility, and physical abuse might be characterized by a belief such as "Other people cannot be trusted." Such a client, then, would be likely to interpret kind words from others in a negative light, perhaps even to the point of misperceiving that a sexual attraction has been expressed or an SBV has occurred. Another client with a history of rejection by others might be characterized by a belief such as "I'm unlovable." Such a client, then, might interpret kind but innocent words from others as an expression of the love or desire for which she has longed.

Cognitive behavioral therapists are cognizant of detecting subtle signs that their clients are interpreting their behaviors toward them in a way that might be misconstrued, or that might even set the stage for an SBV. Furthermore, they also recognize the fact that they, like their clients, are human beings who carry their own unique personal histories that have shaped their own underlying beliefs. They are encouraged to be particularly aware of beliefs that can affect their own therapeutic work with clients and compromise the clinical decisions that they make. For example, a therapist whose parents were cold and who withheld affection could be characterized by the belief that he is unlovable, which could set the stage for inappropriate behavior with a client who shows attention and admiration, thereby compensating for that painful belief. Thus, underlying beliefs, when activated, can serve as cognitive vulnerabilities that have the potential to put clients and therapists alike at risk for an SBV.

In addition to these cognitive vulnerabilities, it is important to recognize that therapists can hold beliefs about their work with clients, and clients can hold beliefs about their work with therapists, that provide a context for an SBV to unfold. For therapists, it is not difficult to imagine that narcissistic beliefs about their own importance and abilities, about the degree (or lack of degree) to which ethical guidelines apply to them, or about the need for patients to be subservient to their authority could increase the likelihood that they would act on urges and commit an SBV. In addition, therapists who doubt their own ability to be assertive or interpersonally effective, or who worry about being too confrontational with or off-putting to clients, could recognize that a situation is ripe for an SBV but fail to take appropriate action to address it in a preventive manner. Further, therapists who believe they need to "save" their patients could be blind to warning signs that the dyad is moving toward conditions that are conducive for an SBV to occur.

The therapeutic relationship is unique as relationships go because therapists can be privy to clients' innermost feelings, fears, insecurities, or vulnerabilities (Wenzel, 2019). Many clients therefore share a unique trust and bond with their therapist that might be unlike those with which they have had with romantic partners. It is not difficult to imagine that some clients would misinterpret therapists' care, concern, respect, and unconditional regard for romantic feelings. In addition, clients who carry the belief that their therapist is an authority figure or who is a person who should be trusted to make decisions for them could be vulnerable to an SBV if the therapist make advances, and they believe that they do not have the power to stop it. Moreover, clients who believe that therapists' professional standing makes them especially attractive or desirable may be at an increased likelihood to experience sexual or romantic feelings toward their therapist.

A logical question to ask is when these issues would reach a threshold that they compromise the therapeutic relationship. There are no available empirical data or, more generally, any scholarly discourse to guide cognitive behavioral therapists in answering this question. However, cognitive behavioral therapists are strongly encouraged to ensure that they are applying the principles that they teach and model to their clients to have keen awareness when they are experiencing beliefs associated with emotions and behaviors that could interfere with anything but the highest level of care for their clients. If therapists find themselves engaging in behaviors in which they would not engage with other clients, they must ask themselves whether such behavior is explained, at least in part, by beliefs that increase the likelihood of the occurrence of an SBV. Similarly, they must also be aware of instances in which client behavior is outside of the realm of the typical therapeutic relationship and could increase the likelihood of the occurrence of an SBV. If the cognitive behavioral therapist acknowledges something in either domain, then they must make a determination as to whether therapy in its current form can proceed.

CBT INTERVENTIONS

Collaboration, transparency, and *prevention* are among the fundamental tenets of CBT. Collaboration means that the therapist and client are equal members of a team, and both contribute actively to sessions by deciding the issues that will be addressed and sharing viewpoints in an open, honest, genuine, and nonjudgmental manner. Transparency means that they conduct themselves in an "above-board" manner, communicating with clients about cognitive behavioral principles underlying the way in which they are conceptualizing an issue and sharing honest viewpoints about their clients' clinical presentation. Prevention means that therapists and clients work together to identify and address risk factors that could bring on or exacerbate symptoms, poor decisions, and/or maladjustment to mitigate their effects. These principles hold true for addressing factors that could put the dyad at risk for an SBV such that, when indicated, the therapist and client work together to identify circumstances or behaviors that have the potential to be inappropriate and apply cognitive behavioral strategies to prevent an SBV from occurring. That said, it is always the responsibility of the therapist (and not the client) to maintain appropriate and professional boundaries and to avoid dual relationships.

PREVENTION WITH CURRENT CLIENTS

An SBV, by definition, is an issue that interrupts the cultivation of a healthy therapeutic relationship because it is unequivocally unethical and harmful for therapists to engage in sexual relations or other inappropriate intimate behavior with their clients (including comments, gestures, or social media contacts). Thus, this section is geared toward the prevention of SBVs by using the CBT framework to recognize and alleviate issues within the therapeutic relationship that could increase the likelihood of the occurrence of an SBV.

Recognizing Warning Signs

Warning signs for an array of problematic symptoms and behaviors that can lead to an SBV may take many forms, including cognitions (e.g., thoughts, fantasies, interpretations), emotions (e.g., warmth, attraction, lust or longing, obsession, discomfort), behaviors (e.g., subtle or overt inappropriate expressions of affection or self-disclosure; Somer & Saadon, 1999), and life circumstances (e.g., divorce, other loss; Perlman, 2009). As mentioned previously, cognitive behavioral therapists are encouraged to be aware of their own personal vulnerabilities in their clinical work and in their life circumstances so that they can quickly "catch" one or more cognitive, emotional, or behavioral warning signs that could provide context for an SBV. In DBT, a well-known specific type of CBT that was originally developed to work with clients with borderline personality disorder who engage in self-injurious behavior, therapists are strongly encouraged to participate in peer consultation to address their reactions toward these (often) challenging clients that could interfere with the delivery of effective therapy (Linehan, 1993). Although I generally encourage cognitive behavioral therapists to participate in some sort of regular consultation or peer support with their full array of clients, when they recognize a warning sign within themselves that could signal risk for an SBV, it is imperative that they bring it to their consultant for discussion (cf. Somer & Saadon, 1999). A central issue in consultation is an honest and ongoing assessment of whether the therapist can provide effective and uncompromised treatment to the client.

Therapists should also be alert for the same sorts of warning signs in their clients. When cognitive behavioral therapists notice their clients responding to them in a certain way that could increase the likelihood of an SBV, using the principles of collaboration, transparency, and prevention, they might make observations and ask questions such as "I notice that you reacted in a certain way when I [insert therapist's behavior]. Tell me what was running through your mind when that happened" or "Tell me what that means to you." Such questions elicit clients' thoughts about the therapeutic relationship and the associated beliefs that might be activated. Cognitive behavioral therapists are encouraged to adopt an accepting, nonjudgmental stance regardless of what their clients might say in these circumstances because indicators of alarm or disapproval could send the message that the client is doing or feeling something wrong (which has the potential to reinforce other beliefs that might be the target of treatment, such as a belief of inadequacy or worthlessness). They should, however, make it clear to the client, as necessary, that the feelings are not wrong but that acting them out would be, and therefore professional boundaries will be maintained.

Modifying Thinking

A central intervention in many specific CBT packages is *cognitive restructuring*, or the process through which therapists help their clients acquire skill in recognizing thinking associated with emotional distress or poor behavioral choices (as described earlier), evaluating the accuracy and helpfulness of their thinking, and modifying their thinking to be more balanced and adaptive (i.e., a balanced or adaptive response). Therapists who notice warning signs in themselves that increase the likelihood of an SBV should be alert to *permission-giving thoughts* (e.g., "The client says she is just as interested in me as I am in her, so there is no harm in pursuing this relationship because it is consensual"). Helpful reframes that they can apply to themselves might include the recognition that (a) feelings toward the client could be indicative of unmet needs that the therapist should work toward meeting in healthier ways and (b) although it is part of being human to experience romantic and sexual feelings toward others, acting on these feelings toward a client is unethical and could result in serious professional as well as personal repercussions. Therapists who notice narcissistic or grandiose thoughts (e.g., thoughts of deserving the relationship because of one's professional accomplishments), like clients who have such thoughts, often will not regard such cognitions as problematic or enabling; however, peers or supervisors who provide consultation can reshape them by encouraging the therapist to think about implications of harm toward the client or his or her professional reputation and personal life. Conversely, other therapists will view warning signs as a professional or personal failure and experience self-deprecating thoughts that make them question their clinical decision making (e.g., "I'm a terrible therapist who should not be practicing"). In these cases, cognitive restructuring can be helpful to normalize their feelings, give themselves credit for recognizing their feelings in order not to act on them, recall the many instances over their career in which they handled delicate clinical situations with grace and wisdom, and develop a sense of hope that a resolution will be achieved. Cognitive restructuring used in this manner is preventive because it is applied to decrease risk factors for the occurrence of an SBV.

Clients who express romantic or sexual feelings toward their therapist will likely be experiencing an array of accompanying feelings, such as confusion, guilt, shame, trepidation, and even, at the same time, exhilaration (Somer & Saadon, 1999). To help clients achieve a balanced, adaptive cognitive response to thoughts of attraction to their therapist, cognitive behavioral therapists can provide psychoeducation to normalize feelings of closeness toward another person who demonstrates care, concern, and unconditional positive regard. In other words, a balanced, adaptive response that clients can adopt will include the notion that they have not necessarily done anything wrong and that, in fact, it is a sign of growth and maturity that they are able to discuss their feelings openly and honestly in a safe environment. At times, therapists work with clients who behave inappropriately, such as a client who continues to make provocative or invasive comments despite the therapist setting appropriate limitations. In these instances, the therapist can help the client identify the meaning and gains associated with making such statements and move toward a balanced, adaptive response that will incorporate respect for others. These cognitive interventions are also preventive because they are aimed at lowering the likelihood of the occurrence of an SBV.

Social Problem Solving

The identification and adjustment of thinking in both the client and therapist are essential to soften the guilt, shame, and anxiety over romantic or sexual feelings within the therapeutic relationship so that these emotional experiences do not exacerbate the client's psychopathology (or contribute to undue distress in the therapist). Nevertheless, in light of the seriousness of this issue, cognitive restructuring pertaining to the issue must be accompanied by a problem-solving intervention to ensure ethical behavior on the part of the therapist and the safety of the client. According to D'Zurilla and Nezu (2007), who developed and have honed PST over the course of the past 30 years, *social problem solving* is defined as "the self-directed cognitive-behavioral process by which a person attempts to identify or discover effective or adaptive solutions for specific problems encountered in everyday living" (p. 11). PST interventions include those that focus on the acquisition of problem-solving skills (i.e., problem identification and definition, generation of alternatives, decision making, solution implementation and verification) and the modification of a negative problem orientation (i.e., an attitudinal set characterized by a resistance toward and generally negative view about the occurrence of problems). Therapists who identify warning signs within themselves for behavior consistent with an SBV can apply this framework to develop a course of self-remediation, perhaps by working with a mentor who can provide supervision and oversight of the case, as well as to address any needs in their own lives that are not being met. Moreover, therapists can apply this framework with their clients to achieve many of the same aims in a preventive manner to decrease the likelihood that an SBV will occur.

The paramount question that must be addressed is whether the dyad can continue to work with one another when conditions that put them at risk for an SBV are identified and acknowledged (but when no SBV has yet occurred). A fundamental assumption with which both the therapist and client should be working is that a romantic or sexual relationship is "off limits." Both parties should feel free to conclude that they can no longer reasonably work with the other. If this decision is primarily driven by the therapist, the client's reactions to this decision should be considered using the CBT framework so that the client can exit the therapy arrangement with the most balanced, adaptive response possible. There will likely be the recognition that this is a profound event in the client's life that very well might need to be addressed in a course of therapy with a new therapist. If this decision is primarily driven by the client, the therapist should validate the client's wishes and, in fact, frame the decision as one that is sound and thoughtful and that facilitates the client's self-care. In both instances, the therapist will work diligently to facilitate a referral to a trusted colleague who will be able to see the client in a timely manner.

Effective communication is essential for solving problems, and many cognitive behavioral therapists routinely incorporate communication skills training into CBT work with clients (e.g., Wenzel, 2013). Sensitive situations in which it is recognized that the dyad is at risk for an SBV are likely to be uncomfortable for the client and therapist alike. Nevertheless, the cognitive behavioral therapist can model the implementation of effective communication skills when addressing any observed warning signs, and they can coach their clients in using such skills to achieve the aims of social problem solving.

WORKING WITH CLIENTS WHO HAVE EXPERIENCED A PREVIOUS SBV

Many clients who have experienced a previous SBV and who present for a subsequent course of psychotherapy request to process it and address its aftereffects. Cognitive behavioral therapists are encouraged to be alert for cognitions indicative of a false sense of personal responsibility (e.g., "I'm to blame for this happening," "It's my fault if the therapist loses his license") or a sense of personal shortcoming (e.g., "Something is wrong with me," "No one will want to work with me now"). Therapists might provide psychoeducation about the role of therapists and the ethical code to which they are bound to normalize clients' reactions to the previous SBV and understand that they are not to blame; they might use cognitive restructuring to reframe distorted cognitions that are contributing to the client's emotional distress. Attention to building a sound, warm, and appropriate therapeutic relationship is paramount in these cases for the client to have a corrective learning experience, seeing that a healthy therapeutic relationship can be much different from the previous one in which the SBV occurred. While this relationship is being cultivated, therapists are encouraged to seek regular feedback from patients regarding the "feel" of the therapeutic relationship to maximize the likelihood that the new course of psychotherapy is a positive experience, to identify and remedy anything happening in the therapeutic relationship that is uncomfortable or activating for them, and to reframe any unhelpful or distressing thoughts that occur in the context of the therapeutic relationship. A social-problem-solving approach might be adopted for clients who are working through whether and how to disclose the SBV to others and even file a complaint with the transgressor's state licensing board.

Exposure is an empirically supported behavioral intervention for clients who demonstrate posttraumatic stress symptoms, which could certainly comprise the sequelae of an SBV that the client experiences as traumatic. Imaginal exposure is typically used for survivors of sexual transgressions, such that they work with their therapist to create trauma narratives that they write down, speak out loud, and often record vivid descriptions of the trauma so that they can consult them for homework in between sessions. In addition, sessions with a new therapist could constitute in vivo, or "real-life," exposure. Regardless of the particular modality of exposure that is used, it facilitates what is called *emotional processing* so that clients habituate to the distress associated with memories and reminders of the trauma (Foa et al., 2007) and also so that they learn that they can tolerate discomfort and continue to live their lives the way that they want.

CONCLUSION

Cognitive behavioral therapists believe strongly that their clinical practice should be guided by results from empirical research. However, there is a notable lack of empirical investigation of risk factors and interventions for SBVs in the literature. In the absence of such empirical guidelines, cognitive behavioral therapists conduct themselves strategically as "practitioner-scientists," meaning that their clinical decisions are guided by (a) a cogent case formulation based on established cognitive behavioral principles, (b) related scholarly discourse that is relevant to the client's clinical presentation (e.g., literature about exposure), and (c) observational "data" collected across the course of treatment (Wenzel, 2013). In addition, cognitive behavioral therapists also conduct themselves in a collaborative and transparent manner, with an eye toward prevention and a focus on helping clients generalize the learning that has occurred to other areas of and relationships in their lives. Above all, cognitive behavioral therapists recognize that they, like their clients, carry their own unique histories and even "baggage" that could form underlying beliefs that shape the way in which they respond to their clients in session. Making the commitment to conduct themselves with the utmost ethical attention to the care and safety of the client paramount, cognitive behavioral therapists recognize and remedy any warning signs that increase the likelihood of an SBV, and they create a corrective learning environment for clients who have experienced an SBV in the past.

REFERENCES

Beck, A. T., Rush, A. J., Shaw, B. F., & Emery, G. (1979). *Cognitive therapy of depression*. Guilford Press.

Clore, G. L., & Ortony, A. (2000). Cognition in emotion: Always, sometimes, or never. In R. D. R. Lane, L. Nadel, G. L. Ahern, J. Allen, & A. W. Kasniak (Eds.), *Cognitive neuroscience of emotion* (pp. 24–61). Oxford University Press.

D'Zurilla, T. J., & Nezu, A. M. (2007). *Problem-solving therapy: A positive approach to clinical intervention* (3rd ed.). Springer.

Ellis, A. (1994). *Reason and emotion in psychotherapy* (Rev. and updated ed.). Carol.

Foa, E. B., Hembree, E. A., & Rothbaum, B. O. (2007). *Prolonged exposure therapy for PTSD: Emotional processing of traumatic experiences*. Oxford University Press.

Hayes, S. C., Strosahl, K. D., & Wilson, K. G. (2012). *Acceptance and commitment therapy: The process and practice of mindful change* (2nd ed.). Guilford Press.

Knapp, S. L. (Ed.). (2011). *APA handbook of ethics in psychology* (Vols. 1 and 2). American Psychological Association.

Linehan, M. M. (1993). *Cognitive behavioral therapy for borderline personality disorder*. Guilford Press.

McCullough, J. P. (2000). *Treatment for chronic depression: Cognitive behavioral analysis system of psychotherapy (CBSAP)*. Guilford Press.

Nezu, A. M., Nezu, C. M., & D'Zurilla, T. J. (2013). *Problem solving therapy: A treatment manual*. Springer.

Perlman, S. D. (2009). Falling into sexuality: Sexual boundary violations in psychotherapy. *Psychoanalytic Review, 96*, 917–941. https://doi.org/10.1521/prev.2009.96.6.917

Resick, P. A., Monson, C. M., & Chard, K. M. (2017). *Cognitive processing therapy for PTSD: A comprehensive manual*. Guilford Press.

Somer, E., & Saadon, M. (1999). Therapist–client sex: Clients' retrospective reports. *Professional Psychology: Research and Practice, 30*(5), 504–509. https://doi.org/10.1037/0735-7028.30.5.504

Sookman, D. (2015). Ethical practice of cognitive behavior therapy. In J. Z. Sadler, K. W. M. Fulford, & C. W. van Straden (Eds.), *The Oxford handbook of psychiatric ethics* (pp. 1293–1305). Oxford University Press.

Wells, A. (2009). *Metacognitive therapy for anxiety and depression*. Guilford Press.

Wenzel, A. (2013). *Strategic decision making in cognitive behavioral therapy*. American Psychological Association. https://doi.org/10.1037/14188-000

Wenzel, A. (2019). *Cognitive behavioral therapy for beginners: An experiential learning approach*. Routledge. https://doi.org/10.4324/9781315651958

Young, J. E., Klosko, J. S., & Weishaar, M. E. (2003). *Schema therapy: A practitioner's guide*. Guilford Press.

7 GOING BEYOND THE CONTACT BOUNDARY

A Gestalt Therapy Perspective

MONIQUE N. RODRIGUEZ

Gestalt therapy is a body-oriented approach with its philosophy grounded in holism and phenomenology. The therapy process involves a client who is reorganizing their experiences and way of being in the world through full contact and resistance processes, and at times these experiences happen through the relationship with the therapist. Although most gestalt therapy training programs today focus their training on the relational field, the use of touch, and the immediate here-and-now sensory experience of the therapist as well as the client, there seems to be little to no dialogue about the danger of sexual boundary violations and how it is being addressed in therapy. In academic or professional settings

> where the risks of misunderstanding, litigation, and even prosecution are increasing, it can only become harder to find the space to talk about what it might mean to be sexually attracted to a client and how it might be managed as an issue of the psychotherapeutic process. (O'Shea, 2000, p. 14)

Given the physical focus and the use of touch in gestalt therapy, it becomes the gestalt therapist's obligation to address the risk of sexual boundary violation.

https://doi.org/10.1037/0000247-007
Sexual Boundary Violations in Psychotherapy: Facing Therapist Indiscretions, Transgressions, and Misconduct, A. Steinberg, J. L. Alpert, and C. A. Courtois (Editors)

My own experience as a gestalt therapist began with my teachers and mentors at the Gestalt Institute of Cleveland. It was through my work as a student, trainee, and colleague of Jim Kepner and Michael Clemmens that I began to explore gestalt therapy as an embodied approach. My interest in the embodied dimensions of gestalt therapy has led me to train in different approaches to somatic work and movement. Reflecting on my own training in gestalt therapy, I have been surprised by how little attention has been given to erotic experiences and boundary violations with clients. Perhaps this is related to the misconduct of Fritz Perls or the shame and embarrassment we as gestalt therapists might carry. I urge us as gestalt therapists to acknowledge the risks of sexual boundary violation as we often use ourselves as a vehicle to healing our patients. My intention and focus in this chapter is not only to contribute to what has been written on the erotic field in gestalt therapy, but to make its presence and its power more explicit; to provide a perspective on what emerges in the cocreated field between client and therapist, supervisor and supervisee, trainer and trainee, to explore challenges that can and do arise in gestalt therapy; and to highlight aspects of our work such as the use of touch and somatic processes that present unique challenges. This is an invitation to generate a dialogue around the experience, for us, as gestalt therapists, of emotional involvement and the real and genuine therapeutic *use of self* that could potentially lead to a sexual boundary violation.

HISTORICAL BACKGROUND

To fully understand the box in which gestalt therapists find themselves—to understand the silence around sexual boundary violation—a historical understanding of gestalt therapy and Fritz Perls is imperative. Gestalt therapy is a "third-wave" humanistic approach to psychotherapy encapsulating existential–phenomenological and process–experiential theoretical foundations. It came into general awareness in 1951 with Fritz S. Perls, Laura P. Perls (uncredited), Ralph F. Hefferline, and Paul Goodman's seminal work, *Gestalt Therapy: Excitement and Growth in the Human Personality* (Perls et al., 1951). Although this book was a collaborative effort, only Fritz Perls remained committed to the movement. It is he, and to a lesser extent his wife, Laura Perls (Feder, 2004), who are most popularly associated with it. Gestalt therapy is based on an integrative theory that was, in many ways, born as a reaction to traditional psychoanalysis, in which both Fritz Perls and Laura Perls were trained as practicing analysts. Perls et al. (1951) devoted a large portion of their text to the discussion of the modifications of classical psychoanalytic principles and concepts. Gestalt therapy emphasized the obvious in contrast to psychoanalysis' emphasis of the hidden. Gestalt therapy focused more on direct human-to-human physical contact in contrast to classical psychoanalysis, which emphasized on projection onto the analyst, where physical contact was prohibited because it supposedly had a negative impact on the processes of transference and countertransference. Fritz helped change the direction of psychotherapy. In *An Intimate Portrait of Fritz Perls and Gestalt Therapy*, Martin Shepard (1975) described his experience of Perls:

> He led many of us away from a preoccupation with the past to a concentration on the present, away from blaming parents to accepting responsibility for oneself, away from the narrow confines of the libido theory into the broad awareness of myriad numbers of needs, away from an *analysis* of one's condition and toward a *satisfaction of one's desires*. (p. 13, italics in original)

During the early days of gestalt therapy (the 1950s, 1960s, 1970s) and within the human potential movement, some of the things that would be seen as boundary crossings and violations today were not seen as such. Touching became an accepted practice used to improve the therapeutic alliance and to effect change. This was true across therapies with their roots in the humanistic tradition. The movement was formed around the concept that there is extraordinary potential untapped in all people, and through the development of "human potential," humans can experience an exceptional quality of life filled with happiness, creativity, and fulfillment when they strive to reach their full potential; this included sexual liberation. Those latter decades were a time of societal rebellion (Vietnam War protests, women publicly rebelling against proscribed roles and practices, race riots, the flower children) and experimentation. One could turn on the TV, if not step out into the street, and see all of this. Fritz Perls was declaring that his group therapy sessions had no rules, Paul Bindrim (1920–1997), with the support and approval of Abraham Maslow (1908–1970) who was considered the father of humanistic psychology and was then president of the American Psychological Association, was leading nude group marathons around the country, and Martin Shepard (1971) was advocating sex with clients (E. Smith, personal communication, March 2019).

All of this fit nicely with the sexual revolution (1960s–1980s) and the flower child movement, and for a while, gestalt therapy was enormously popular, partly as a result of its flagrant espousal of all types of dual relationships, promulgated by both Fritz Perls and Paul Goodman (Stoehr, 1994). "Therapist and client were friends, lovers, playmates, comrades, and whatever came to mind, including supervisor and trainee. If the client got hurt by this, then it was his/her job to take care of himself/herself" (Feder, 2004, p. 137). When Fritz Perls found that his marriage was no longer fulfilling, he began engaging in affairs. One in particular was with a woman who attended individual therapy with Perls about 3 to 5 days a week. According to Shepard (1975), Perls had been giving her friendly supportive kisses at the end of each session until during one session, the kiss became erotic. This encounter evoked a dream for the client that was processed with Perls during a subsequent session. It was after she explored the dream that she decided to become Perls's lover. Perls was known for his solicitation of patients at social occasions, his fraternization with other patients, and his open sexual enjoyment of both men and women (Shepard, 1975). He had a negative reputation and turned off most of the therapeutic community. Robert Resnick (2015) described Perls as follows:

> Perls's disregard for professional boundaries created a lot of confusion in discriminating between Gestalt therapy and Perls's personality, resulting in a bad reputation in some quarters for Gestalt therapy. For instance, Perls's sexual escapades with women, his sometimes-outrageous behavior, and his unpredictable, strong reactions were often erroneously attributed to Gestalt therapy when they actually reflected Perls's complex and contradictory personality. His deficits sometimes detracted from his genius, creativity, sweetness, and generosity. Gestalt therapists, as other professional therapists, follow the ethical codes of their professional organizations. (p. 764)

While Perls was notorious for womanizing, poor boundaries, and other concerns, his personal foibles and misconduct were never a part of gestalt therapy. Of course, as with any model of psychotherapy, there are always a few individuals who take advantage of their power as therapist or trainer, so it is not that there are no gestalt therapists who have (or are) doing this. However, this is in contradiction to the official ethos and ethics of gestalt therapy. There may have been those who heard a lecture and then from that point on called themselves a "gestalt therapist" with no training and took gestalt therapy as a mandate to do "whatever you feel." These untrained people were calling themselves gestalt therapists, violating ethical boundaries, and thereby reflecting poorly on gestalt therapy. Therapists, including no doubt gestalt therapists, were not exempt from the field conditions at this time, some of which supported "free sex," LSD, "make love not war," "do what you feel" (with little regard to others or consequences), and so on. These individuals sullied the waters of gestalt therapy and have never represented the official view of gestalt work. Although one cannot know how much the hippie movement also influenced this behavior, gestalt therapy has since struggled with carrying the weight of its history.

With the hippie movement quieting down, the field called for a more responsible and ethical position (Feder, 1980; Melnick et al., 1994). Today gestalt therapists are trained to be more aware of client's needs, and it is the therapists' ethical obligation to do no harm.

GESTALT THERAPY AND THE CONTACT BOUNDARY

Contact is the ability to be fully present with all aspects of ourselves—our sensing, emotional, intellectual, behavioral, sexual, and spiritual being. We are always in contact, but we modulate the level of our contact by creatively adjusting to the sensory experience of our environment to maintain homeostasis. We make contact by seeing and looking, touching and feeling, tasting, smelling, sound, gesture, language and movement (Mann, 2010). Contact is central to the gestalt therapy process; "it is that which occurs at the boundary between organism and environment, at the meeting of self and other" (Kepner, 2008, p. 165). The contact boundary is the location where we meet and withdraw from our environment. In gestalt therapy, arriving at the contact boundary is the experience in which the therapist or the client, or both, meets the situation and the situation meets the other, the experience of "me" in relation to what is not "me." In other words, awareness of arriving at the contact boundary is awareness of the experience of me, the experience of you, and the difference between the two.

The term *boundary* in this regard is not a fixed point, but rather a fluid, ever-changing space between two human experiences. Healthy functioning is the capacity to move along a permeable–impermeable continuum in relation to a present situation (Mann, 2010). In gestalt therapy, for healthy functioning to occur in the therapeutic relationship, contact boundaries need to be permeable enough to allow nourishment and intimacy, and sufficiently impermeable to maintain autonomy and to resist what could be damaging to the relationship in the environment. The therapist uses a variety of awareness experiences and experiments to facilitate awareness and expand the client's contact boundary. The basic intent of focusing on awareness techniques is to restore a person to his or her potentially whole or integrated personality. It is also critical for therapists to be aware of their own contact boundary. The awareness of the client–therapist contact boundary is an important element in the discussion of boundary violations. Gestalt therapists must maintain awareness of this boundary throughout their work to be aware of an experience that may lead to a transgression.

BOUNDARY VIOLATIONS AS AN EMERGENT EVENT AT THE CONTACT BOUNDARY

Despite boundary problems and sexual misconduct ranking highest in complaints to licensing boards, adequate training in boundary crossing and violations remains lacking in gestalt therapy training. Hunter and Struve (1998) stated that it is mostly the extreme cases in which a therapist has violated professional standards and become sexual with a client, and these are the cases cited as examples of unethical behavior; however, little attention is focused on helping clinicians understand the intricacies of how such encounters between therapist and client come to be—and most important, the degree to which any therapist may have personal vulnerabilities for an erotic transgression with a client. O'Shea (2000) argued that what gestalt therapy trainers fail to do is acknowledge the actuality of sexual attraction and boundary violation, which is deflective and diminishes any real dialogue and exploration of possible transgressions.

It is important to make the distinction between what gestalt therapy considers boundary crossing and a boundary violation. Traditionally, there is a contract between therapist and client about when, where, for what fee, and in what general way the therapeutic interaction will take place. Any deviation from this contract is likely to constitute a dual relationship or boundary crossing. Boundary crossings can sometimes be helpful to the client and relationship. In contrast, a boundary violation is entering into a dual relationship for the primary purpose of serving the therapist (Feder, 2004). Boundary violations are harmful and usually exploitive of clients' needs, using them to feed the therapists' narcissistic, dependent, sexual, or other needs. It is important to place as much emphasis on boundary crossings as on boundary violations, as well as sexual and nonsexual boundaries. Alpert and Steinberg (2017) argued that

> nonsexual boundaries are more common that sexual ones and therapist–client sex may be the result when there is a violation of nonsexual boundaries. This is the "slippery slope" in which boundary violations that begin as inconsequential and nontoxic rocket to major and destructive ones. (p. 144)

In gestalt therapy, "dual relationships were initially practiced indiscriminately, and no doubt often harmfully" (Feder, 2004, p. 144). Since then, there have been efforts to shift the way clinicians are trained to manage boundaries around dual relationships. Gestalt therapists hold a sense of responsibility while engaging in these kinds of contacts with clients. It is our responsibility to uphold behaviors, whether implicit or explicit, that are consistent with the philosophical, aesthetic, and ethical principles of the gestalt approach.

EROTIC CO-TRANSFERENCE AS A FIELD PHENOMENON

Gestalt therapy's history with the theory of transference and counter-transference is a topic of further consideration, although not one that can be fully explored given the limited space this chapter permits. One approach to understanding transference and countertransference within a gestalt therapy context is found in the conceptualization of "co-transference" (O'Shea, 2000; 2003). O'Shea (2003) described co-transference as a process of mutual influence between the therapist and client. She draws on the work of intersubjective theorists who have taken the step of eradicating the split between transference and countertransference, which is viewed as being more consistent with the gestalt approach. According to O'Shea (2003), sexual attraction within the client–therapist dyad can be more usefully understood as a function of the cocreated client–therapist field rather than a client's transference or therapist's countertransference. From a field theoretical perspective, it is not possible to see the transferential process as something that "just" happens to the therapist because of what the client thinks, feels, or does. Moreover, it is a cocreated experience.

Little has been written about sexuality and erotic co-transference from a field-dependent position. O'Shea (2000) argued that "trainees need to be able to understand, speak about, and work with the complex web of erotic co-transference" (p. 18). Psychoanalytic literature gives attention to erotic transference; however, there is danger in viewing transference as something the client does and countertransference as a therapist's response. "Understanding the transference process from a field perspective means seeing it not as a cause and effect phenomenon, but as a function and consequences of the therapeutic relationship itself" (O'Shea, 2000, p. 19). As gestalt therapists, we must not ignore how and what we contribute to the experience of erotic tension and take responsibility for and recognize our reactions as being part of what we bring to the therapeutic process. It is also our responsibility to safeguard boundaries and take responsibility when violations do occur.

USE OF TOUCH IN GESTALT THERAPY

Although psychotherapy professionals acknowledge that erotic touch is inappropriate and a boundary violation, gestalt training programs routinely fail to address the complex dimensions of this topic. Several years ago, when I started to collect material on the ethical use of touch in psychotherapy,

I was surprised to find that little exists on this subject. I was training in gestalt body process psychotherapy (Kepner, 2008) and the use of touch as a therapeutic intervention. I learned that only well-trained and experienced clinicians should use touch in their work. This includes not only training in gestalt therapy but also expanding your range of body awareness through modalities such as Alexander and Feldenkrais work, movement and dance therapies, and body–mind centering, to name just a few. I was aware of my own embodiment, and throughout my training, I became increasingly aware of my yearnings, desires, arousals, and responses in my interactions to others in my training group. I began to explore my own personal history with touch while witnessing the range of different experiences in the group. This sparked my interest in how Gestalt trainers teach beginning practitioners to use touch in gestalt therapy and how I bring my own body's history to the process of using touch with clients.

Kepner (2008) wrote,

> If therapists are to understand the use of touch in therapy and so be able to create for their clients an atmosphere that makes the use of touch safe, comfortable and natural, we must first examine our own nature and attitudes. We must come to understand how we embody the cultural, as well as personal beliefs, and attitudes that make touch forbidden or frightening. The understanding of one's self and biases is a prerequisite for any therapeutic application, but is even more essential for such intimate and directly contactful work as touch. (p. 74)

Purposes of Touch in Gestalt Therapy

Touch can serve different functions and purposes in gestalt therapy. The most common is to promote increased awareness of some aspect of embodiment (Kepner, 2001). Touch can be done by the therapist or by the client touching their own body. An example of this could be asking the client to touch certain parts of their own body, and by doing this, they can heighten awareness of their body sensations. Hands-on, nonsexual touch by the therapist is to be used with caution and only with the client's assent. Examples of hands-on nonsexual touch include expressive/emotional touch, supportive touch, or touch for catharsis, for example. A client can feel overwhelmed or extremely vulnerable when working through difficult emotional experiences and sometimes unable to coherently consent to the therapist's touch.

Touch can bring awareness to what is physically happening here and now, bringing the client more in touch with their body. Kepner (2001) explained how he utilizes direct physical contact through movements to revitalize or enliven specific parts of the body. Bodily touch can bring clients into the here and now and foster awareness of a different experience. Although they might feel frightened or alone, they can see this is not a dangerous situation.

Touch can also support a client to stay with their experience longer to allow for more awareness when working through difficult emotional experiences. For example, during a piece of boundary work, Mary wanted to voice her "NO!" to her mother for violating her as a child. She wanted to feel supported and safe while doing this, and this was achieved by the therapist putting a hand on her back as she exclaimed "NO!"

For some clients, touch as a positive, nonabusive way of contact can be a new experience; they may be unable to recall positive touch experiences in their personal history (Eyckmans, 2009). In my work with touch, I often find that clients have an empowering experience when they realize that they can say no to the possibility of touch without a negative consequence. For example, Jane was a client with a history of sexual abuse and came to work on the challenges of being intimate with her husband. When I first introduced the concept of raising awareness of the contact boundary between her and her husband, I offered an experiment where I stood on the opposite side of the room and took steps toward her while reaching for her as if I were going to touch her. The moment Jane began to feel sensations in her body that were unsafe I instructed her to tell me to stop. She decided every step of the way how close I would be to her, and if she wanted to be touched by me. The cocreation of this experiment allowed her to be in control and in more contact with her sensate experience and access her "no" when I stepped too close. Furthermore, the therapist's ability to maintain a sense of self-awareness throughout experiential interventions with touch is crucial. For example, if Jane had not said no and I sensed that she was overwhelmed or dissociative, I might have slowed down, stopped, and checked with her to determine if she was indeed sure about her invitation for my touch. If I was still unsure within my own embodiment about how to proceed, I might continue assessing the situation with Jane or determine that the use of touch is not appropriate at that time. Keep in mind that this depth of sensory awareness can only occur with highly experienced and trained clinicians.

Touch and Power in the Therapeutic Relationship

Understanding power dynamics between client and therapist is essential in gestalt therapy, and especially critical when using touch. Within the constructs of most Western cultures, touch is linked with images and feelings ascribed to power. Therefore, touch illuminates and enforces the existing power hierarchies that characterize relationships (Hunter & Struve, 1998).

Gestalt therapy often emphasizes balancing the relational dynamics between client and therapist, to the extent that can at times lead therapists to ignore the power differential that does and must continue to exist for treatment. Gestalt therapists must take responsibility for the power we hold in the therapeutic relationship and the implications that this has for intimacy and nurturance, as well as exploitation and abuse (O'Shea, 2000). Touch increases intimacy in any relationship, and with increased intimacy, there is increased vulnerability and risk of boundary violation. Differentiating nonsexual touch from the sexual or erotic is also important to distinguish.

Touch as Ethical Practice

The use of touch as a therapeutic intervention places the client and therapist in a position of unusual closeness and intimacy, and this discussion would not be complete without noting ethical considerations and challenges. In his article "Touch in Gestalt Body Process Psychotherapy," Kepner (2001) described the ethical mandate to "do no harm":

> Ethics are not only about moral prudence, they also help me form the relational frame that can hold the work. Contrary to those who find ethical principles to be a restriction of therapeutic freedom, I find that they help me create the clarity of purpose and boundaries. (p. 109)

A confluence of factors foster an ethical practice of using touch in gestalt therapy. A therapist must consider the client's issues, what is known about the client's history of touch, the client's particular dilemmas and patterns of self-organization, the therapist's training and skill level and personal comfort with touch, and the setting, which can also include the social field. That is to say, it is a relational and personal-environmental field question of whether the use of touch is appropriate with each individual client (Kepner, 2001). Establishing clarity around the intention of touch is critical. It is the responsibility of the therapist to recognize the interface of their own needs when using touch and assessing the readiness of the therapeutic relationship for an intervention as risky and intense as physical touch is crucial throughout the assessment process.

CONCLUSION

To date, there remains little to no published literature on sexual boundary violations in gestalt therapy. Leanne O'Shea (2000, 2019) has made a significant contribution to beginning this dialogue by acknowledging the silence around sexuality and the erotic in the gestalt community. Her chapter "Erotic Ground: Always and Already There" (O'Shea, 2019) provides an important perspective on embodiment and the constant presence of eros. However, to date, nothing has been written by gestalt practitioners on the subject of sexual boundary violations. Gestalt therapy carries centuries of historical baggage of Perls' sexual behavior and misconduct, much of which has dirtied the waters of gestalt therapy. Perhaps this has contributed to the silence of sexual boundary violation in the field, leaving the challenges of Perls's misconduct unaddressed while disowning of risks we face as gestalt therapists in transgressing against our patients.

Sexual boundary violations can be a source of much confusion, distress, harm, and profound injury and shame, supported by silence and isolation. For these reasons, I encourage gestalt therapist to continue not only to dialogue about sexuality and boundaries, but to dialogue, write, and research about boundary violations and transgressions in gestalt therapy.

REFERENCES

Alpert, J. L., & Steinberg, A. (2017). Sexual boundary violations: A century of violations and a time to analyze. *Psychoanalytic Psychology, 34*(2), 144–150.

Eyckmans, S. (2009). Handle with care: Touch as a therapeutic tool. *Gestalt Journal of Australia & New Zealand, 6*(1), 40–53.

Feder, B. (1980). Responsibility in gestalt therapy. *The Gestalt Journal, 1*, 46–50.

Feder, B. (2004). Dual relationships: A gestalt therapy perspective. *Gestalt Review, 8*(2), 135–145. https://doi.org/10.5325/gestaltreview.8.2.0135

Hunter, M., & Struve, J. (1998). *The ethical use of touch in psychotherapy.* Sage Publications. https://doi.org/10.4135/9781483328102

Kepner, J. (2001). Touch in body process psychotherapy: Purpose, practice, and ethics. *Gestalt Review, 5*(2), 97–114. https://doi.org/10.5325/gestaltreview.5.2.0097

Kepner, J. (2008). *Body process: A gestalt approach to working with the body in psychotherapy.* The Gestalt Press.

Mann, D. (2010). *Gestalt therapy: 100 key points and techniques.* Routledge.

Melnick, J., Nevis, S. M., & Melnick, G. N. (1994). Therapeutic ethics: A gestalt perspective. *British Gestalt Journal, 3*, 105–113.

O'Shea, L. (2000). Sexuality: Old struggles and new challenges. *Gestalt Review, 4*(1), 8–25. https://doi.org/10.5325/gestaltreview.4.1.0008

O'Shea, L. (2003). The erotic field. *The British Gestalt Journal, 12*(2), 105–110.

O'Shea, L. (2019). Erotic ground: Always and already there. In M. Clemmens (Ed.), *Embodied relational gestalt: Theory and applications* (pp. 123–168). Routledge. https://doi.org/10.4324/9780429330858-4

Perls, F. S., Hefferline, R. F., & Goodman, P. (1951). *Gestalt therapy: Excitement and growth in the human personality.* Julian Press.

Resnick, R. W. (2015). Perls, Fritz. In E. S. Neukrug (Ed.), *The SAGE encyclopedia of theory in counseling and psychotherapy* (pp. 762–765). Sage Publications. https://doi.org/10.4135/9781483346502.n271

Shepard, M. (1971). *The love treatment: Sexual intimacy between patients and psychotherapists*. Peter H. Wyden.

Shepard, M. (1975). *Fritz: An intimate portrait of Fritz Perls and gestalt therapy*. Saturday Review Press.

Stoehr, T. (1994). *Here now next: Paul Goodman and the originals of gestalt therapy*. Jossey-Bass.

8 THE ART OF HELPFUL SEX TALK IN THERAPY

A Psychoanalytic Sex Therapist Speaks

ELIZABETH GOREN

I entered one of the country's first behaviorally oriented doctoral clinical psychology programs at Rutgers University in 1971. My training included formal training in sex therapy. I arrived on the scene in what is now considered a period of "first wave" feminism, the dawning of the sexual liberation era at a moment when sex therapy was gaining public popularity and when psychoanalysis was starting to be debunked in the field of psychology. The terms *sexual boundary violations* (SBVs) and *risk management* had yet to enter professional discourse. One of my first sex therapy courses involved a series of role-playing exercises, including one of taking turns giving and receiving massage, a standard sex therapy homework assignment. We were clothed, and touch was restricted to the kind of back, neck, arms, and hands massage now offered in airports and nail salons. As we were role-playing patient and therapist, we talked about our bodies and sexuality in a very personal and detailed way with one another. This was a teaching tool that could never be a part of a professional curriculum today with our deepened sensitivity to the subtleties of sexual exploitation and abuse in society and overarching focus on risk management, legal regulation, and liability in training and education.

https://doi.org/10.1037/0000247-008
Sexual Boundary Violations in Psychotherapy: Facing Therapist Indiscretions, Transgressions, and Misconduct, A. Steinberg, J. L. Alpert, and C. A. Courtois (Editors)

I offer this vignette in the spirit of bringing my perspective as a sex therapist from a time in our field not yet marked by a singular focus on not committing an actual SBV. In this chapter, I hope to highlight how key aspects of a sex therapy approach, when informed by and integrated with basic psychodynamic precepts, can help therapists in all models of psychotherapy practice develop greater comfort and confidence in working with the intense and complex matters of sex and sexuality in the consulting room. One needn't be a sex therapist to broaden knowledge and skill in talking about sex in realistic yet intimate terms in all its subtleties, personally and interpersonally. Nor does one need to be a psychoanalyst to recognize and responsibly explore with our patients their sexual and romantic feelings, fantasies, and impulses and to be committed to the self-reflection and self-examination of romantic and sexual feelings that we may experience and struggle with in relation to our patients.

The challenge for all therapists in working in the heat of the powerful intimacy of speaking about sex is to find a psychological position that enables us to speak openly, directly and explicitly about this in a way that is reassuring and invites more openness while not being confusing or disturbing to the patient. Just how can a therapist convey openness and speak directly and explicitly about this most profoundly intimate aspect of self—one's sexual feelings, impulses, fantasies, and desires—in such a way that doesn't inadvertently foster being misconstrued as seductive, provocative, or, alternatively, as teasingly depriving by the patient? Similarly can our reluctance to bring up sexuality or our efforts to respectfully not respond to a patient's erotic, romantic intimations or their explicit sex talk be experienced by them as our being detached, critical, or judgmental?

Most challenging for every one of us therapists regardless of our experience or training is talking about sex with a patient when it directly pertains to us. This calls for a delicate balancing act between over- versus underresponding. Helpful communication about sexual feelings and issues between therapist and patient requires that the therapist does not accidentally silence the patient, as a conscious or unconscious expression of our own anxiety, or, unwittingly, subtly drawing the patient into stronger erotic feelings, again out of our own anxiety or other unacceptable feelings, like our own erotic feelings for the patient.

That universal fear of falling prey to the dreaded slippery slope down into actual romantic or sexual involvement, although understandable, can paradoxically make us more vulnerable to actually falling down that slope. The importance of distinguishing helpful from harmful "sex talk" with patients cannot be overstated. Genuine comfort and competency in communication about sexual issues is a key preventative for actual SBV.

WHAT ETHICS CODES CAN TEACH US

Responsible and skilled communication requires that the therapist not feel anxious. Although this is obvious, I think that anxiety around matters of sex and sexuality in professional relations runs much higher than we might want to think for multiple reasons. Between the #MeToo and movement and professional emphasis on risk management practices, clinicians tend to be anxiously focused so much on liability concerns and not committing an actual SBV that they do not feel free to raise the subject of sexual issues between them and their patients with supervisors and are also less likely to seek consultation when needed. Unfortunately, today's legalistic culture and violation-oriented professional ethics codes leads clinicians to be more anxiously focused on the "letter of the law" and the "Do Not's" (Goren, 2017) than on recognizing and working effectively with underlying or subtle sexual issues in general, especially as they relate to the relationship between therapist and patient. Here I am referring to the inherent and long-term power the person of the therapist can hold over the patient—and therefore the power that the therapist's unconscious can exercise on the patient. Specifically, the patient will pick up on both the implicit and overt content and tone of the therapist's communications. Therapists' lack of self-awareness can cloud their judgment and thereby influence and cloud the patient's judgment. Further, we know that the impact of therapists' power over a patient can last long after therapy has terminated.

With its fundamental belief in the role of the therapist's unconscious (broadly defined countertransference) as well as patients' unconscious (broadly defined transference), the code of ethics of the American Psychoanalytic Association, the largest organization representing psychoanalysts, takes a simple position that prohibits any romantic sexual involvement between "former" as well as "current" patients. This highlights the unequivocal importance that the therapist's unconscious can play in what they see as the inherent and lifelong hierarchical nature of the therapist–patient relationship.

Similarly, while leaving room for the personal discretion and judgment of the psychologist "after a 2-year interval" posttermination, the American Psychological Association (APA; 2017) *Ethical Principles of Psychologists and Code of Conduct* also unequivocally states that the psychologist must *"bear the burden of demonstrating that there has not been exploitation* [emphasis added]," pointing to the profound, nonspecific but powerful impact that the therapist has on the patient even after termination of therapy. We also see that the National Association Social Workers (NASW), the professional organization for licensed social workers whose practice, like that of psychologists, includes but is not limited to psychotherapy, holds to the principle that "Social workers should not engage in sexual activities or sexual contact with former clients because of the potential for harm to the client," and if a social worker does so, "*because of extraordinary circumstances*, it is social workers—not their clients—who assume the full burden of demonstrating that the former client has not been *exploited, coerced, or manipulated, intentionally or unintentionally* [emphasis added]." Both organizations govern professionals working from multiple theoretical points of view in diverse settings.

Finally, the primary code of ethics governing sex therapists, the American Association of Sex Educators Counselors and Therapists (AASECT) not only prohibits sexual romance between therapist and patient "in perpetuity" (posttermination) but also makes a point of including certain nonphysicalized verbal interactions in definitions of abuse that relate to sexual communication and related interaction between patient and therapist: "Sexual misconduct is also sexual solicitation, physical advances, or *verbal or nonverbal conduct that is sexual in nature* [emphasis added]." Like the APA and NASW, AASECT does not privilege concepts of the unconscious or transference countertransference but strongly emphasizes the power that therapists wield in the hierarchical power dynamics between therapist and patient and thereby the power of therapists' conscious and less conscious feelings to affect their judgment. These differing professions concur on the crucial importance of therapists working to prevent exercising excessive or otherwise inappropriate power over the patient.

So in the muddy and often tumultuous waters of sex, sexuality, and romance in therapy, how can we improve therapist self-awareness and limit self-deception, while maintaining full and deep engagement with patients in these matters? I believe by combining key elements of precepts and training from sex therapy with psychoanalysis and other therapeutic orientations.

WHAT SEX THERAPY CAN OFFER

Sex therapy education is geared to teaching therapists the importance of their own "sex-positive" attitudes and communication, along with developing expertise in human sexuality. Training is oriented around therapist modeling and guiding patients in respectful positive communication and attitudes about sex in such a way that I believe reduces the therapist's as well as the patient's anxiety and resultant vulnerability to acting out.

Seared into sex therapy training, which can easily be misconstrued by laypeople and professionals alike, is the principle that no matter how intimate the patient–therapist relationship may be, no matter how much the patient brings the therapist into his or her personal intimate life, regardless of how explicit and detailed the sex talk is on an ongoing basis, the professional boundary of the patient–therapist relationship is sacrosanct and never involves sexual contact between them or any behavior or tone that could be construed as sexual. In fact, the founders of sex therapy, William Masters and Virginia Johnson, were the first professionals to publicly declare therapist–patient sexual involvement as not only unprofessional but criminal—in fact referring to it as rape (Pope, 2001).

Of course, therapists in all models and forms of practice are trained about the crucial importance of boundaries, but they are not typically trained in how to construct clear-cut boundaries while delving into sexuality and sexual issues in personal detailed ways. The fact is, patients' feelings and attitudes about sex are quietly but indelibly marked by what their therapists feel about sex and how they then talk about sex. It is a basic assumption in sex therapy that a therapist's personal conflicts, attitudes, and general ease with sexual matters determine the tone and effectiveness of therapy.

Because this is seen as a nonspecific but key therapeutic element, sex therapy training includes (a) ongoing opportunities for therapists to practice open, appropriately boundaried talk about sex, with respect for individual sexual anxieties and values; (b) education that focuses on every dimension of sex and sexuality for the individual at all stages of development and for relationships, with an eye and ear for familial, sociocultural influences and evolving societal norms; and (c) a focus on helping therapists develop greater comfort with discussing sex. The very nature of sex therapy—that is, the therapist thinking and talking about the details and mechanics of sex and the many variations of sexual practices—fosters an accepting attitude about sex on the part of patient. The therapist manifesting in a natural, matter-of-fact way in and of itself has an ameliorative effect on sexual anxieties, guilt, and embarrassment. This way of communicating also mitigates risk for therapists' miscommunication (based on anxiety or conflict) in a potentially stimulating, shaming, or otherwise nonhelpful manner.

A basic tenet of sex therapy is nonjudgmental acceptance and appreciation of all sexual desires, variations in practice and fantasies, within the boundary and frame of basic human rights and the primacy of consent. Sex therapy training thereby includes helping therapists confront their own biases and prejudices about sex. Thanks to the progress the women's and LGBTQ+ movements have brought to society over recent decades, most contemporary psychotherapy training now includes recognition and greater respect for sexual diversity and variations in sexual and gender expression.

But sex therapy, with its historic role in the depathologizing of many cultural restrictive beliefs and attitudes about sex, continues to prioritize broadening notions of "healthy" sexuality. This means working with therapists in training to challenge themselves and their patients to examine their personal values and predilections, and for the therapists to work through personal prejudices that can inevitably find their way into the consulting room. As a cognitive behaviorally oriented form of therapy, sex therapy seeks change via the conscious self.

In contrast, because psychoanalysts recognize that we cannot assume that "a cigar is just a cigar," we don't take a patient's expressed attitudes and feelings about sex at face value. We consider potentially important underlying meanings and feelings surrounding sex and sexuality, including unconscious issues operating for both patient and therapist. A therapist needs to be able to recognize how the patient is "seeing" the therapist as a result of the patient's history and personality (i.e., *transference* in psychoanalytic terms). Therapists also need to examine their own unconscious feelings about sex in relation to the patient and the therapy interaction. This is crucial if one accepts the idea that therapists' unintended thoughts and feelings can get expressed towards or experienced by their patients in their interaction in ways that can significantly influence the therapy. This means that therapists need to be able to constructively self-reflect and explore their own personal feelings, issues related to their own history and personality separate from the patient and then those that they may be feeling in response to specifics with the patient, broadly defined in psychoanalytic terms as *countertransference*. These factors hold true regardless of the form of therapy being practiced, which is why psychoanalytic understanding and training may be helpful.

WHAT PSYCHOANALYSIS CAN OFFER

Analytic therapy is all about using the therapist experience as a therapeutic tool to deepen understanding of the patient and the interpersonal dynamics operating in the consulting room in a way that moves the therapy process forward so that this knowledge can be applied to the patient's life outside the consulting room. This entails therapists focusing on, identifying, and using their reactions and feelings toward the patient in the course of the therapy process. Training involves learning how to attend to one's own state of mind while maintaining focus on the patient, the specifics of their interaction, and the therapy goals. Through didactic and experiential training, therapists learn to track how their ongoing feelings are affecting their communication patterns and how patients are responding to them. This emphasis on therapist self-awareness and self-exploration builds competency in working with the kind of intense emotional and interactional vicissitudes that happen around such emotionally and interpersonally vulnerable topics as sex, especially what's happening between therapist and patient.

Although psychoanalytic recognition of the inevitability of counter-transference helps therapists accept their own missteps—particularly when it comes to the "hot" issues around sex when it arises during therapy, therapists hold extremely high, sometimes unrealistic ideals (Slochower, 2003). We try to help our patients accept their own humanness, yet we can sometimes have trouble acknowledging our own human limitations. This makes us vulnerable to dealing with some of our less-than-ideal feelings and reactions to a patient by trying to manage them in one way or another, potentially compromising the therapy.

Finding that balance between being oversexualizing and under- or desexualizing, between being too avoidant of the subject or being inappropriately stimulating or voyeuristic can end up being hurtful, even harmful to the patient. This balancing act is most difficult when we find ourselves caught in the throes of intense transference–countertransference dynamics involving sexuality; naturally, this most often occurs when we least expect it and feel least prepared to deal with it. We can become flummoxed if not outright rejecting of our own less-than-ideal or outright antitherapeutic feelings by denial or trying to manage them in a way that may have inadvertently confusing or negative impact on the patient and the therapy.

Feeling sexually attracted to one's patient is the most common and difficult challenge for therapists to grapple with, even though we rationally know that it's natural and normal to feel sexually attracted to certain patients. It is crucial for therapists to accept their feelings while exploring the basis of these feelings in his or her own life, and how their attraction is affecting the patient and therapy. The therapist needs to consider how the patient may be either consciously or more often unconsciously evoking these feelings, such as whether they are being seductive or in some other way provoking the therapist to relate in a sexually responsive way. It is clearly therapists' responsibility to be aware of and control how their feelings are being expressed and how the patient, at varying degrees of awareness, may be reacting to the therapist. Seductive speech and manner is the most obvious way that therapist attraction manifests.

We have to remember that, as Davies (2013) succinctly put it, "*talking sex can be as exciting or even more exciting than *doing* sex*" (p. 172) and, I would add, as potentially harmful when not acknowledged or managed in a way that helps a therapist accept and learn how to control his or her own strong and confusing sexual and related feelings, such as fear or anger, that can arise with a sexually or aggressively provocative patient.

A second pattern, less often focused on by therapist, supervisor, or patient, is when the therapist becomes more distant than before and possibly in a clinically contraindicated way. To feel more in control of the situation and try to be more "clinical," the therapist will shift and become less personal and intimate, leaving patients potentially confused, rejected, or feeling suddenly humiliated, questioning themselves about whether they've been the one to have done something wrong that made the therapist withdraw. In this situation, patients may question their own judgment about having felt close and trusting of the therapist.

A related therapy dynamic is when the patient, correctly or incorrectly, interprets the therapist as being sexually interested when in fact the therapist is actually feeling anxiety and a great deal of discomfort or worry about the patient. For instance when a patient is being sexually provocative, a therapist might make efforts to be respectfully affirming and nonrejecting of the patient while trying to maintain control of the therapy situation (Jørstad, 2002; Renn, 2013) in such a way that can leave the patient confused about the therapist's feelings, and potentially feeling ashamed of their own strong sexual feelings.

Another interactional risk is when therapists start to have strong negative feelings toward the patient or therapy. Because the image of a good therapist today is that of a caregiver, a person who wants to help and heal, it is sometimes difficult for a therapist to accept and reflect on negative emotions toward a patient. This can lead to unconscious, defensive transformation, a kind of reaction formation, of these feelings to more acceptable feelings, from hate or fear to love, from disgust to desire. Why is this so?

The nature of sexual arousal often involves an admixture of fear, lust, and aggression. One can feel an enticing attraction toward or desire for that which scares or disturbs us. This is analogous to people's love for rollercoasters, horror movies, and other nonsexual play that includes elements of fear and aggression. So too, we therapists are humanly vulnerable to being sexually drawn to emotionally confusing states of arousal—that is, being turned on in the face of frustration, worry, and even resentment of the patient, such as can occur when a therapist fears a patient's suicidality, feels unable to reach a patient, or feels disgust or anger at a patient's provocative aggressive behavior. Combined with a need to deny having such negative nontherapeuticlike feelings—we want to feel we love, not hate, our patients—we become understandably vulnerable to counterproductive erotic feelings toward patients. Further, given therapists' prime motivation to help—we can be prone to strong rescue impulses with patients in their desperation and then our own, such as in the face of patients' active suicidality, personality-disordered demanding provocative behavior toward us, their hostility, or their seemingly intractable unresponsiveness to our efforts to help them.

Gabbard (2001) heroically reported on a case in which he described the how's and why's of his working through an erotic countertransference that he developed with a patient with a thorny erotic transference that was unresponsive to his efforts. After a prolonged period of his patient adamantly insisting "I told you before—I cannot talk about sex" in person without feeling deep shame, Gabbard allowed the therapy to proceed via email correspondence in which the patient's expressions of lust and related desires became so intense that Gabbard reported finding himself feeling "embarrassed" by how excited he had become: "There was a part of me that felt I needed to close my door while I read her messages. . . . I felt like I was reading pornographic communications. . . . I would feel a pressing need to delete her emails. . . . to avoid discovery." Few therapists are in a position to feel safe enough to talk about, much less write about, their erotic countertransference. But with his stellar reputation as the founding leader in the psychotherapy movement to address the egregious problem of SBVs in the field, Gabbard was in a unique position to acknowledge and address that to which we are all vulnerable. That is, to find ourselves embroiled in a sexually charged enactment to which each of us has our own unique reasons for being vulnerable (in Gabbard's case, the risk to his reputation as a leader in SBV) and that repeats, or is resonant with, the patient's own particular history. The abundance of research and literature on SBV throughout psychology, as represented in the varied chapters in this book, attests to the potential vulnerability every therapist has to becoming embroiled in erotic transference–countertransference dynamics. They can become seriously problematic without therapist skill and commitment to ongoing self-examination and willingness to seek the help of trusted colleagues.

In sum, therapists have the challenge of trying to manage their own intense feelings for and about the patient and therapy without being so "objective" that the patient ends up feeling rebuffed, ashamed, humiliated, or rejected—which paradoxically can intensify a patients' sexual longings, pushing them toward acting out with the therapist. In these various ways, by privileging and training therapists in the art and skills of acknowledging, accepting, and knowing how to confront and work through one's own less-than-ideal therapeutic reactions and feelings, psychoanalysis has much to contribute to therapists working with sex and sexuality in all therapeutic modalities.

CONCLUSION AND RECOMMENDATIONS FOR TRAINING

My sex therapy training endowed me with a relaxed and open attitude about sex and talking about even the most exquisitely personal and intimate matters of sex with patients. But because of its behavioral focus on sex "out there" in the patient's life, it did not have much to offer on the "how-to's" of working with sex and romance when it came to the subtleties of my relationship with the patient. Thankfully, my psychoanalytic training armed me with ways of thinking about the multiple dynamics operating in the consulting room and learning how to use my own feelings in a respectful and constructive way to forward patient growth.

To summarize, professional training and education on this subject tends to focus on ethics and boundary violations and consequently can end up feeling so morally freighted as to compromise appeal and utilization. Experientially based training, separated from the specter of SBV, because of its association with danger, failure, and immorality, will be far more welcoming to clinicians at all career stages. For our patients to feel greater comfort and skill in addressing their sexuality, we therapists need to feel more comfortable with our own sexuality, inside and outside the consulting room. For as Freud (1963), the founder of psychotherapy, taught, "The behavior of a human being in sexual matters is often a prototype for the whole of his other modes of reaction."

REFERENCES

American Psychological Association. (2017). *Ethical principles of psychologists and code of conduct* (2002, amended effective June 1, 2010, and January 1, 2017). https://www.apa.org/ethics/code/index.aspx

Davies, J. M. (2013). My enfant terrible is twenty: A discussion of Slavin's and Gentile's retrospective reconsideration of "Love in the Afternoon." *Psychoanalytic Dialogues, 23*(2), 170–179. https://doi.org/10.1080/10481885.2013.772479

Freud, S. (1963). *Sexuality and the psychology of love.* Touchstone.

Gabbard, G. O. (2001). Cyberpassion: E-rotic transference on the internet. *The Psychoanalytic Quarterly, 70*(4), 719–737. https://doi.org/10.1002/j.2167-4086.2001.tb00618.x

Goren, E. (2017). A call for more talk and less abuse in the consulting room: One psychoanalyst–sex therapist's perspective. *Psychoanalytic Psychology, 34*(2), 215–220. https://doi.org/10.1037/pap0000092

Jørstad, J. (2002). Erotic countertransference: Hazards, challenges and therapeutic potentials. *Scandinavian Psychoanalytic Review, 25*(2), 117–134. https://doi.org/10.1080/01062301.2002.10592737

Pope, K. (2001). Sex between therapists and clients. In J. Worell (Ed.), *Encyclopedia of women and gender: Sex similarities and differences and the impact of society on gender* (pp. 955–962). Academic Press.

Renn, P. (2013). Moments of meeting: The relational challenges of sexuality in the consulting room. *British Journal of Psychotherapy, 29*(2), 135–153. https://doi.org/10.1111/bjp.12017

Slochower, J. (2003). The analyst's secret delinquencies. *Psychoanalytic Dialogues, 13*(4), 451–469. https://doi.org/10.1080/10481881309348751

9 SEXUAL MISCONDUCT IN THE FEMINIST THERAPY REALM

LAURA S. BROWN AND CHRISTINE A. COURTOIS

Feminist therapy was developed beginning in the late 1960s as a corrective against the sexism and misogyny of psychotherapy as practiced. It also developed in acknowledgment of the increased number of women who were becoming psychotherapists at the time, the result of the impact of the nascent women's liberation movement on women's educational and professional aspirations. As more women became psychotherapists, they began to look closely at the dominant models, which they heavily critiqued and sought to expand and change. Feminist therapy has evolved in the subsequent five decades into a technically integrative multicultural model of liberatory practice with a focus on exploration of power dynamics arising from gendered narratives as they intersect with other aspects of identity (Brown, 2018). Although it was originally developed by cisgender women for working with cisgender women, it has become a therapy by and for people of all gender orientations and expressions in which the question of gender is central, although often not in the foreground. It also attends very directly to issues of cultural and racial diversity and to intersectionality because these also involve gender and power differentials. Liberation from discrimination and

https://doi.org/10.1037/0000247-009
Sexual Boundary Violations in Psychotherapy: Facing Therapist Indiscretions, Transgressions, and Misconduct, A. Steinberg, J. L. Alpert, and C. A. Courtois (Editors)

oppression leading to personal empowerment and social justice are incorporated into treatment plans and ways of conducting treatment.

Feminist therapy is defined as follows:

> The practice of therapy informed by feminist political philosophies and analysis, grounded in multicultural feminist scholarship on the psychology of women and gender, which leads both therapist and client toward strategies and solutions advancing feminist resistance, transformation and social change in daily personal life, and in relationships with the social, emotional and political environments. (Brown, 1994, pp. 21–22)

Because it is technically integrative, there are few, if any, specific feminist therapy techniques. Consequently, fidelity to the underlying liberatory model of the therapy relationship is one of the first ways in which a therapy can be constructed as feminist.

CONSTRUCTS OF FEMINIST THERAPY

One of the central constructs of the feminist frame for psychotherapy is that of the *egalitarian relationship*. This construct arises from the earliest feminist analyses of power dynamics and inequalities in psychotherapy (Chesler, 1972). The predominant therapeutic orientation of the time was psychoanalytic–psychodynamic, although cognitive behavioral and humanistic theoretical models and treatment methods were being developed during that same period. Whatever the treatment type, the therapist (most often a cisgender male) was established as dominant in authority and power/status and the client (mostly cisgender female) as having lesser power and influence. In the psychoanalytic method, the therapist was the identified expert who proffered interpretations of the client's symptoms and verbalizations. The client was the recipient who was expected to accept the interpretations made by the authority figure in their quest for healing. In cognitive behavioral applications, the therapist offered information and exercises to the client to identify, correct, and change cognitions and behaviors underlying their symptoms, in the process diminishing their hold over the client. Humanistic therapists were often charismatic men who exercised a great deal of influence on their followers and clients, many of them female, often in nontraditional settings and with nontraditional methods that both crossed and violated boundaries (e.g., therapists might simultaneously be clients of the leaders, clients and therapists would be mixed together in groups and other settings, nude encounter groups involving therapists and clients were developed, transcendent and experiential methods were explored, and so on; see Chapter 7).

All of these newer formats created environments in which therapists could easily abuse their power and authority in a number of ways, including sexually (although this was less likely—but not completely absent—in the cognitive behavioral tradition due to its brevity and focused, less exploratory, and relationship-based treatment; see Chapter 6). In contrast, in a more egalitarian, liberatory relationship, the therapist attempts to structure the treatment to systemically lessen the imbalance of power between client and therapist. An unintended consequence may have been to underemphasize the overarching responsibility of the therapist for establishing the treatment frame and maintaining professional and safe boundaries within which to conduct the psychotherapy.

The feminist tradition has also historically supported the *presence of role and life overlaps between clients and therapists*. Rather than therapists and clients leading very separate lives, early feminist therapy thinkers bowed to the realities of practice in small social communities such as LGBT or communities of color, or in rural or other isolated or closed settings. While acknowledging that overlap of lives could and likely would occur for many feminist therapists, early feminist thinkers saw this as benign, or mostly so. Seeing one's therapist at a women's music concert or other community events, the grocery store, or at an equal rights demonstration would, it was thought, assist in the construction of the egalitarian relationship. Feminist therapy theory posits that no therapist, no matter what their theory, can be neutral or objective or pretend to be invisible to their clients. Instead, the reasoning went, the therapist would be more transparent in ways that were helpful to clients, creating a sense of solidarity, a "consciousness-raising group of two," to quote one of those early authors (Kravetz, 1978). Yet again, any potential risks or problems with such overlaps were underrecognized and underemphasized.

Consistent with this frame of role overlap as inevitable and possibly valuable was a support of the use of *self-disclosure* in therapy. This stance was also espoused as a corrective to the dominant psychoanalytic treatment of the time. In classic psychoanalysis, the analyst's role was as a silent, unseen, noninteractive and relationally abstinent figure who, by design, was mostly unknown to the client and who made the occasional pronouncement and interpretation about the client's free associations. In a similar vein, while behaviorists were more interactive, their focus was largely the assessment and change of cognitions and behaviors over the course of the treatment. And in the more open humanistic environments, clients and therapists were often well known to one another, as they were encouraged to be self-exploratory and open to others in the therapeutic community. Again, the rationale for supporting therapist self-disclosure was ostensibly to equalize the power between the parties. The therapist would no longer be a mystifying powerful figure, like the Wizard of Oz behind the curtain. Instead, therapists would be more genuine, more human, more transparent in their own human struggles. Self-disclosure could, it was argued, be validating; the therapist could say "Hey, me too" as a strategy for assisting clients to know that they were not alone. Self-disclosure could reduce the stigma of a history of abuse, of struggling with a marriage, with infertility or sexual arousal challenges or being lesbian; all components of therapists' identities that had been invisible, and thus not known to clients, would be seen. Although the rationale for such disclosure was clear, its benefit to the treatment was not. Even today, self-disclosure is one of the elements of the treatment process that seems promising but is in need of additional research (Norcross & Lambert, 2018). Also, excessive self-disclosure of the therapist's life and especially their personal problems has been found to unbalance the treatment and to be among the preliminary and the primary risk factors on the slippery slope to therapist sexual boundary violations (SBVs). Often, a role reversal ensues with the client becoming the therapist's helper, as attention shifts to the therapist's needs. For some clients (most of them female) who have been conditioned into a caretaker role, this scenario sets up an opportunity to engage in that role rather than to explore and potentially change or realign it. It also sets the stage for additional boundary crossings and other incursions that may lead to sexualization of the relationship.

During this time period, feminist researchers and theorists were also documenting the inequities produced by highly prescribed gender beliefs and roles (including those for females, such as compliance, overdependence on males, and caretaking of others, and what were often the inverse for males) that, for females, led to ongoing gender-based discrimination and oppression in all major life settings. As these issues were more deeply investigated, researchers uncovered astoundingly high rates of physical and sexual abuse of women and female children in the family (in the form of incest and child sexual abuse, physical and emotional abuse, and spousal violence) and in the community (rape and other forms of assault, sexual harassment in the workplace and the community) due in large measure to the playout of gender-related stereotypes, including their power imbalances. In terms of incest and child sexual abuse and incest, this led them to repudiate Freud's Oedipal theory, one of the main tenets of classic psychoanalytic theory and treatment. They wrote that in favoring fantasy and wish on the part of the child for sexual contact with the opposite sex parent, the theory negated the reality of abuse for innumerable women who sought treatment for their symptoms, which were explicated by Gelinas (1983) as secondary elaborations of the original untreated effects of the abuse.

Simultaneously, feminists were challenging the status quo by examining and differentiating the roles of males and females and by emphasizing the positives associated with "women's ways of knowing and growth in connection" the latter the title of an influential book authored by Jean Baker Miller and colleagues at the Stone Center (Jordan et al., 1991). Carol Gilligan (1982) contributed another book, titled *In a Different Voice*, that heralded women's strengths and resources that had previously gone unidentified or been minimized, especially their relationship and communication abilities. Women's autobiographical and narrative histories were encouraged, as were their voices in expressing themselves. Women were emboldened to find their personal truths and to make them known by speaking them. This became another hallmark of the feminist treatment of the time: to *stop the silencing of women* and *to give them and their experience a voice equal to that of men's*. They were inspired to appreciate their own inner strengths and resources, their personal narratives, and those of other women. These and other writings became highly influential in efforts to transform traditional forms of psychotherapy to a relational-cultural rather than an abstinent stance on the part of the therapist and based on the emerging recognition of the power of the relationship in treatment efficacy.

These various ways in which early feminist therapists attempted to equalize power in the psychotherapy relationship had potential to in fact empower clients and to make the therapeutic relationship one that was more collaborative. Yet they also created risks that went largely unseen and were inadequately acknowledged at the time.

SBVs IN FEMINIST THERAPY

In the initial 2 decades of its development, the world of feminist therapy was rocked by scandals in which several charismatic therapist–teacher–supervisors in the emerging feminist therapy world chose to interpret these framework issues as permission to be sexual with clients. Most of these relationships were between two women; the therapists in question argued that because that was so, this was not abuse, as was the case when the therapist having sex with a client was a man. Instead, the rationale was that *because* there were egalitarian power dynamics in these therapies, the client was free to choose to be sexual with the therapist. Note that in such an explanation, there was little or no acknowledgment of the differential power between therapist and client based on the therapist's role and ultimate fiduciary and professional responsibility for the treatment and its outcome.

The first author (LS) served as a forensic expert witness for former clients in two cases (one in Seattle, Washington; one in Boulder, Colorado) where the client reappraised the sexual relationship as an abusive boundary violation and filed a civil lawsuit against the therapist. In one other case in the Minneapolis–St. Paul area, she was asked to consult with local therapists who were attempting to challenge the therapist–leader–teacher who was sexualizing therapy relationships. In each of these cases, the offending therapist was strongly identified in her local community (and in the instance in Boulder, nationally) as a leader in the field of feminist therapy. Sadly, many other similar cases are known to both authors.

Our discussion in this chapter derives from having read sworn testimony (depositions, witness statements) in these cases, spoken with or read the testimonies of corroborating witnesses, and reading or hearing testimonies of the therapists involved. Although the two lawsuits were matters of public record, in the interests of privacy for the women who were sexually abused in therapy, we do not refer to case titles. Notably, in each case, the therapist did not deny having been sexual with her client. Rather, she rationalized it by extending the constructs of the egalitarian relationship in feminist therapy.

Many, not all, of these relationships occurred in the context of an organized community of feminist therapists in which the leader–teacher had become central. Thus, the sexual contact happened within a social reality in which people sought to be in the favor of and to gain the approval of the therapist–teacher–leader, much like the dynamics that are seen in cults with charismatic and usually narcissistic leaders (Shaw, 2014). These cases began to become known more broadly in the world of feminist therapy when one or more courageous women in each group became willing to break silence and expose what was happening. These were the days when the "first wave" of sexual abuse of (female) clients and supervisees by their (male) therapists and supervisors (as well as charismatic leaders of therapy groups and traditions) was starting to emerge. Such sexual involvements were beginning to be identified as abusive and unethical and as having high potential for far-reaching damage, as discussed by Ken Pope, a pioneer in the field, in his introduction to this book in which he discusses the history of professional and legal attention to SBVs by therapists.

Both cognitive dissonance and hypocrisy became apparent when feminist therapists decried the exploitation of women clients by male, but not by female, therapists. And, similar to the usual response of organizations to reports of abuse, especially when they allege it at the hands of a higher status, powerful, revered, or charismatic leader (a process now identified as organizational betrayal; see Chapter 17) and as organizational cowardice that often undergirds organizational betrayal (Brown, 2020). It was usually the case that the women making the disclosures were shunned and ostracized from the group surrounding and supporting the identified therapist, losing friends and professional networks in the process. The victim was typically disbelieved or blamed, or both—a process that caused further emotional damage. Both of these responses are in line with what typically happens to the truth-teller victim or to other reporters and disclosers in many organizations, a process so commonplace that Freyd (1997) developed the acronym DARVO, standing for Defend-Avoid-Reverse-Victim-and-Offender, to describe it.

The larger community of feminist therapists was for the most part critical of these boundary-violating therapists and did not support their rationalizations. A collective response to these cases emerged within the Feminist Therapy Institute (FTI), an international organization of advanced and experienced feminist therapists that met annually from 1982 through the early 2000s and sponsored the publication of a number of books that were central to the development of theory and practice in feminist therapy.

Early in the organization's life, it became clear in discussions among the membership that, because of these cases, there was a necessity for organized groups of feminist therapists to explicitly disavow the rationale that an egalitarian relationship in therapy could include sexual contact between client and therapist. FTI's organizational response to the problem was through the development of its own ethics code.

DEVELOPMENT OF THE FTI CODE OF ETHICS

The FTI Code of Ethics was conceived of as an aspirational code, additive to the enforceable codes and jurisdictional laws under which licensed therapists within many different disciplines practiced, given that FTI lacked the apparatus with which to do ethics investigations and impose penalties. By the time FTI began to develop its code in the late 1980s, nearly every major professional association had spelled out clearly that it was unethical for a therapist to have sexual contact with a client. This unambiguous definition of intratherapeutic sexual contact as unethical had not existed before then, although most codes had warned against dual relationships of which sexual contact was the most obvious sort (see Chapter 2 for a discussion of the development of the American Psychological Association [2017]

Ethical Principles of Psychologists and Code of Conduct and the state statutes regarding sexual contact between mental health and other professionals and their clients).

The FTI code (FTI, 1990) took on the issues of the egalitarian relationship that had been used by sexually offending therapists to justify their actions. It, too, made it unmistakable and clear that sexual contact between therapist and client was a violation and a form of abuse, entirely inconsistent with the values, norms, and practice of feminist therapy. Moreover, it supported the important notion that as much as an egalitarian relationship was aspired to in feminist psychotherapy, the reality was that a power differential did exist between the parties, evident in the fiduciary responsibilities and legalities inherent in the therapeutic role. In the code and in the two books of commentary that accompanied it, FTI discussed the ethics of egalitarian relationships, role overlap, and the use of self-disclosure. This was important because for some therapists, these forms of egalitarian relating had apparently resulted in "slippery slope" issues, that is, issues that increased vulnerability to ever more serious boundary violations. If the frame of therapy required strict abstinence, then these strategies for egalitarian relationships were a violation of the frame. Sexual contact was, in that way of thinking, simply another step in throwing aside the piece of an already broken frame.

In response, the FTI Code of Ethics created a well-defined frame for egalitarian feminist practices, such as self-disclosure and role overlap, while clearly spelling out that sexual contact either during or after the ending of therapy was a violation not only of general therapeutic ethics but specifically of the ethics of feminist practice. This created a clear-cut ethical holding environment for feminist practice that had not previously existed. By 1990, there was a feminist frame for best practice that was grounded in this ethics code; that frame, in turn, became the seed from which feminist therapy theory developed (Brown, 1994, 2018).

Even though few feminist therapists were members of the organization that wrote that code, the code itself was broadly disseminated through the publications of FTI, at the national conferences of the Association for Women in Psychology (AWP) and at many local feminist therapy workshops and organizations. For example, in Los Angeles, a group of feminist therapists who had been dealing with their own charismatic therapist–leader–teacher committing sexual misconduct organized a conference and developed consensual local standards that, like the FTI code, banned sexual contact while supporting a feminist frame of role overlap and self-disclosure as long as these were in the client's best interest. It was acknowledged that personal overdisclosure on the part of the therapist could become a hindrance rather than a benefit to the treatment and even create a role reversal between the parties. Moreover, indiscriminate self-disclosure could lead to any number of problematic and nontherapeutic responses in the client and, once made, could not be taken back. The FTI code became a consensus standard of practice among self-identified feminist therapists because it so effectively stopped the abuse of feminist therapeutic principles in the service of therapeutic sexual abuse while empowering feminist therapists to understand more deeply how to enact principles of egalitarian relationship.

In the ensuing 3 decades, there had been no more such large-scale cases of SBV in the feminist therapy community (although one was recently disclosed to the second author by a distraught friend who was the supervisor and mentor of an unethical therapist–leader of a feminist organization who reportedly had had several sexual relationships with her clients and with supervisees). The friend was dealing with her personal reactions of disbelief, outrage, disgust, sadness, and personal betrayal—what Courtois (2017) identified as colleague betrayal (see also Chapter 17). To the authors' knowledge, there have been fewer individual cases of sexual abuse by self-identified feminist therapists, although it should be noted that the prevalence of female abusers of both female and male clients has risen over these past decades as more women have become psychotherapists. This points to the role of the abuse of power—and to personal and professional vulnerability to succumbing to it over the course of a treatment. This is illustrated by the following case example:

> Chloe survived an extremely brutal childhood. She was repeatedly physically and sexually abused by her sadistic father and brother and routinely emotionally abused and treated as less-than by her family due to her gender and appearing to be a tomboy. Her mother opted not to notice and "not know" and did not intervene or protect her. Her brother modeled his behavior on their father's and continued his attacks into adulthood. Chloe reacted by becoming defiant and oppositional, and from age 10, she would fight her tormentors and violently attack others, even when she would get injured in the process and would receive punishment from her parents. She refused to back down and was considered a delinquent from her teen years and into adulthood. She joined a notorious motorcycle gang, where she was considered "one of the boys." She became heavily tattooed, drank to excess and used street and prescription drugs, engaged in frequent self-injury, and was often suicidal. She identified as a lesbian and would routinely get into physical fights with partners because that was how she knew to engage with others, but that behavior ended up costing her relationships that she valued.
>
> Chloe finally sought treatment with a cisgender feminist therapist who was well known in her South American country and saw her for several years. They had many ups and downs in the treatment based on Chloe's mistrust and the

severity of her behavioral issues, but ultimately Chloe felt that the therapist had truly helped her to the point of saving her life. Her knee-jerk violence diminished, she learned to avoid her brother and distance herself from other family members, she developed life goals, and she was much more able to engage productively with others. She began a relationship with an American woman, which prompted her decision to emigrate to the United States to be with her.

After her therapy ended, she reports that her therapist shocked her by telling her she *expected* them to have a sexual relationship going forward. The therapist disclosed an ongoing intense attraction to Chloe and justified her solicitation of sex because the treatment was now ended. She was seeking to "learn about how to do lesbian sex." Additionally, she felt that Chloe "owed her" because of how hard she had worked on her behalf over many years and because she had provided her treatment on a sliding scale. Chloe angrily refused and years later, she is still shocked, angered, and saddened by the actions of her formerly admired and idealized therapist. She is also contemptuous of her therapist's ongoing status as a feminist therapy leader in her country and sees her as a major hypocrite who used her status to prey on her and possibly on other clients. Chloe continues to consider whether she should report her therapist for her misbehavior or take other action against her. Her partner, now her wife, strongly counsels against it as she feels it will be too upsetting to Chloe and will disrupt their stable family life.

A MORE SOPHISTICATED UNDERSTANDING OF ABUSES OF POWER

Feminist therapists began to discuss other ways in which power could be abused in therapy and have become more sophisticated and complex in their thinking about how to create egalitarian relationships between the parties. The naive notion that was present in the very early days of feminist therapy that therapist and client were equal in power was set aside in favor of a more nuanced appreciation of how the unconscious and manifest dynamics of power affected client choice and consent, not only in the realm of sexuality. Because of the clarity with which the FTI code associated SBVs with violations of feminist ethics, and because of the specificity with which other kinds of boundary and role overlap and crossing were described and allowed, the FTI code appears to have served as a highly effective corrective against sexual misconduct within the community of those identifying with feminist practice.

What feminist therapy does, by identifying power imbalances as inherent in the therapeutic relationship, is draw attention to the ways in which a therapist can exploit or abuse those imbalances that have nothing to do with sex. This, in turn, invites feminist therapists to focus their thinking on the subtle manners in which their power manifests itself in relationship to clients. As the first author has discussed (Brown, 1994, 2016, 2018), abuse and exploitation of power in therapy does not begin nor end with sexual violations. Instead, power can be taken in problematic ways, starting with the process of diagnosis and labeling of the client (Ballou & Brown, 2002). It is taken in the very structure of therapy (where and when therapy takes place, no matter how inconvenient for clients; when and how therapy ends; how available—or not—a therapist chooses to be); all of these are not inherently problematic, nor are they violations. Yet they are ways in which power is asserted by a therapist; thus, they are all ways in which feminist therapists attempt to think through the taken-for-granted assumptions about how the therapeutic relationship will be arranged.

These are all in addition to a more fine-tuned understanding of the power inherent in the treatment relationship itself and how that power can be used by naive, unscrupulous, and predatory therapists to further their own needs, whatever they may be. Clients, due to their dependence on the treatment relationship and possibly their idealization of the therapist, may all too easily come under the influence of a needy and unethical therapist who would seduce or otherwise use them. Clients who have a previous history of childhood abuse, trauma, and polyvictimization are especially susceptible. The grooming process through which therapist abusers engage and confuse their clients is becoming ever more evident based on study of the dynamics involved as reported primarily by clients, but also by some of the therapists themselves, and by the study of these dynamics. In 2017, an entire issue of the *Journal of Trauma & Dissociation*, edited by Warwick Middleton, Adah Sachs, and Martin Dorahy, was devoted to the topic of victim–perpetrator dynamics in all sorts of abuse. (See Chapters 14 and 15 for descriptions of the grooming process.)

Additionally, the psychotherapy field has undergone major changes over the past few decades based on scientific findings from developmental psychology and the neurosciences and from research examining psychotherapy process and outcome. New theoretical and treatment models have developed—especially in the treatment of trauma—many of which place more emphasis on somatic and experiential approaches and relational strategies that attend to attachment and developmental/neurobiological issues. Therapists have moved away from the role of authority figure who *does to* the client through interpretation or manualized cognitive-behavioral strategies (referred to as a one-person psychology) to one who is, in fact, more equal as a coinvestigator *with* the client of the client's inner world of reactions and experience (in a two-person psychology). This shift is based on the stance espoused early on by the relational feminists mentioned earlier and the research findings regarding the significance of various relational elements, such as reflection and response, attunement, prosody, and mirroring on the part of the therapist to the successful outcome of treatment. Moreover, this relational shift has the effect of lessening the power disparities between parties while not erasing the therapist role or responsibilities.

SUMMARY

SBVs became a problem for feminist therapy because, initially, the field and its practitioners made overly simplistic assumptions about what constituted abuse and power dynamics. It was mistakenly seen as the sole purview of men to abuse; women were the targets of abuse, not its perpetrators. This has changed. Women are no longer idealized and valorized, as a group, as being beyond the capacity to abuse power. Just as feminist therapists now know that women can be abusive to women in intimate partner relationships; that women can perpetrate sexual abuse and harassment on other women, men, and nonbinary individuals; that women can behave in the larger political arena in ways that are oppressive and even violations of basic human rights, so feminist therapists know that a therapist who is a woman and who identifies herself as a feminist can abuse power and sexually violate a client. Although FTI is now defunct as an organization, it made major contributions to the field of feminist theory and treatment by developing a stringent code of ethics, followed by two explanatory casebooks.

REFERENCES

American Psychological Association. (2017). *Ethical principles of psychologists and code of conduct* (2002, amended effective June 1, 2010, and January 1, 2017). https://www.apa.org/ethics/code/index.aspx

Ballou, M., & Brown, L. S. (Eds.). (2002). *Rethinking mental health and disorder: Feminist perspectives*. Guilford Press.

Brown, L. S. (1994). *Subversive dialogues: Theory in feminist therapy*. Basic Books.

Brown, L. S. (2016). *Essentials of the feminist psychotherapy model of psychotherapy supervision*. American Psychological Association.

Brown, L. S. (2018). *Feminist therapy* (2nd ed.). American Psychological Association.

Brown, L. S. (2020). Institutional cowardice: A powerful, often invisible manifestation of institutional betrayal. *Journal of Trauma & Dissociation*. https://doi.org/10.1080/15299732.2020.1801307

Chesler, P. (1972). *Women and madness*. Doubleday.

Courtois, C. A. (2017). Colleague betrayal: Countertrauma manifestation? In R. B. Gartner (Ed.), *Trauma and countertrauma, resilience and counterresilience: Insight from psychoanalysts and trauma experts* (pp. 251–281). Routledge, Taylor & Francis Group.

Feminist Therapy Institute. (1990). *Feminist Therapy Institute Code of Ethics.*

Freyd, J. J. (1997). Violations of power, adaptive blindness, and betrayal trauma theory. *Feminism & Psychology, 7*(1), 22–32. https://doi.org/10.1177/0959353597071004

Gelinas, D. J. (1983). The persisting negative effects of incest. *Psychiatry, 46,* 312–332. https://doi.org/10.1080/00332747.1983.11024207

Gilligan, C. (1982). *In a different voice.* Harvard University Press.

Jordan, J. V., Kaplan, A. C., Miller, J. B., Stiver, I. P., & Surrey, J. I. (1991). *Women's growth in connection: Writings from the Stone Center.* Guilford Press.

Kravetz, D. (1978). Consciousness-raising groups in the 1970s. *Psychology of Women Quarterly, 3*(2), 168–186. https://doi.org/10.1111/j.1471-6402.1978.tb00532.x

Norcross, J. C., & Lambert, M. J. (2018). Psychotherapy relationships that work III. *Psychotherapy, 55*(4), 303–315. https://doi.org/10.1037/pst0000193

Shaw, D. (2014). *Traumatic narcissism: Relational systems of subjugation.* Routledge, Taylor & Francis Group.

PART **III** UNIQUE
SETTINGS AND
POPULATIONS

10 SEXUAL BOUNDARY VIOLATIONS IN PASTORAL COUNSELING

CHRISTINE A. COURTOIS AND ARLENE (LU) STEINBERG

As noted throughout this book, sexual boundary violations (SBVs) of adults can occur in helping and training contexts outside of psychotherapy. In this chapter, we discuss abuse by members of the clergy in their roles as providers of spiritual care and pastoral counseling to adult congregants/clients. We discuss both common factors and unique issues found across religious communities, as well as the vulnerabilities of clergy, congregants, and adherents that may lead to sexual and other boundary violations. We also address the aftereffects on all parties, including family members of the victims, others in the church, synagogue, temple, meeting house, or ashram community; the broader organization and community; and the religion itself. Finally, we look at ways to identify the problem and its scope, with attention to various efforts that are underway to prevent further occurrences and to provide assistance to all who are affected. The common goal of numerous organizational efforts is to ensure the safety of all congregants and adherents from inappropriate coercion and incursions into forbidden sex. We address boundary violations when priests, ministers, rabbis, imans, elders, and other spiritual teachers or agents serve in formal or informal counseling roles. Although

https://doi.org/10.1037/0000247-010
Sexual Boundary Violations in Psychotherapy: Facing Therapist Indiscretions, Transgressions, and Misconduct, A. Steinberg, J. L. Alpert, and C. A. Courtois (Editors)
Copyright © 2021 by the American Psychological Association. All rights reserved.

we focus mainly on Roman Catholicism, various Protestant and Christian denominations, as well as Judaism, which are the religious traditions we were raised in and, therefore, are most informed about, we alert the reader that boundary violations can and do occur in all religious organizations, congregations, sects, and communities. No religion is immune.

To date, the type of abuse perpetrated by members of the clergy that has received the most attention and publicity involves children and adolescents, while the abuse of adults has remained obscured. Despite this, clergy abuse of adults—although mainly between male clergy and female congregant/ clients, there are incidents of same-sex abuse by men and abuse by female clergy of both male and female congregants—has been frequently reported. At least one credible source has reported that the prevalence of clergy sexual abuse of adult congregants is greater than abuse of adults by other psychotherapists (Cooper-White, 1991), and that it occurs at much higher rates than clergy sexual abuse of children (https://www.adultsabusedbyclergy.org).

A preliminary study of adult survivors of abuse by Roman Catholic clergy who volunteered to respond to a survey (making it a nonrandom and noncontrolled study) yielded surprising results. If these results hold up in more scientifically sound studies, they open another window into the dimensions of clergy abuse. According to the survey, 51% of survivor respondents were female; 40% of clergy predators were not on any diocese "list"; 90% of the survivors were abused by priests, brothers, and/or nuns; and approximately 10% were abused by lay (nonclergy) employees and volunteers. Finally, the survey indicated that women do not come forward due to victim blaming, perpetuation of "rape myths" by clergy, disenfranchisement in the legal system, lack of female attorneys representing victims, and a belief that many attorneys only represent male victims (Casteix, 2020). Although a number of these survivors were abused in childhood, some of them were abused as adults.

When sexual misconduct has come to light, it has usually been blamed on the neediness, seductiveness, or disturbance of the (often, but not always) female congregant/client and not on the clergy member, who is typically not judged by the same standard due to his stature, and who is frequently exonerated (or may be forgiven through the sacrament of confession). The abuse is most often labeled as an affair that the *female client (rather than the male clergy)* "should have known better than to engage in" rather than seen as the clergy member's violation of a sacred and fiduciary duty. In addition, although the civil law recognizes clergy abuse regarding children, it is less clear or specific when recognizing parallel violations of duty to adults in the care of clergy. This is a lacuna that may allow predator clergy to go undetected and their behavior to go uncurbed (Tobin & Helge, 2013), providing serial perpetrators with the occasion to abuse again.

Clergy have a high degree of influence in the lives of their congregants and adherents, who trust them as valued, and often unquestioned, sources of spiritual and secular guidance. As Matthews (2012) stated regarding Christian clergy: "Persons not only tend to put their trust in their pastor as a loving and trusted father figure, they often come for help from the pastor when they are in emotional need and vulnerability" (p. 17). In all faiths and religious traditions, clergy are frequently the first point of contact for those seeking help for a variety of life circumstances. In addition to spiritual guidance and other faith-related and existential issues, these can include marital and child-rearing stresses and distress, other relationship or family issues, medical and mental health problems, and career and financial woes. In fact, it has been estimated that approximately 40% of individuals in distress initially seek help from clergy rather than from other professionals (Bisbing et al., 1995). This puts them in the position of providing guidance or counseling as part of their pastoral role. One study reported that clergy spend between 25% and 60% of their time in counseling-type relationships (Bisbing et al., 1995).

TERMINOLOGY: CLERGY SEXUAL ABUSE OF ADULTS

In the executive summary of the Baylor University School of Social Work, Clergy Sexual Misconduct Study, the following definition of *clergy sexual misconduct* was offered: "Ministers, priests, rabbis, or other clergypersons or religious leaders who make sexual advances or propositions to persons in the congregations they serve who are not their spouses or significant others" (Garland, 2009, para. 3; see also Chaves & Garland, 2009). Concerning the *abuse of power* involved, the study authors wrote the following:

> Religious leaders are, by definition, community leaders who carry spiritual as well as organization and community leadership roles. They are expected to be compassionate, ethical, and moral leaders. The differential of power between religious leader and a congregant is like that of a physician and patient or counselor and client, although with the added dimension of their responsibility being a sacred trust. Because of the power the leader holds and the attachment of congregants to them, the congregant has much less power to say "no" to sexual overtures, rendering the concept of "consent" virtually meaningless. Any sexual relationship between a religious leader and a congregant is thus more accurately described as "abuse of power" rather than "affair," which implies mutual consent. (Chaves & Garland, 2009)

Clergy leaders who identify as pastoral counselors can come from a variety of training backgrounds. There are traditional religious and spiritual leaders, who utilize prayer and religious ritual in counseling congregants on spiritual and/or secular issues; modern pastoral counselors, whose traditional leadership roles include counseling methods that integrate religious and secular approaches and may or may not have formal training in counseling (typically not, but this may be changing in some clergy training); and finally clergy who have more formal secular counseling training (including an organized course of study, supervised practice, certification, and degrees) and may apply both religious and secular methods to their work. Some in this latter group may obtain licensure as psychologists, psychiatrists, or other mental health practitioners; serve as faculty in professional training programs; or teach and/or practice in other settings apart from their congregations. There are also teachers and gurus who function as clergy within Eastern or less traditional Western groups, and who may be perceived as spiritual leaders from whom adherents/counselees seek enlightenment.

The overlap between communal leadership responsibilities and individual counseling or spiritual guidance can present inherent role conflicts and easily lead to the formation of dual relationships, particularly as the boundaries between the two may lack definition and, therefore, be quite diffuse. A situation comes to mind of a rabbi asking loudly from the communal setting of a synagogue's steps regarding a confidential matter that a congregant had divulged in a more private setting, which caused embarrassment to the congregant. Although it was not a sexual transgression, a serious lack of discretion and confidentiality occurred. For reasons related to the risk of these kinds of situations leading to the development of dual relationships, some religions and congregations consider it inadvisable for clergy to provide individual counseling to their own congregants and instead are encouraged to refer them to others.

Sexual abuse by clergy is now recognized as an abuse of power that constitutes a crime in many jurisdictions. It is so highly egregious that clergy SBVs have been referred to as "soul stealing" (Cooper-White, 1991) and betrayal of the deity (Schoen, 2013), and the perpetrator referred to as a "slayer of the soul" (Rossetti, 1990) and "wolf in shepherd's clothing" (Garland, 2009; see also Chaves & Garland, 2009) to account for the additional role transgressions and major moral/spiritual dereliction of duty involved. Marie Fortune (1989), an early researcher in this area, wrote a book she famously titled "Is Nothing Sacred?"

Although many similar factors leading to SBVs have been found in clergy members as those found in other professionals, clergy have unique vulnerabilities in their roles, and common risk factors have been identified beyond those identified for secular psychotherapists. For example, in different religions, clergy may be viewed as divine representatives; conduits of divine power; chosen and anointed ones; as interpreters of scripture, religious arbiters, and moral leaders; or as elders who possess specialized knowledge or historical tradition with each designation giving them special influence, discretion, power, and even reverence. In addition, God is frequently viewed as male in many monotheistic religions structured around patriarchal traditions and gender roles, and most male clergy are being afforded many gender-based prerogatives. Moreover, female congregants are frequently encouraged into conservative roles of compliant wives/mothers and caretakers of others, as well as other roles that require them to be deferential to male authority figures, including their husbands, fathers, and members of the clergy. These designations afford male clergy enormous power and influence that can be used to pressure, compel, and rationalize sexual contact and forbidden sex, especially with the most vulnerable. This is discussed in more detail in this chapter.

Yet, because members of the clergy are human, they themselves are susceptible to human needs, frailties, pressures, temptations, opportunities/situations, and to their own characterological issues and deficits. Their role requires them to provide extensive spiritual, religious, and administrative guidance to their adherents, as well as to counsel individuals on an as-needed basis, usually without much, if any, specialized training in counseling and mental health issues outside of the standard clerical preparation. Not infrequently, they are overworked and underpaid for their services. They often function rather independently and sometimes in isolated and isolating circumstances, without ongoing supervision or interaction with peers. Furthermore, many entered seminary or other religious preparation and training during adolescence, a maturational epoch when personal identity (including sexual identity and functioning), self-worth, peer and social relationships, and skills are shaped. Certain rigid or repressive religious belief systems and teachings may place limits on such self-exploration and self-definition as it may potentially lead to "free thinking" and away from religious dogma, teachings, and values.

Additionally, clergy training may have occurred without exploration of the trainee's reasons or personal discernment for choosing a clerical and spiritual path or without exploration of temperament, personal beliefs, needs, personality deficits, and psychopathology—including an exploration of the trainee's relational and intimacy history, sexual history including sexual functioning, sexual difficulties, and questions about sexual and gender identity and orientation. In fact, some individuals may even seek to become clergy to distance themselves from sexuality, as when a previous history of unacknowledged or unresolved sexual trauma (sometimes at the hands of clergy when candidates were in childhood or adolescence) had taken place. Some with this background may be seeking a way to be purified as well as manage ongoing shame brought on by the previous abuse. And, it is an unfortunate observation that some abused individuals have identified with their perpetrator, becoming abusers themselves, usually in an attempt at mastery or reenactment of their own abuse (Middleton et al., 2017). Additionally, some individuals may become clergy to meet the expectations and needs of others, especially parents or other relatives who may encourage a religious vocation as a means of bringing special respect and pride to the family or as an intergenerational legacy and expectation. It also may be a way of gaining approval and standing within the nuclear and extended family, which for some may add to the pressure of their position and may lead to later acting out of unacknowledged or unexpressed feelings.

Finally, as detailed in an article with the provocative title of "Why Predators are Attracted to Careers in the Clergy," there are some who may even enter religious organizations due to their desire for power, status, and authority over others, enticed by the availability and accessibility of victims who are usually individuals in distress or need, coupled with the protection accorded by relatively lax organizational standards and responses when sexual misconduct is suspected, observed, or disclosed/reported (Navarro, 2014). Navarro noted that, unlike in many other service professions, he was able to find no religion or sect that screened for signs of psychopathy in its clergy.

Some religions require clergy to take vows of celibacy, to abstain from intimate relationships, and to be chaste and modest in interactions. Others may encourage traditional heterosexual marriage, emphasizing large families with multiple children starting soon after marriage, often when the couple is still quite young. Children are raised to adhere to a traditional heterosexual viewpoint, with circumscribed roles for males and females.

Homosexuality in clergy and in congregants is not accepted in most religions, and, even when it is, it remains controversial. This issue of homosexual clergy is so divisive in some religions that it has led to recent schisms in the Anglican/Episcopal Church and the United Methodist Church between supporters and dissidents, some of whom have gone on to found splinter groups or congregations with others who hold similar beliefs. Despite the general nonacceptance of homosexuality among clergy, there are indications that a high percentage of Roman Catholic clergy may be homosexual, frequently hiding their orientation and presenting themselves as heterosexual. This high percentage has facilitated the misattribution of the sexual abuse of boys as due to homosexuality, rather than as due to pedophilia, a major way the Roman Catholic hierarchy has sought to defend the church and its reputation. Homosexual clergy may be found in other Christian denominations and among other faiths as well, often hidden within heterosexual marriages. In some cases, these clergy lead a bisexual lifestyle that is kept secret from their spouses. In some especially tragic and shocking situations, wives may only find out that their husbands have been leading a bisexual lifestyle, when they are diagnosed with a sexually transmitted disease or HIV/AIDS as a result of their husbands' extramarital same-sex activities.

Regarding cultural or ethnic religious groups, none is immune. Matthews (2012) conducted a study of the sexual abuse of power in African American Christian churches that documented an extensive history of sexual contact between pastors and congregants in some churches. He believes that traditional heterosexual beliefs and power dynamics underlie much of this misconduct (as do characterological issues in some pastors and a passive bystander mentality among congregants when abuse is disclosed or reported). He has been active in urging African American churches to address these issues and to enact change. There have been similar reports in Filipino and other Asian churches, as well as among other religious groups, particularly where clergy are held in the highest esteem and are believed to be unable to do wrong. Stories such as these abound in all religions and denominations—none are spared.

CHARACTERISTICS OF CLERGY SEXUAL ABUSE OF ADULTS

A cursory review of the literature on clergy sexual misconduct and the ever-increasing media reports (many related to "#MeToo" disclosures) across multiple faiths, denominations, and sects yields a wealth of information. We have easily found information on clergy abuse of congregants/clients in the following religions, denominations, and sects including: American or Western Buddhism; Asian Buddhism; Amish; The Family International; Greek Orthodox; Roman Catholic; Hindu; Jewish (all denominations); Muslim; Pagan; and Protestant Christian denominations (including Adventist, Anglican/Episcopal, Baptist, Church of Christ, Church of the Nazarene, Lutheran, Methodist, Mennonite, Mormon, Pentecostal, Presbyterian, Seventh Day Adventist, Southern Baptist, and United Church of Christ). No doubt, there are many others that we have missed or that have not yet become public. For example, as noted previously, abuse by charismatic leaders who are clergy or have clergylike roles are also reported in less traditional but spiritually-affiliated or -based traditions and settings (e.g., meditation and yoga groups and in leader-based cults and sects, including psychotherapy cults).

Violations take place in a variety of different settings and locations, including the church, mosque, synagogue, meeting place, temple, ashram, and other place of worship where clergy work or in religiously-affiliated or freestanding pastoral counseling offices, private residences, on campuses, in training programs, hospitals, and military and other settings where clergy members serve as chaplains. They can also take place in the client's home, in a clergy or community-owned beach house, retreat house, wilderness cabin, or camp setting, or in a more neutral location like a hotel. Clergy abuse of adults also occurs in countries around the globe or, as noted on one website, occurs as "boundary violations without borders." A more accurate picture regarding the scope and prevalence, quantitative research about cases, dynamics, locations, specific religions, and religious contexts has been lacking and is needed (Shupe et al., 2000).

To date, the Roman Catholic Church has received the most media attention and approbation for child sexual abuse committed by its priests and others in church-affiliated roles, as well as for its systematic cover-up by the church hierarchy. More recently, abuse of teenage or young adult seminarians by their teachers and mentors, including some of the highest level Church leaders, as well as the related cover-ups, have created the latest scandal leading to resignations of bishops and cardinals, including the first defrocking of a cardinal—Theodore McCarrick, of Washington, DC, who reportedly abused multiple seminarians and young priests under his authority in vacation settings, abbeys and seminaries, and in diocesan offices. As part of these revelations, sexual perpetration both of children and of adult men and women by men and women in religious orders has come to light. In fact, there even have been cases of sexually abused congregant/counselees and nuns who became pregnant and bore children. Most often, these children are left in a netherland existence, shrouded in shame, their paternity denied or hidden from them. In some cases of admitted paternity, their priest/father may help care for them or shun them or alternate between the two. The Church, when made aware of these situations, has rarely offered more than limited or subsistence financial support, leaving the mother/victim on her own to raise and provide for the child.

Many justifications are offered by perpetrators in defense of their transgressions. As an example, in a notorious case in California, a self-described Christian therapist working in a New Life Treatment Center said he was following "higher laws" than those of the state when he developed a sexual relationship with and impregnated a former client 40 years his junior (Marquis, 1994). Accordingly, he showed a total lack of remorse.

Contributing to the problem, it is often the case that when abuse suspicions are raised or problematic interactions revealed, many congregants, clergy, and even family members have been passive bystanders who do not attempt to intervene or offer assistance. Some actively blame, shun, and otherwise mistreat the victim, while at the same time exonerating the abuser and, in the process, enabling the behavior. The clergy member is likely a powerful and influential individual who is feared, revered, or both. Recent media reports of such behaviors have included extensive cover-ups in many faith communities which are geared exclusively to protecting the accused and maligning the accuser.

CLERGY-CONGREGANT/CLIENT VULNERABILITY FACTORS ACROSS RELIGIONS

Although clergy share many of the vulnerabilities with other professionals who provide mental health counseling or psychotherapy, elements of the clergy–congregant relationship may exacerbate them and create additional risk. These elements include the congregant's blind trust, veneration, or idealization of the clergy member's position and authority as a spiritual leader, and a transferencelike phenomenon that creates and reinforces an especially strong power imbalance. As noted above, the imbalance is exacerbated by the clergy member being perceived either as having a unique divine connection, as found in several Christian theological settings, or as a prestigious scholar and interpreter of Jewish philosophy, text, and law in Jewish community settings. Similar dynamics occur in other religions and religious contexts. In addition, awareness of the possibility for and risk of dual relationships—where the clergy is also spiritual advisor, pastoral counselor, administrator, CEO, friend, and even employer—is crucial, as it can become exploitative, leading to an atmosphere of emotional and sexual harassment and to other coerced sexual contacts by the clergy and other affiliated individuals. Clergy must be ever mindful of this potential as part of their "coat of armor," as discussed in Chapter 3.

It is solely the clergy member's ethical and moral responsibility to avoid conflicted roles and maintain boundaries that create safety from sexual misconduct for all congregants, especially for the congregant/clients they counsel.

Many religious communities are vulnerable because of their insularity or isolation from a larger community. When suspicions are aroused or abusive behavior is observed or reported, the institutional response is typically one of denial and disbelief, driven by leaders and congregants wishing not to bring shame on their leader or community by identifying or stirring up a scandal. This extends to avoidance in confronting the alleged violator, and thereby, in the process, colluding with him. When the issue is brought up for discussion or investigation, violators typically lie as to its occurrence and otherwise dissimulate and deny. If they do admit to their transgression, then they may minimize, identify it as an aberration, and vow never to repeat it. With no formal or informal education or policies about the significance of professional boundary maintenance or a system in place to foster best-practice intervention in cases of reported sexual exploitation, religious leaders and hierarchies may be hard-pressed to respond in a standardized and appropriate way. Patterns of denial/disbelief and a resulting reluctance to question the clergy's authority or to report the abuse outside of the community are often the norm. The unfortunate result is twofold: (a) it can leave the victim without recourse and to fend for themself in conditions that are generally accusatory, nonsupportive, and shaming; and (b) it conveys to the abuser that the behavior will not be questioned or challenged, leaving them to continue sexually abusive behavior with impunity and without fear of negative repercussions.

The job of clergy is a special calling that is enormously satisfying and fulfilling for many; however, as noted above, it may be highly stressful, with many responsibilities and pulls on the individual for spiritual, religious, and administrative/organizational leadership, as well as congregant guidance, advice, and other services. Among other things, these involve ongoing exposure to the vulnerable and needy in the congregation, sometimes including immersion in their private lives and access to their home, and given the communal nature of their position, little separation between the clergy's own private life and that of their congregants.

Clergy members can find themselves stretched very thin by the sheer number of responsibilities, in terms of their own spouse and family and their professional obligations. Some gain stature over the course of their careers, not infrequently at the expense of their marriages and families, a situation exacerbated by the lack of demarcation between their communal and home-lives. In some cases, homelife may seem like an additional burden rather than a source of support and reprieve. The ongoing stresses, lack of personal and professional support, lack of adequate opportunities for rest and respite and, at times, alienation from spouses (who may be experienced as unhappy, demanding, unappreciative, and unsupportive) may have become a part of a mutual alienation.

Spouses may feel responsible for maintaining their husband's reputation and remain silent, perhaps feeling trapped and fearing being disbelieved if they suspect or report their husband's unethical behavior or seek help. Problems of this sort can lead to cynicism, despair, and burnout in both spouses as they struggle with the toll of infidelity and the hypocrisy involved in keeping up a good front and maintaining secrecy. What's more, in such circumstances, when clergy have characterological, personal/psychosexual, and professional issues (including spiritual crises) to contend with, there are far too few mechanisms in place to which they can turn for personal ventilation, support, supervision, and consultation. Circumstances such as these can make a highly appreciative congregant/counselee a major source of gratification (and temptation) for a depleted, cynical, and/or alienated clergy member and spouse. Such scenarios present fertile ground and great risk for SBVs, as clergy may be more susceptible to seek outside sources of relief or support, which then may lead to more intimate personal and ultimately sexual encounters and relationships.

Because clergy are unlikely to have received education in human development, mental health, or individual or couple counseling in their clerical training, it is unlikely that issues of intimacy, sexuality, and sexual functioning have been discussed. This results in clergy being ill-equipped to address these issues, except from a religious perspective. Many religions are quite conservative or even repressive regarding issues of sexuality, with sex considered primarily a means of reproduction occurring within traditional male–female marriage, rather than enjoyed for its own sake. Such viewpoints and spiritual directives may discourage any discussion of sex or sexual difficulties. As a result, clergy may be singularly unprepared for a sexually tempting situation to develop and not know how to handle it in an appropriately healthy way for both parties. Additionally, if a clergy member is experiencing difficulties regarding personal sexual functioning, satisfaction, or sexual orientation/identity, they may be more at risk, as there are few places to go to safely and confidentially address them. In such a void, clergy may experiment with and act out their sexual concerns and desires instead of managing them.

TYPES OF CLERGY SEXUAL BOUNDARY VIOLATIONS

As discussed throughout this volume, the range of motivations and behaviors involved in adult sexual abuse is widely diverse and spans a continuum. It ranges from the situational or more spontaneous and unplanned circumstance at one end of the continuum to the premeditated, highly planned coercion and assault at the other, with many variations in between. Sexual contact might be disguised as treatment, training, or what has been identified as "sexual fraud" in some jurisdictions. It can also involve religious behaviors, rituals, and traditions. This is illustrated by the case of a nationally esteemed and influential rabbi in Washington, DC, who utilized the traditional Mikvah bath, a sacred ritual in a sacred space, to surreptitiously photograph unclothed women students/congregants. This went on for many years before he was apprehended due to a camera discovered in the Mikvah and pictures of the victims on his personal computer. Many of the victims expressed feelings of shame, humiliation, and mortification, as well as enormous betrayal, by this esteemed religious leader (Boorstein & Bahrampour, 2018). After the fact, many victims reported having experienced grooming as part of their religious studies with the clergy member, during which he strongly encouraged them to engage in the Mikvah tradition. As another example, in a number of reported Roman Catholic cases, the sacrament of confession and the confessional have been used as both an excuse for and a location for sexual misconduct. Other items and rituals considered sacred have also reportedly been used in abuse, further mortifying or intimidating/subjugating the congregant/victim or as a means of maintaining silence and secrecy. Victims have even been told that no one would believe them, especially if their report involves abuse that is so aberrant and desecrating.

The progression of behaviors, including outright grooming, resembles the typical pathway of sexual misconduct in psychotherapy discussed throughout this volume, especially in Chapters 14 and 15; however, additional issues compound clergy abuse. As the relationship progresses and the congregant/client becomes increasingly emotionally responsive and dependent, the relationship becomes mutually dependent and emotionally entangled. As with other forms of SBVs in psychotherapy, this may lead to increasing self-disclosure of personal circumstances and needs by the pastoral counselor and ultimately lead to longer, more frequent sessions with ever more intimate discussions and disclosures. Both parties become increasingly enmeshed and dependent. It may then escalate to include ongoing obsession and compulsive contact through between-session texts, emails, phone calls, and perhaps contact outside of the counseling or the religious setting. Over time, casual physical contact increases and becomes more urgent, progressing to more intimate forms. The grooming may even include the use of religious rationalization—increasingly intimate expressions of needs and desires may be couched in religious obligations, as a blessing or a special gift from God, or have other religious connotations and justifications.

Transference and countertransference issues inevitably enter the relationship that confuse and entice both parties. Without specific training in recognizing and working with these and related dynamics more common to religious roles and settings, clergy and pastoral counselors may be prone to act them out, rather than to identify them, maintain safety and propriety, and behave within the teachings of their faith. In this, as in other types of sexual abuse, the counselee/victim is likely enjoined to secrecy. If they try to end the relationship or break away, the victim may be blamed and shamed in the interest of either denying its occurrence, rationalizing it, or to keep it going. The usual tropes found in other types of therapist abuse may be used—that is, that it was wholly the client's fault, in that they were seductive, irresistible, available, needy, responsive, an answer to a prayer, etc., etc. The client/congregant may also be threatened with losing their standing and the respect of the faith community, as well as being shunned and shut out by other members— a stinging rebuke that may not extend to the clergy abuser. A Roman Catholic case exemplifies the divided loyalties that can develop: after a disclosure of abusive sexual interactions, the congregants split in terms of who they believed (this was despite the fact that the priest's housekeeper had found the victim's earring in Father's bed, which was a fact disclosed to the congregation), with the priest's supporters fundraising for his defense when he was subjected to a civil lawsuit by the victim! She received no similar support and instead needed to relocate to another parish where she was unknown to other church members.

CHARACTERISTICS OF CLERGY MEMBERS WHO ABUSE

Mosgofian and Ohlschlager (1995) cautioned against an overly reductionistic understanding of clergy who sexually violate and of counselees who are violated, stating that "helpers who violate sexual boundaries in counseling do so for various and complex reasons" (p. 53). They distilled a broad range of violators into three primary typologies of risk that are on a continuum similar to the one mentioned above: the *vulnerable violator* (who is likely to get caught in situational forms of abuse), the *mixed violator* (who shows traits and dynamics of those at both ends of the continuum), and the *predatory violator* (whose abuse is preplanned and intentional and who may be serially predatory). Premeditated sexual contact and its justification usually involve grooming behavior of the sort found in SBVs committed by other therapists and counselors as described in Chapters 14 and 15; however, as noted, clergy perpetrators may additionally use religious beliefs, scriptures, rituals, and their status as spiritual (and often charismatic, highly sensitive, and/or powerful) authority figures to coerce, confound, and confuse the client/victim. Like those clients abused in secular forms of psychotherapy, many victims in clergy cases describe their confusion about the relationship and questioning how they became involved and entrapped. Many describe their behavior as against their values and morals and end up disgusted with themselves for their spiritual as well as personal weakness.

Clergy therapists quite frequently invoke their religious beliefs and traditions to justify their sexual transgressions to themselves and to the victim. As noted above, some may tell their client/victim that the sexual behavior is divinely sanctioned, a means of connection, purification, enlightenment, sacrifice, punishment, bringing one closer to God, or supported by scripture— anything to justify or rationalize it. Such justification further confounds the situation, creating other types of emotional and spiritual damage and betrayal trauma for the victimized client. As both parties become caught up in the seduction and become sexual, their behavior can take on an addictive and compulsive quality, involving a cycle of anticipation/need/engagement/ reward/relief (fueled by the sexual excitement and the thrill associated with being involved in a secret and taboo activity) and a counter cycle of regret/ shame/recrimination/blame (often fueled by religious injunctions, shame and guilt) that repeats itself. At times, the clergy member may be able to acknowledge and have some insight into their behavior, perhaps bemoaning the personal lack of control, and feeling guilt and remorse for their moral and religious failures. However, it is also possible that some will project blame for the failings onto the victim as discussed previously. More extreme abusive clergy, who are in the predator category, may even seek out access to victims' families as a means of blackmailing or threatening the client/victim or other family members. Brenneis (2001) reviewed the available literature describing the personality characteristics of both healthy, well-functioning clergy and their psychologically "impaired" and abusive counterparts in an attempt to identify differences between the two. The more impaired group were found to have psychiatric issues, including substance abuse, compulsive or impulsive disorders (including those that were sexual), affective disorders, and psychosexual and personality pathology. Some additionally showed issues with authority and tendencies to easily experience emotional abandonment and betrayal by others. It can be said that they had intimacy disorders. Intellectualized defenses were often used "in the service of reducing or blocking awareness of painful inner states, which included emotional and social vulnerability, sexual identity confusion and aggressive or hostile impulses" (Brenneis, 2001, p. 28). In recent years, discussions of ways to prevent clergy abuse have focused attention on the problematic character-istics that can place individual congregants and whole communities at risk (Blau, 2017a, 2017b; Dratch, 2017). Researchers further discovered that most religions (with some exceptions) do not require broad-based psycho-logical preassessment of their clergy trainees, or follow-up assessment of clergy members over the course of their careers, to determine whether they have any of the identified impairment characteristics, nor do they routinely assess the quality of their functioning in their positions or their degree of career fit and satisfaction. Although some members of the clergy are highly trained and undergo a period of apprenticeship that helps them to become habituated to their role and position, others have had little or no formal training, "learning by doing," a less than ideal way of learning such a complicated and responsible role.

In addition to being a proponent of the religion in question who can represent its tenets and beliefs, the major requirement for the clergy in some religious traditions seems to be that he (and less often she) have a charismatic personality that is highly appealing to others. This allows the clergy member to be able to influence and lead followers/congregants as a respected authority figure and moral leader. If their personality is in the narcissistic range, there may additionally be mutual satisfaction derived by both parties, because such attention may satisfy their craving for attention and approval. In some communities, the clergy member's success as a fund-raiser is also valued, a situation that in some more extreme circumstances can become a slippery slope to corruption, fraud, and scandals.

CONGREGANT/SEEKER/COUNSELEE CHARACTERISTICS

Other researchers have commented on the characteristics of the congregant/client that may contribute to greater susceptibility to both spiritual and sex-ual abuse. As noted earlier, most adult victims are female and transgressors male, but the inverse also occurs (see Chapter 13 for discussion of SBVs in same-sex and LGBTQ+ dyads). Also as noted previously, gender-based expectations for women congregants requiring deference and obedience to male authority figures is one contributory factor, especially given that the clergy member may be endowed with divine attributes or seen as important, perhaps even exclusive purveyors of enlightenment. This bestows on them an even more powerful status. As part of gender norms and conditioning, many female congregants have been trained as caregivers in their mostly patriarchal families—respectful and deferential to all in authority, especially males and members of the clergy. A history of prior interpersonal trauma in childhood (especially incest and child sexual abuse), may also have accustomed them to dual and transactional relationships, making them more susceptible to boundary transgressions and exploitation. A counselee's feelings of attraction can become sexualized, leading to sexual fantasies and perhaps even contact; however, over time and with the need to keep the relationship hidden from others (including spouses and members of the congregation), other more mixed feelings, including confusion, moral/ spiritual reservations, entrapment, and despair may emerge, along with feelings of betrayal. The counselee may feel increasingly guilty when infidelity on the part of either or both parties is involved and be unable to disengage or disclose.

In some congregations, the relationship is an "open secret," known to a select few or to many. Even when it is known, there may be no attempt to question, interrupt, or otherwise intervene, which is an abandonment of both parties. It is often viewed as an affair rather than abuse, blamed on the female victim/client for having been seductive (even with evidence to the contrary), and considered a private issue to be worked out between them (and their spouses). Attempts to end the relationship by reporting it to other congregants or the leaders of the congregation or to the religious hierarchy not infrequently result in denial/disbelief/incredulity. If abuse is admitted, abusive clergy may get a proverbial slap on the wrist, maintain their position—often without other intervention, be sent for treatment, or be moved or reassigned elsewhere (usually with no record of the transgression)—later to repeat the behavior with someone else. In all religions and faiths, expectations and standards for any rehabilitation, including ongoing monitoring and supervision, are generally lacking.

DAMAGE TO VICTIMS OF CLERGY-CLIENT SEXUAL ABUSE

Just as the power dynamics between the clergy member and congregant/ client are highly asymmetrical, the effects seem to be as well. However, the prototypic client/victim generally suffers much more serious consequences than the clergy therapist. The violator may hide behind their position and deny the accusation and be assisted in this by a variety of enablers in the community, some of whom "don't see" what is evident, don't ask, or actively cover it up. If the transgression is admitted, they may place the blame squarely on the victim, a ploy that many religious authorities and congregants are all too willing to accept, because it both maintains their own innocence and denial while keeping their view of the clergy person as a revered and powerful figure. The counselee will likely be viewed as the seductive one, an adult capable of consenting to the sexual involvement, which is a stance that totally ignores the power inequality, the clergy member's power and influence, the hypocrisy and violation of the clergy's role and its responsibilities, as well as the effectiveness of the grooming process in confusing and confounding the client/victim. In this way, the grooming process can extend to the entire spiritual community.

Deficient and ineffective responses of this type on the part of other congregants and adherents (many of whom were considered friends and spiritual allies of either or both parties) are usually described by victims as worse than the sexual behavior itself. The congregant victim is thus additionally betrayed by this gross misunderstanding of the dynamics of abuse, which further isolates, shames, and humiliates. Moreover, the victim may not only lose reputation and standing in the congregation, but could lose their marriage and family (including custody of the children) as well as their religious communal life and faith. This and many other emotional and psychosocial aftereffects (which are detailed in other chapters of this volume) experienced by clergy abuse victims can be compounded by damage to spirituality and religious beliefs. The pain and trauma caused by abuse at the hands of a religious figure can overtake the victim, causing them to withdraw into shamed self-protective isolation, in the process destroying what were once integral aspects of their life and identity. They may also become depressed, highly anxious, and even self-harming and suicidal in response. A crisis of faith commonly results from this spiritual and communal betrayal.

As with other types of sexual abuse, the damage of clergy abuse is often exacerbated by exposure due to the witnessing, disclosure, or reporting of the abuse, with some victims experiencing disbelief, invalidation, personal attacks, and shunning on the part of others, including members of their own family. Because it is viewed by many as salacious and taboo, it can generate unwanted and intrusive attention (including mismanagement of the report and extensive social or more traditional media attention) further compounding the humiliation and trauma. This is more likely if a report was made outside of religious channels to secular authorities due to a legal reporting mandate, and thus it is not under the victim's control. Even in such a circumstance, the victim may be perceived as tainted and as having lost their soul. The congregant may be labeled as disloyal—to the clergy member, to their own family, to the congregation. Some victims have been barred from attending services or participating in rituals or have been forced to leave their congregations, and what were often their lifelong neighborhoods and spiritual and social communities, when both the clergy member and the victim are in the same location. A victim and their supporters may even be shunned, trolled, threatened, or stalked in person or through social media by those who disbelieve or cast blame. An additional insult to the injury occurs for victims who are painfully disavowed and abandoned by their spouses (who may divorce them and even cause them to lose child custody), and sometimes by their children and other members of their nuclear and extended families who maintain their primary allegiance to the religion and faith community. In this, the losses are acute and cumulative, and the victim is made to feel expendable even to those closest to them.

COLLATERAL DAMAGE

It is not only the individual victim who suffers consequences. There is collateral damage to spouses and partners, children, parents, members of the nuclear and extended family, colleagues and friends of both parties, along with other members of the congregation and faith community, all of whom may experience serious repercussions. First and foremost, their religious beliefs may be profoundly shaken or even shattered. The marriages or intimate relationships of one or both parties may fray or end, and families may be blown apart due to the infidelity and sexual betrayal, erroneously blamed on both parties, negating that the congregant/victim lacked the ability to give true consent. Family members too may take sides, becoming alienated from one another and leading to some finding themselves shunned or unwelcome by parents and other close relatives. Thus, alienation may be extreme and punitive.

The community needs to find ways to recover after a violation has been exposed. As discussed, congregations frequently are torn by split loyalty, and they struggle with their identification with and response to both parties, as well as to other congregants. Common communal reactions include denial and avoidance of discussing the sexual misconduct as a way to maintain secrecy and normalcy at all costs, as well as to protect the congregation, its reputation, and its integrity. This type of reaction often leads to attempts to cover up the behavior and to deal with it internally (i.e., not involving others outside of the individual congregation or the religion or its hierarchy, especially secular authorities and the criminal justice system). Other typical reactions include fear of family and community conflict, loss of valued relationships and membership, feelings of abandonment, anguish, betrayal, helplessness, disbelief, outrage and anger, with difficulty dealing constructively with these feelings. It is not uncommon for a communal spiritual crisis or even a schism to develop. It can cause the disintegration of a congregation and great damage to the standing of a religion. This can be seen with the Roman Catholic Church and its ongoing mismanagement of the clergy child sexual abuse scandal. (See Chapter 17 for discussions of betrayal trauma—from the individual to the organizational level.)

Despite mandatory reporting requirements in many jurisdictions, likely only a minority of communities are transparent about reporting sexual misconduct and abuse to outside authorities. They accept the reality of its occurrence and invite members to work together to express their reactions and heal the rifts in the community caused by the transgression. They try to keep its occurrence in open awareness and to deal with its aftermath, including the establishment of measures to assure the safety of all members going forward, especially the most vulnerable. By considering an SBV a serious misconduct and a betrayal of the clergy role and responsibility, they hold the clergy member (or other religious representative) accountable by reporting it to outside authorities who are expected to be better trained and prepared to conduct a less biased investigation. They further seek ways for the perpetrator to get needed assessment, assistance, and treatment, to determine (a) whether the clergy member can be rehabilitated and can resume clerical and counseling duties under supervision, (b) whether the clergy member should be removed or should resign from the clergy, or (c) whether imprisonment is called for following criminal charges and a trial. They attempt to assist and support the clergy member's spouse and children and any other impacted family and community members. They further provide ongoing support and assistance to the client/victim, rather than blaming and shaming.

COMMUNITY REMEDIES

Historically, there has been a relative lack of religious and institutional remedies for SBVs. Now as the problem and its extent have become more evident, religions and their affiliated groups and congregations are beginning to institute policies, procedures, and standards. Foremost, they must begin by acknowledging not only that abuse is possible but also that it occurs with some degree of regularity and frequency. They must engage in soul searching, examining their own structures and attitudes and the ways that those may directly or inadvertently contribute to the problem. Were there signs that weren't seen, other motivations that may have blinded them to what was going on, were they coerced to "toe the line," perhaps by a need to protect an individual or organization from liability or potential image tarnish? Perhaps they saw some signs and dismissed them, possibly because clear standards and policies were not in place to facilitate intervention or to better protect a vulnerable/susceptible client. Was there due diligence in hiring clergy members and others that included deep background (including criminal) checks? Is it enough for religious institutions to independently do all these steps or are more generally applicable standards needed? Much as we have laws at the broader level (state or federal), general organizational policies might lead to greater applicability and accountability.

Especially in the absence of clear acknowledgment on the part of a religion and its leaders (and related neglect or mistreatment of the client/victim in the aftermath of a report), many victims have turned to judicial remedies, most of which involve civil suits against the transgressive clergy member, their affiliated institution (e.g., parish, synagogue), and the overarching religious organization that allege negligent hiring, inadequate supervision, neglect, and malpractice for which damages are sought (Bisbing et al., 1995). Many of these suits have been initiated by victims of clergy child sexual abuse, but these actions are now being initiated based on the abuse of adults. Spouses, as well as victims, have filed suits alleging marriage interference. Torts and damages as a result of clergy malpractice have only relatively recently been recognized (Tobin & Helge, 2013). There is currently little uniformity between the states as to the definition of clergy malpractice, but that situation is slowly changing.

Indeed, First Amendment concerns have limited the law's standardization around these issues, because a standard of care for clergy implies to some a restriction of religious freedom. A way to circumvent this, especially regarding SBVs in pastoral counseling, has been to use standards from other mental health professions, including psychology, social work, and psychiatry. Yet some have questioned the applicability of these standards that are, on average, more strict, given the disparities in education and training between clergy and mental health professionals. Standardized mental health training as a component of clergy preparation remains limited; however, recent programs combining pastoral and licensed mental health counselor training may be reducing the disparities. When clergy practice in more secular capacities or settings than in more strictly pastoral ones, legal remedies seem to be more applicable (Tobin & Helge, 2013). As more clergy receive secular training in counseling, there is a greater possibility for and emphasis on regulation and accountability.

EXAMPLES OF RESPONSES IN CHRISTIAN AND JEWISH COMMUNITIES

Christian Communities

Roman Catholic

To date, the best-known initiative in identifying the scope of Roman Catholic clergy abuse, calling for appropriate, responsible response and prevention, is the John Jay Survey (John Jay College of Criminal Justice, 2004). The survey was undertaken after the 1992 *Boston Globe* expose regarding the widespread scope of clergy abuse. It was a result of the efforts of the Survivors Network of Those Abused by Priests (SNAP), whose members picketed churches and dioceses locally, nationally, and internationally for years, and of Bishop Accountability, which has developed an extensive database of abusive priests, including their names, location, credibility of the accusation, and status. Additionally, the Pennsylvania Attorney General's report, released 2 years ago after a multiyear investigation, documented shockingly widespread abuse in Pennsylvania dioceses at all levels of the church hierarchy and routine cover-up and reassignment of priests to different parishes. Since the report's release, many other states have followed Pennsylvania's initiative by empaneling their own investigative task forces, and many have or are currently debating extending the statutes of limitations for civil torts cases and updating their criminal statutes.

Advocacy and investigative groups are different from those that develop policies and procedures. The church hierarchy, involving the Vatican, the College of Cardinals, and the bishops, has made efforts to develop a church-wide method of response (i.e., the Conference of Catholic Bishops, which took place in Dallas in 1992) that has thus far not yet satisfied critics nor been effective in providing congregants with needed standards and adequate protection. Although Pope Francis has decried abuse in strongly worded statements, he is yet to develop an effective plan of intervention and prevention, for which he has been highly criticized. However, Voice of the Faithful, composed of groups of congregants across parishes and dioceses who have remained members of the church, are working to respond to and decrease the possibility of future abuse at the local level.

Protestant

Thus far, in most Protestant denominations, church responses have been piecemeal rather than organized, and they remain a work in progress. This is no doubt related to the fact that

> the Protestant world includes tens of thousands of denominations, plus thousands more nondenominational churches, ministries, mission boards,

and subcultures. Unlike the Catholic Church, there is no Vatican, no shared leadership connecting say, Calvary Chapel's 1,600 churches with the Southern Baptist convention's 46,000. No common standards apply but the authority of scripture, which is interpreted differently from church to church, school to school, mission to mission. [Yet], even with its tightly controlled hierarchy, the Catholic Church has responded abysmally to sex abuse. (Shoebat, 2014)

However, despite this, resources and initiatives have developed across denominations and in various congregations and communities, often in interfaith efforts. Many of these can be found online.

An organization named GRACE (Godly Response to Abuse in the Christian Environment), which is an independent group of evangelical lawyers, pastors, and psychologists founded in 2004 by Boz Tchividjian, an attorney and grandson of Billy Graham, serves as a model of a multidisciplinary effort. Through his work as a prosecutor, Tchividjian had come to believe that the problem of child sexual abuse in Protestant churches rivals and possibly exceeds that in the Roman Catholic Church (Shoebat, 2014). Until recently, Protestants have tended to assume immunity to the abuse perpetrated by Roman Catholic priests, but over the course of the past decade, a number of exposes chronicling extensive child sexual abuse across the Protestant world have been published that challenge this assumption. These exposes have now extended to the sexual abuse of adult congregants.

GRACE has the identified mission of educating Protestant churches about sex abuse and the ways in which religion can be used to minimize or deny it. It has developed individualized education and training programs for organizations through their Safeguarding Certification Initiative and have further developed a seminary curriculum to educate future ministry leaders on issues of abuse and victimization. Additionally, it provides independent investigations and organizational assessments, as well as serves as a repository for educational resources. Since its founding, GRACE has trained more than 150 churches and ministries, consulted with many others on prevention policies, and helped implement abuse awareness programs at several Christian colleges and universities. They have been hired to conduct major investigations for a variety of prestigious Christian organizations and reported findings that were so shocking they led to some suppression efforts.

Tchividjian has also participated in an interfaith effort with a Jewish colleague resulting in a handbook, *The Child Safeguarding Policy Book*, (Tchividjian & Berkovits, 2017). It is authored and edited by a multidisciplinary team of child abuse experts and is designed to help different faith communities formulate policies and procedures to protect children and deal with possible child abuse in their ministries, schools, and synagogues. No doubt, these can be extended in response to the abuse of adult congregants.

Jewish Communities

Sexual boundary violations have been noted in reform, reconstructionist, conservative, and Orthodox congregations and communities. No Jewish community is immune. Blau (2017a, 2017b) cites an article in 2005 on the prevalence of sexual abuse in the orthodox Jewish community; it reported that the percentage of sexually abused women was essentially the same as in the general population. Despite this, the prevalence and risk have continued to not be sufficiently acknowledged and have continued to be minimized in many Jewish communities (Lev, 2003; Neustein, 2009). Although more and more rabbinic seminaries are providing training and courses in pastoral counseling, it is a relatively new phenomenon. Rabbinical training, until now, has rarely included specific training in addressing abuse or boundary violations. In some states, Rabbis are even mandated reporters of abuse, yet many are not aware that they carry that duty nor have they received specific training about how to make such a report.

In some Jewish communities/congregations, there is an additional concern: the fear of reprisal if secular authorities are brought in to address clergy abuse. This fear is in keeping with "mesira," a historical taboo regarding reporting a fellow Jew to the secular authorities (Blau, 2017b; Brofsky, 2017). This taboo stems from historically anti-Semitic periods, when reporting could lead to the torture or even murder of one's fellow Jews at the hands of secular and other clerical authorities. However, many renowned historic rabbis, including Maimonides, the twelfth-century Torah scholar, physician, and philosopher, and the current Rabbinical Council of America have asserted that not reporting abuse when someone is in danger is proscribed and likened to the biblical injunction of standing idly by when one's neighbor is being hurt (Blau, 2017b; Brofsky, 2017). So, from this perspective, one must report, including to secular authority, to assist someone who is being endangered or hurt and to prevent a future occurrence.

Another Jewish teaching is the avoidance of Lashon Hara (the prohibition against speaking evil of others). This prohibition, however, can unfortunately lead to minimization, denial, and cover-ups of concerning and suspicious behaviors. Well-known rabbis have noted that suspecting is not the same as accepting damaging information and that relaying concerns is not commensurate with accusing. But misunderstandings such as these have contributed to the lack of acknowledgement and the silencing of victims.

Although many renowned rabbis encourage reporting, individuals and communities remain hesitant or resistant to doing so for many reasons, including denial, shame, and fear of negative publicity; this leads them to instead attempt to handle the matter from within the organization. These efforts have generally been limited and unsuccessful, due to lack of appropriate training in assessment and intervention; dual relationships involving bias and divided loyalty; and the insularity of some of these communities.

Offending rabbis are often not referred to appropriate treatment or may be forgiven and even reinstated but then not monitored or supervised on a sufficient or ongoing basis. Of course, for the repeat violator who remains in the throes of addictions/compulsions and other personality, personal, or spiritual issues or crises that have not been addressed or treated, recidivism and additional sexual misconduct is likely. Unfortunately, it is also routine for the victim's status and needs to not get acknowledged or addressed sufficiently; rarely are they offered supportive resources.

An American organization called Sacred Spaces has recently been organized to focus on instituting more standardized policies within American Jewish organizations, including synagogues and schools. Founded by psychologist–attorney Shira Berkovits, who has studied the specific sexual abuse risk factors within Jewish communities and partnered with Tchividjian on *The Child Safeguarding Policy* book, Sacred Spaces works with individuals, congregations, and other groups to establish standardized policies that are individualized. The need for more accepted communal standards regarding response to abuse has been spurred by cases where an abusive rabbi was able to leave one school after being reported internally but not to secular authorities, only to be hired by another school because there was no formal record of the previous misconduct. Many stories such as these are easy to find across all religions.

Sacred Spaces observed characteristics typical of Jewish communities (many of which are consistent with those found in other religious groups) and used applied social psychological concepts to understand and explain communal reactions to abuse reports. For example, the well-known concept of cognitive dissonance helps to understand denial in response to allegations involving a highly respected and well-entrenched rabbi or clergy member. Others in the community typically reject the evidence at hand by holding onto prior beliefs about the individual because not doing so would create too much cognitive dissonance. The clergy member, in turn, is likely to use their influence, power, and aura of respectability to deny the allegations and to camouflage grooming behaviors and actual abuse. As another example, all-or-nothing thinking, a common cognitive error, may also apply. The responses of community leadership and congregants may range from total denial, disavowal, or minimization that an allegation could be true to total demonization of the clergy member when an investigation determines that it is founded. Victims can receive similar dualistic responses. As discussed elsewhere in this chapter and volume, SBVs occur in many ways for many reasons, and it is a mistake to assume they are all the same and require the same response. Berkovits (2017) and her team found that such binary positions overlook more nuanced issues that can open many more possibilities for protecting congregants while supporting all involved individuals.

CONCLUDING REMARKS

We conclude by emphasizing that clergy members, in their pastoral, teaching, and counseling capacities, have unique responsibilities, roles, and personal and situational vulnerabilities. Included among these are that they historically have tended to receive little to no training in counseling or mental health, yet they have been called upon to provide in vivo care on an as-needed basis to individuals who seek them out during crises and times of exposure, with few safeguards or boundaries in place. They have enormous influence and power for both good and evil, due to what Rauch (2009) termed the "trance of religious power," and carry great responsibility for those entrusted in their care. Yet, unfortunately, most have had little opportunity in their training to learn about pastoral and personal vulnerabilities and situations of temptation and how to handle them. When SBVs occur in this context, they create enormous damage to those directly involved, to their significant others, their fellow congregants, and their faith and spirituality and to the religion itself.

Even now, in the face of personal and institutional ignorance and misunderstanding and the mounting evidence of the ubiquity and prevalence of abuse across all religions and associated organizations by members of the clergy or other religiously affiliated individuals, standards of care as well as policies and procedures for response and intervention are weak and ill-defined. In an attempt to rectify this situation, more organized efforts, both within religious groups and as interfaith efforts, are being undertaken by multidisciplinary groups of secular and religious experts instituting programs that include clear, transparent, and consistent institutional standards and policies aimed at prevention, intervention, and cooperation with secular authorities when cases are disclosed and reported. These programs cannot be implemented too soon.

REFERENCES

Berkovits, S. M. (2017). Institutional abuse in the Jewish community. *Tradition: A Journal of Orthodox Jewish Thought, 50*(2), 11–49.

Bisbing, S. B., Jorgenson, L. M., & Sutherland, P. K. (1995). *Sexual abuse by professionals: A legal guide.* Michie.

Blau, Y. (2017a). Guest editor introduction. *Tradition*, *50*(2), 8–10.

Blau, Y. (2017b). Sexual abuse in the Orthodox Jewish community: An analysis of the roots of the failure to effectively respond to the crisis. *Tradition: A Journal of Orthodox Jewish Thought*, *50*(2), 50–59.

Boorstein, M. & Bahrampour, T. (2018, August 30). Victims of voyeur-rabbi with Baltimore ties reach $14.25 million settlement. *The Baltimore Sun*. https://www.baltimoresun.com/news/crime/bs-md-rabbi-bath-settlement-20180830-story.html

Brenneis, M. J. (2001). Personality characteristics of clergy and of psychologically "impaired" clergy: A review of the literature. *American Journal of Pastoral Counseling*, *4*(2), 17–30. https://doi.org/10.1300/J062v04n02_03

Brofsky, D. (2017, September 23). Discussing and reporting abuse—A Halakhic perspective. *Tradition (New York)*, *50*(2), 60–77.

Casteix, J. (2020, September 23). What if women comprised 50% of sex abuse victims in the Catholic Church? *The Worthy Adversary*. http://theworthyadversary.com/5368-what-if-women-comprised-50-of-sex-abuse-victims-in-the-catholic-church

Chaves, M., & Garland, D. (2009). The prevalence of clergy sexual advances toward adults in their congregations. *Journal for the Scientific Study of Religion*, *48*(4), 817–824. https://doi.org/10.1111/j.1468-5906.2009.01482.x

Cooper-White, P. (1991, February 20). Soul stealing: Power relations in pastoral sexual abuse. *The Christian Century*, 196–199.

Dratch, M. (2017). What to do with abusive rabbis: Halakhic considerations. *Tradition (New York)*, *50*(2), 93–106.

Fortune, M. M. (1989). *Is nothing sacred? When sex invades the pastoral relationship.* Harper & Row.

Garland, D. R. (2009). *The prevalence of clergy sexual misconduct with adults: A research study executive summary.* Baylor University School of Social Work. https://www.baylor.edu/clergysexualmisconduct/index.php?id=67406

John Jay College of Criminal Justice. (2004). *The nature and scope of sexual abuse of minors by Catholic priests and deacons in the Unites States, 1950–2002.* http://www.bishop-accountability.org/reports/2004_02_27_JohnJay_revised/2004_02_27_John_Jay_Main_Report_Optimized.pdf

Lev, R. (2003). *Shine the light: Sexual abuse and healing in the Jewish community.* Northeastern University Press.

Marquis, J. (1994, December 3). Therapist's license revoked: Misconduct: James D. Lisle developed a sexual relationship with a former patient he met when he was a contract counselor at a Christian therapy program. *Los Angeles Times*. https://www.latimes.com/archives/la-xpm-1994-12-03-me-4499-story.html

Matthews, D. H. (2012). *Sexual abuse of power in the Black church: Sexual misconduct in the African American churches.* WestBow Press.

Middleton, W., Sachs, A., & Dorahy, M. J. (2017). The abused and the abuser: Victim–perpetrator dynamics. *Journal of Trauma & Dissociation*, *18*(3), 249–258. https://doi.org/10.1080/15299732.2017.1295373

Mosgofian, P., & Ohlschlager, G. (1995). *Sexual misconduct in counseling and ministry.* Word.

Navarro, J. (2014, April 20). Why predators are attracted to careers in the clergy. *Psychology Today*. https://www.psychologytoday.com/us/blog/spycatcher/201404/why-predators-are-attracted-careers-in-the-clergy

Neustein, A. (Ed.). (2009). *Tempest in the temple: Jewish communities and child sex scandals*. Brandeis University Press. https://doi.org/10.26812/9781584656715

Rauch, M. (2009). *Healing the soul after religious abuse: The dark heaven of recovery*. Praeger Publishers.

Rossetti, S. J. (1990). *Slayer of the soul: Child sexual abuse and the Catholic Church*. Twenty-Third Publications.

Schoen, G. (2013). *Buddha betrayed: When spiritual relationships go awry*.

Shoebat Foundation. (2014, May 6). There is more sexual abuse in the Protestant Churches than Catholic. http://shoebat.com/2014/05/06/sexual-abuse-protestant-churches-catholic/

Shupe, A., Stacey, W. A., & Darnell, S. E. (Eds.). (2000). *Bad pastors: Clergy misconduct in modern America*. New York University Press.

Tchividjian, B., & Berkovits, S. M. (2017). *The child safeguarding policy guide for churches and ministries*. New Growth Press.

Tobin, B., & Helge, K. (2013). Clergyperson sexual misconduct with congregants or parishioners: Past attempts to impose civil and criminal liabilities and a proposed criminal law to increase the likelihood of criminal punishment of perpetrators. In C. M. Renzetti & S. Yocum (Eds.), *Clergy sexual abuse: Social science perspectives* (pp. 144–171). Northeastern University Press.

11 SEXUAL BOUNDARY VIOLATIONS IN THE DIGITAL AGE

New Frontiers and Emerging Challenges

FREDERIC G. REAMER

The subjects of boundaries and dual relationships in the behavioral health professions emerged in the 1980s. The pioneering works of Bograd (1993), Brodsky (1986), Epstein (1994), Gabbard (1989), Gutheil (1989), Pope (1988), Schoener (1995), and Simon (1992), among others, laid the rich conceptual foundation for contemporary practitioners' thinking about the complex nature of boundary crossings and boundary violations. Since then, behavioral health professionals—including psychologists, psychiatrists, clinical social workers, mental health counselors, marriage and family therapists, psychiatric nurses, and substance abuse counselors—have sharpened their focus on potential and actual boundary challenges (Celenza, 2007; Reamer, 2020; Syme, 2003).

Until recently, the scholarly literature on boundaries and dual relationships presumed that the clinician and client engaged in traditional face-to-face counseling and communicated in person. The literature is replete with discussions of sexual boundary violations (SBVs) that developed between clinician and client, which had their origins in the intense psychotherapeutic discussions that occurred in the clinician's office (Celenza, 2007; Lazarus &

https://doi.org/10.1037/0000247-011
Sexual Boundary Violations in Psychotherapy: Facing Therapist Indiscretions, Transgressions, and Misconduct, A. Steinberg, J. L. Alpert, and C. A. Courtois (Editors)

Zur, 2002; Peterson, 1992; Pope & Bouhoutsos, 1986; Reamer, 2015, 2020; Syme, 2003).

Recently, however, newer forms of boundary crossings and boundary violations have been emerging as a direct result of behavioral health clinicians' increasing use of digital and other technology to serve and communicate with clients. Clinicians' remote contact with clients, via technology, has expanded the ways in which clinicians can violate professional–client boundaries and have created new opportunities for boundary confusion. As with more "traditional" types of boundary violations, these newer forms that have emerged in the digital age have great potential to harm clients and imperil practitioners' careers. Remote, online, and electronic contact—including clinicians' provision of distance counseling services—have led to unprecedented uncertainty and ambiguity about the elasticity of professional boundaries, including questions about the appropriateness of electronic communications outside of normal working hours and outside the office setting. According to Drum and Littleton (2014),

> because the client and clinician are now capable of communicating through means typically reserved for social and personal interactions with family and friends (e.g., through e-mail, instant-chat, and video conferencing), tele-psychology interactions can occur at any hour of the day or night, and both parties can now virtually enter each other's homes, there is the potential for an increased sense of intimacy between client and therapist which could lead to boundary challenges. (p. 310)

Mental health services emerged on the internet as early as 1982 in the form of online self-help support groups (Kanani & Regehr, 2003). The first known fee-based internet mental health service was established by Sommers in 1995 (Skinner & Zack, 2004). By the late 1990s, groups of clinicians were forming companies and e-clinics that offered online counseling services to the public using secure websites (Skinner & Zack, 2004).

Current psychotherapeutic services include a wide range of digital and electronic options: online, telephone, text-based, video, email, and avatar counseling (Barsky, 2017; Chester & Glass, 2006; Finn, 2006; Graffeo & La Barbera, 2009; Gutheil & Simon, 2005; Kanani & Regehr, 2003; Kolmes & Taube, 2016; Lannin & Scott, 2013; Menon & Miller-Cribbs, 2002; Midkiff & Wyatt, 2008; Mossman & Farrell, 2012; Reamer, 2017, 2021; Recupero & Reamer, 2018; Zur, 2012). Practitioners are using this technology to assist people who struggle with depression, addiction, marital and relationship conflict, anxiety, eating disorders, grief, and other mental health and behavioral challenges. These newer forms of counseling provide novel opportunities for boundary violations, some of which involve sexual content. In addition, clinicians' and clients' pervasive use of social networking sites and online search engines, such as Facebook and Google, have also created new boundary-related challenges.

This chapter provides an overview of boundary issues unique to the digital age, including common themes and patterns. It also summarizes relevant adopted ethics standards and highlights risk-management protocols designed to protect clients and prevent ethics-related litigation and professional discipline.

BOUNDARY VIOLATIONS IN THE DIGITAL AGE: A TYPOLOGY

Novel boundary and dual relationship challenges in the digital age are appearing in three forms: ethical judgments, ethical mistakes, and ethical misconduct (Reamer, 2015, 2019, 2021).

Ethical Judgments

In some instances, in light of potential boundary challenges, competent, principled, and well-meaning clinicians find themselves faced with ethical decisions about whether and how to use technology in their relationships with clients. In these scenarios, clinicians recognize that technology has the potential to enhance their delivery of services to clients—especially during a pandemic, such as COVID-19, and among those clients who have crises, live in remote geographic areas, or struggle with severe disabilities that limit their ability to travel—but that their use of technology may introduce complex boundary issues. These clinicians must make deliberate ethical decisions about how to use technology in ways that maintain clear, ethical professional–client boundaries. Here are several (disguised) examples based on the author's work as an ethics consultant and expert witness in licensing board cases and lawsuits filed against behavioral health practitioners:

- A clinical social worker provided counseling services to a couple that was experiencing marital tension. One of the clinical issues the couple identified was their chronic distress about their lack of sexual intimacy. The social worker, who specialized in sex therapy, considered sending the couple an email message containing links to a number of websites that offer advice on ways to enhance sexual intimacy. The clinician was unsure about whether it was appropriate for her to send clients an online message containing sexually explicit material. The clinician realized that the clients would be able to forward the social worker's message to others electronically, and that other recipients might misunderstand the nature of the relationship and the purpose of the message.

- A clinical psychologist counseled a 16-year-old teen who was struggling with depression and sexual orientation issues. During one session, the teen talked with deep emotion about the intense distress in her life. Later than night, around 10:30 p.m., the psychologist decided to search the client's Facebook site to see whether there was any evidence of suicidal ideation in the teen's online postings. The psychologist was concerned about several postings and sent the client private Facebook messages inquiring about the client's emotional state.

- A marriage and family therapist and his wife wrote sexually explicit novels that are available as e-books online. The therapist uses a pseudonym for these publications in an effort to separate his professional and personal lives. Nonetheless, the therapist is aware that clients may learn of the link, and that this could introduce untoward boundary issues in his clinical relationships.

Ethical Mistakes

In contrast, some competent, principled, and well-meaning clinicians have found themselves in ethics hot water because of technology-related errors that created boundary problems with a sexual component in their relationships with clients. Some of these errors have led to licensing board complaints and lawsuits filed by disgruntled clients or third parties. Here are several actual examples:

- A clinical psychologist received an unsolicited Facebook request from a client who had sought treatment for her anxiety symptoms. The client had searched for the psychologist's Facebook site and discovered several of the psychologist's postings about his recent divorce. The psychologist thought he understood how to use Facebook's privacy settings to limit access to such postings to his closest friends. However, the client was able to access many of the psychologist's postings about his personal relationships. Before the psychologist blocked the client's access to his site, the client had sent the clinician a series of flirtatious, intrusive, and intimate Facebook messages about the psychologist's personal life. Because of these boundary complications, the psychologist decided to terminate the clinical relationship, against the client's wishes, and refer the client to another provider. The client became enraged and filed a licensing board complaint alleging that the psychologist had abandoned her. The licensing board reprimanded the psychologist for failing to maintain proper boundaries online and failing to obtain proper consultation with colleagues. The board required the psychologist to enroll in supplemental continuing education courses on boundary issues and use of technology. The board also required the clinician to consult with a local ethics expert regarding his management of this case, focusing especially on how the psychologist might have processed these boundary issues with his client in order to avoid termination of services.

- In his private life, a mental health counselor was a member of an online creative writing group that included erotica. Group members posted drafts of their work in their Google Docs accounts so that they could be accessed by other group members. Inadvertently, the counselor did not limit access to his Google Docs postings. His client, who sought counseling to help her cope with the breakup of a long-term relationship, searched Google for information about the counselor and was able to open several of the counselor's erotic writings. The client, who had been harboring sexual fantasies about the counselor, told the counselor about how much she enjoyed reading about his sexual fantasies. The counselor was stunned by this boundary crossing and unsure about whether he could continue to work with the client. The counselor sought ethics consultation from his national professional association's ethics office and a local professor who specializes in professional ethics.

Ethical Misconduct

As in all professions, some behavioral health practitioners—a distinct minority—engage in ethical misconduct. A disturbing percentage of misconduct cases involve sexual relationships between practitioners and clients or former clients (Celenza, 2007; Pope, 1988; Reamer, 2015; Syme, 2003).

Clinicians' use of technology has expanded the ways in which unscrupulous counselors can engage in sexualized relationships with clients. In some instances, the unethical conduct is limited to online communications. In others, electronic communications are a prelude to a sexual relationship. In some cases, evidence suggests that electronic communications were part of a deliberate, calculated effort by clinicians to groom clients for an eventual sexual relationship. Here are examples:

- A psychologist at a prominent outpatient mental health clinic provided counseling services to clients with co-occurring symptoms (substance use and mood disorders). Most of his clients had trauma histories that contributed to their challenges. Over time, the psychologist engaged in sexual relationships with two of his clients. One of the clients disclosed the relationship to the police after the psychologist suddenly ended their intimate relationship. The clinician's arrest was publicized in the local media, after which the second client disclosed her sexual relationship with him. The psychologist was charged in criminal court and sued by the two clients. During the criminal and civil trials, the prosecutor and plaintiffs' attorneys introduced a collection of "electronically stored information," including text messages and email messages between the clinician and his clients containing sexualized content, that provided compelling evidence of the psychologist's unethical conduct. The clinician—who was not aware that his electronic communications left a digital footprint—was convicted, sentenced to prison, lost his professional license, and was found liable for professional negligence.

- A psychiatrist provided medication prescriptions and brief counseling to a woman who struggled with symptoms of depression and anxiety. During the course of the counseling, the patient's husband died, which exacerbated her symptoms. The patient often talked about her intense loneliness. The psychiatrist told the patient that he could help fill the emotional void in the patient's life and began sending her text messages, allegedly to check on her well-being. Over time, the text message exchanges between the pair became increasingly informal. On several occasions, the pair met for coffee, and eventually, they began a sexual relationship. During this period of time, the psychiatrist continued to prescribe psychotropic medication to the patient. The intimate relationship ruptured and the patient filed a licensing board complaint. The board suspended the psychiatrist's license.

- A counselor worked at a school sponsored by a mental health center. The school served adolescents who had difficulty functioning in traditional high school settings, and all of the students struggled with behavioral health issues. The counselor spent most of an academic year counseling a 17-year-old student who became clinically depressed following the sudden death of his father in an automobile accident. Over time, the counselor and student developed an intense emotional connection; at times, the counselor shared with the student details about her marriage and children. The counselor encouraged the teen to text her for support when he was feeling despair. One day, the teen sent the counselor a text message in which he shared his "loving" feelings toward her. The counselor responded with her own text message that told the teen how much she cared about him and how special he was to her. Gradually, the counselor and teen spent time together away from the school and, eventually, engaged in a sexual relationship. The teen's mother disclosed the relationship to the school's director, after she discovered inappropriate text messages on her son's phone, including several graphic, explicit photos that the two had exchanged (i.e., "sexting"). The principal fired the counselor and notified her licensing board. The licensing board revoked the counselor's license.

BOUNDARY THEMES IN THE DIGITAL AGE

Research in the behavioral health professions suggests that, historically, there are several patterns in boundary challenges (Herlihy & Corey, 2015; Moleski & Kiselica, 2005; Reamer, 2003, 2020; Zur, 2007, 2017). These include boundary issues related to intimate interactions between practitioners and clients, practitioners' own emotional and dependency needs, personal benefits to practitioners, practitioner altruism, and unanticipated circumstances. More recently, these themes have become evident in emerging boundary issues in the digital age, some of which involve SBVs and crossings.

Intimacy

Many dual relationships between clinicians and clients involve some element of intimacy. The most extreme cases involve sexual intimacy (Celenza, 2007; Lazarus & Zur, 2002; Peterson, 1992; Syme, 2003), but there are other forms as well. Examples include having physical contact (e.g., hugging), providing counseling services to a former lover, and accepting gifts from a client. However, in the digital age, newer forms of intimate contact between clinicians and clients are possible. These include online and other electronic messages and website postings (e.g., on social networking sites) that contain sexual content and images.

Emotional and Dependency Needs

A number of boundary issues arise from personal issues in practitioners' own lives. What many of these circumstances have in common is that they are rooted in the clinician's emotional needs, such as those stemming from childhood experiences, marital or relationship issues, health problems, aging, career frustrations, or financial and legal problems. These various stressors and related transference can impair clinicians' judgment, which may lead to inappropriate dual or multiple relationships and boundary violations.

Historically, one common manifestation has been clinicians' inappropriate self-disclosure to clients during face-to-face counseling sessions (Barglow, 2005; Bridges, 2001; Cornell, 2007; Farber, 2006; Knox & Hill, 2003; Roberts, 2005; Stricker & Fisher, 1990). Recognizing that some practitioners engage in judicious self-disclosure for therapeutic purposes, research suggests that such self-disclosure can be a prelude to sexual relationships that develop between clinicians and clients (Celenza, 2007; Gabbard, 1996; Gutheil & Simon, 1995, 2005; Reamer, 2015, 2020; Simon, 1995, 1999; Syme, 2003). In the digital age, these disclosures are sometimes embedded in text messages, email messages, and online postings that have become part of the practitioner–client relationship. The unique informality of online and digital exchanges can exacerbate boundary confusion and risks in ways that are less likely in traditional office-based encounters.

Personal Gain

Some dual relationships generate a personal benefit for clinicians. Examples include clinicians who receive services (e.g., car or computer repair) or favors from a client (e.g., use of a client's vacation home).

Clinicians who exploit clients sexually also experience personal gain— online and other electronic communications with clients that lead up to and surround such intimate relationships also provide emotional satisfaction and benefit to clinicians.

Altruism

Some boundary issues arise because of practitioners' genuinely altruistic inclinations. The vast majority of behavioral health professionals are dedicated, caring, and principled people who would never knowingly exploit clients. Ironically, clinicians who are extraordinarily kind and humane may unwittingly foster challenging dual and multiple relationships by engaging in informal online and other electronic communications with clients. Digital communications that begin quite innocently, in an effort to provide clients with emotional support and access outside of traditional office hours (including late-night online exchanges), can sometimes lead to intimate exchanges and, eventually, sexual contact. On occasion, altruistic gestures made electronically may be misinterpreted by clients and trigger boundary confusion.

Unanticipated Circumstances

During the course of a clinical career, most practitioners report unanticipated, sometimes unavoidable, dual relationships. These are especially common when clinicians live and work in small communities, such as rural areas or on military bases.

Digital technology has produced novel and unprecedented opportunities for such inadvertent encounters. In one case, a clinician joined an online dating service. To enhance the likelihood of making a match, the practitioner shared considerable information about her personal life. In a remarkable coincidence, the therapist discovered that she matched with a current client.

In another case, a marriage and family therapist who specialized in sex therapy posted links to various websites pertaining to sexual health. Unbeknownst to the therapist, several of the hyperlinks were hijacked and sent users automatically to pornography websites. Some users concluded that the clinician knowingly directed them to these websites. But the clinician was unaware that what is known as "DNS (i.e., domain name server) hijacking," a type of malicious attack in which an individual redirects queries to a web-based domain name server by overriding a computer's settings, was even a possibility.

EMERGING ETHICAL STANDARDS

In recent years, the major behavioral health professions have embarked on development of rigorous and comprehensive standards pertaining to practitioners' use of technology to serve and communicate with clients. A number of these standards address potential boundary crossings and violations.

The standards are beginning to emerge in three distinct, although related, domains: regulatory law, codes of ethics, and standards of professional practice. First, every licensing board operates under pertinent licensing statutes and regulations. A licensing board's duty is to develop, adopt, and enforce standards in order to protect the public, and a growing number of behavioral health licensing boards have adopted new technology-related standards (Greysen et al., 2012).

Further, some national and international umbrella groups of licensing boards (i.e., associations of state and provincial licensing boards) have adopted model regulatory standards related to technology. Examples include standards adopted by the Association of State and Provincial Psychology Boards (2013), Association of Marital and Family Therapy Regulatory Boards

(2016), Association of Social Work Boards (2015), and Federation of State Medical Boards (2012, 2014).

Professional codes of ethics are a second set of critically important guidelines. For example, the National Association of Social Workers (2017) recently completed a substantial revision of its code of ethics for the sole purpose of adding a large number of new standards related to technology, including standards pertaining to boundary issues. The National Board for Certified Counselors (2016) and American Mental Health Counselors Association (2020) have adopted new code of ethics standards concerning telehealth, distance counseling, and the use of social media.

Third, practice-based standards of care are used to train and guide professionals and, when necessary, adjudicate formal disputes about acceptable conduct (especially in the context of malpractice litigation and licensing board complaints). Practice standards specifically pertaining to practitioners' use of technology, sponsored by prominent professional associations and organizations (see, e.g., Joint Task Force for the Development of Telepsychology Guidelines for Psychologists, 2013) are now emerging. For instance, the American Psychiatric Association (n.d.) developed the "Telepsychiatry Toolkit" to educate psychiatrists about the appropriate use of remote or distance psychiatry.

Also, in an unprecedented effort, the four principal national social work organizations in the United States—National Association of Social Workers, Association of Social Work Boards, Council on Social Work Education, and Clinical Social Work Association (2017)—jointly sponsored a task force to develop comprehensive practice standards pertaining to social workers' use of technology. These new guidelines specifically address boundary and dual relationship issues, along with issues related to practitioner competence, informed consent, confidentiality, service delivery, gathering and managing information, collegial relationships, and the use of technology in education and supervision.

These diverse efforts across the behavioral health professions have led to an emerging consensus about the ethical implications of practitioners' increasing use of technology. New standards focus primarily on a number of common core concepts and themes related to technology: provision of information to the public; designing and delivering services; gathering, managing, and storing information; collegial relationships; and educating students and practitioners. This crosscutting pattern reflects emerging consensus thinking across key national organizations about current "best practices" when practitioners use technology. Importantly, a number of these standards focus explicitly on newer forms of boundary issues, including sex-related communications. Common themes address the need for practitioners to maintain clear professional boundaries in their relationships with clients when they provide services remotely; develop a social media policy that they share with clients; consider the implications of their use of personal mobile phones and other electronic communication devices for work purposes; be aware that posting personal information on professional websites or other media might cause boundary confusion, inappropriate dual relationships, or harm to clients; and be aware that personal affiliations may increase the likelihood that clients will discover practitioners' presence on websites, social media, and other forms of technology.

PREVENTING HARM: RISK MANAGEMENT IN THE DIGITAL AGE

Behavioral health professionals who violate boundaries in conjunction with their use of digital and other technology can cause great harm to clients and, as well, expose themselves to the risk of litigation, licensing board complaints, and criminal charges. Disgruntled clients—who are likely to be former clients by the time they decide to litigate—may file a lawsuit against their clinician alleging professional negligence. In ordinary civil suits, the standard of proof required to find practitioners liable is a preponderance of the evidence. This means that the evidence suggests that, more likely than not, the clinician was negligent. Negligence can include inappropriate digital and other electronic communications with clients, including text messages, email messages, and postings on social networking sites that constitute boundary violations.

Lawsuits brought against practitioners typically allege both negligence and malpractice. In general, malpractice occurs when evidence exists of the following:

1. At the time of the alleged malpractice, the practitioner owed a legal duty to the client.

2. The practitioner was derelict in that duty, either through omission (the failure to perform one's duty, such as maintaining clear clinician–client boundaries when communicating electronically) or through commission (an action taken by the practitioner, such as inappropriate text or online communication that led to sexual contact).

3. The client suffered some harm or injury.

4. The practitioner's dereliction of duty was the direct and proximate cause of the harm or injury.

A preponderance of the evidence is also used in cases before the licensing board regarding alleged violation of licensing standards. Licensing boards typically draw on standards in prominent national codes of ethics and practice standards, directly or indirectly. Some licensing laws explicitly cite psychology, social work, psychiatry, mental health, marriage and family therapy, and other codes of ethics. Other licensing boards draw heavily on pertinent code standards without citing them explicitly. Increasingly, national codes of ethics are adding or strengthening standards that explicitly address boundary issues associated with practitioners' use of technology.

In extreme cases, behavioral health practitioners may be charged in criminal court because of their conduct. Criminal codes in a number of jurisdictions consider sexual relationships between a mental health professional and client to be a felony. In contrast to civil proceedings, the evidentiary standard in criminal court cases requires proof beyond a reasonable doubt (as opposed to a preponderance of the evidence). Clinicians' sexualized email messages, text messages, and postings on online social networking sites may be introduced as formal evidence against them.

Clinicians who engage in unethical conduct involving digital and other electronic communications fall into two groups (Reamer, 2015, 2020). First, some clinicians slide into boundary confusion unwittingly and without malice. Their elastic sense of boundaries leads them to engage in informal, chatty, seemingly innocuous, electronic communications with clients. These may include after-hours exchanges that resemble messages shared between friends about personal challenges, social events, recreational activities, restaurant visits, vacations, and family intrigue. These practitioners often have the capacity to learn from their descent down the digital slippery slope, especially when their attention has been sharply focused after being named as a defendant in a lawsuit or a respondent in a licensing board complaint. With the benefit of competent ethics consultation and therapy—which are frequently required as elements of a licensing board resolution and consent order—these clinicians are often able to gain impressive insight and move on to productive careers once they sweep away the ashes.

The second group, however, includes a much more challenged and challenging group of practitioners. These clinicians are exploitative and use clients to meet their own needs. Extracurricular electronic exchanges with clients are often a deliberate, calculated, and self-serving effort to groom vulnerable clients, luring them with cleverly worded, seductive messages of endearment, support, and praise. These clinicians often struggle with narcissistic instincts and other personality disorder traits listed in Cluster B of the *Diagnostic and Statistical Manual of Mental Disorders* (American

Psychiatric Association, 2013). True insight and rehabilitation, although certainly possible, can be elusive.

Not surprisingly, some of these clinicians struggle with impairment. Research on impairment among professionals suggests that many struggling practitioners do not seek assistance, and colleagues who are concerned about them may be reluctant to share their concerns (Kilburg et al., 1988; Reamer, 2015; Sonnenstuhl, 1989). Some impaired professionals may find it difficult to seek help because of their mythological belief in their competence and invulnerability; they believe that an acceptable therapist is not available or that therapy would not help; they prefer to seek help from family members or friends, or to work problems out by themselves; they fear exposure and the disclosure of confidential information about their struggles; they are concerned about the amount of effort required and about the cost; they have a spouse or partner who is unwilling to participate in treatment; or they do not admit the seriousness of the problem. Licensing boards and professional associations that discipline practitioners who violate boundaries (including digital and online boundary violations) sometimes encourage or require them to enroll in outpatient or residential programs designed specifically to treat impaired behavioral health practitioners.

On occasion, behavioral health professionals become aware of a colleague's inappropriate use of technology in their relationships with clients. They may learn directly or from third parties of colleagues' unwise or salacious Facebook postings or text and email message exchanges, for example. Ideally, practitioners who learn of colleagues' unethical conduct should approach them for frank discussion about the behavior and its implications. Supervisors, especially, should broach these issues when they arise and address them directly. In some instances, supervisors may develop contracts with supervisees that acknowledge these issues and include a detailed protocol to address them.

Prominent codes of ethics exhort colleagues and supervisors to address problematic boundary issues manifested by colleagues and supervisees. Understandably, practitioners sometimes find it difficult to confront a colleague. These awkward conversations can be contentious and emotionally taxing. As VandenBos and Duthie (1986) noted following their research on psychologists' attitudes toward confronting colleagues who engage in questionable conduct:

> The fact that more than half of us have not confronted distressed colleagues even when we have recognized and acknowledged (at least to ourselves) the existence of their problems is, in part, a reflection of the difficulty in achieving a balance between concerned intervention and intrusiveness. As professionals, we value our own right to practice without interference, as long as we function

within the boundaries of our professional expertise, meet professional standards for the provision of services, and behave in an ethical manner. We generally consider such expectations when we consider approaching a distressed colleague. Deciding when and how our concern about the well-being of a colleague (and our ethical obligation) supersedes his or her right to personal privacy and professional autonomy is a ticklish matter. (p. 212)

Some circumstances warrant what Sonnenstuhl (1989) regarded as "constructive confrontation" with colleagues who appear to have engaged in, or are engaging in, boundary violations. Ideally, misbehaving practitioners would be willing to engage in comprehensive and therapeutic efforts to address their poor judgment and personal challenges that led to their unethical use of technology. Practitioners who are responsible for addressing colleagues' boundary violations can follow a series of constructive steps (Reamer, 2015; Schoener, 1995):

- Gather data about the practitioner's professional training, professional work history, and personal history (including noteworthy ups and downs), and the nature of the practice-related complaint (boundary violation involving technology).

- Generate hypotheses about causal factors that may be involved in the boundary violation.

- Formulate a rehabilitation plan, when feasible.

- Coordinate the rehabilitation plan with the licensing board, professional association, and practitioner's employer.

- Implement the corrective action (e.g., psychotherapy, supervision, consultation, continuing education) and, when necessary, appropriate sanctions (e.g., license suspension or revocation, expulsion from professional association).

- Evaluate the practitioner's progress with regard to the possibility of permitting reentry to practice and the profession.

Studies have shown that ambitious, skilled treatment of offending practitioners can be effective (Gutheil & Brodsky, 2008; Reamer, 2015; Simon, 1999). Prospects are less encouraging for practitioners who have been diagnosed with serious personality disorders (Schoener, 1995; Simon, 1999).

One practical way to minimize the likelihood of boundary problems arising out of practitioners' and clients' use of technology is for clinicians to develop a social media policy that they review with clients. Social media policies inform clients about their clinician's professional use of social networking sites, email, text messaging, electronic search engines, smartphone applications, blogs, business review sites, and other forms of electronic communication (Kolmes, 2010). A typical social media policy informs clients that their clinician cannot be their "friend" on social networking sites (e.g., Facebook) and why this is important in order to maintain clear professional boundaries.[1] Such policies also set limits on practitioners' and clients' use of text messaging and emails. Further, typical policies inform clients that electronic communications may not be confidential and can be subpoenaed as part of legal proceedings.[2] Broaching the subject of digital and online communications can heighten both clinicians' and clients' awareness of potential boundary challenges. It is important for practitioners to document their efforts to address these issues with clients.

Social media policies also summarize practitioners' policy about conducting online searches for information about clients without their knowledge or consent. Prominent codes of ethics and practice standards advise practitioners to refrain from conducting such online searches for information about clients in order to respect their privacy, with an exception for emergency or other compelling circumstances; these may include when a practitioner feels compelled to search for information about a high-risk client who has disappeared from care or who poses some other serious safety threat (Reamer, 2017).

In addition, practitioners should develop keen instincts about when they should consult with knowledgeable colleagues and supervisors about ambiguous boundary challenges, especially those related to sexual boundaries. Practitioners' malpractice insurers also can offer practical guidance. When necessary, practitioners should consult an attorney who specializes in defending behavioral health professionals in malpractice and licensing board matters.

---

[1]Practitioners should also think carefully about engaging with *former* clients on online social networking sites. As with in-person social relationships with former clients, electronic relationships with former clients can produce boundary confusion. One possible consequence, among many, is that former clients who have developed online social relationships with their former clinician may forfeit the possibility of returning to that clinician for counseling because of the changed nature of the relationship. That may not be in the client's best interest.
[2]Keely Kolmes has developed a widely used social media policy template, which can be found online (https://drkkolmes.com/product/my-updated-and-annotated-social-media-policy/#.Xz7AYuhKhPY).

CONCLUSION

Boundary violations in behavioral health professionals are not new. As in every profession, a relatively small group of practitioners crosses the proverbial line and engages in conduct that contravenes widely embraced ethical standards. Such conduct causes profound harm to clients and imperils practitioners' careers.

The advent of digital technology has introduced novel and unprecedented opportunities for boundary violations. Informal, casual, and spontaneous electronic communications between clinicians and clients—in the form of text messages, email messages, online postings, and private messages on social networking sites—can lead to a loosening of what would otherwise be tight boundaries in the clinical relationship. In the digital age, practitioners must be careful to avoid casual electronic exchanges that may confuse professional–client boundaries—maintaining a professional tone is critically important.

The fact that digital and other electronic communications can occur so easily outside of customary work hours and the context of face-to-face counseling can enhance both clients' and professionals' uncertainty and confusion about the nature of their relationships. Although most clinicians use digital and other electronic communication options responsibly, some do not, and this can be a prelude to boundary violations.

Some clinicians engage in extracurricular electronic communications with well-meaning intent, perhaps to enhance clients' access to services and to offer emotional support to clients. What may start out as truly innocent communications may lead to boundary ambiguity and, ultimately, inappropriate contact, both electronic and physical. In extraordinary instances, unscrupulous clinicians use electronic communications with clients as a manipulative tool, and as a calculated grooming strategy designed to seduce clients.

We now know that the digital age has brought with it new and unprecedented boundary-related risks and perils, along with many benefits in behavioral health practitioners' efforts to assist people who struggle. Going forward, our task is to be mindful of technology's two-sided coin, be alert to potential risks, be earnest in our efforts to educate practitioners about the responsible use of technology, and be diligent in our efforts to prevent and confront misconduct.

REFERENCES

American Mental Health Counselors Association. (2020). *AMHCA code of ethics*. http://connections.amhca.org/HigherLogic/System/DownloadDocumentFile.ashx? DocumentFileKey=d4e10fcb-2f3c-c701-aa1d-5d0f53b8bc14

American Psychiatric Association. (n.d.). *Telepsychiatry.* https://www.psychiatry.org/psychiatrists/practice/telepsychiatry

American Psychiatric Association. (2013). *Diagnostic and statistical manual of mental disorders* (5th ed.).

Association of Marital and Family Therapy Regulatory Boards. (2016, September). *Teletherapy guidelines.* https://amftrb.org/wp-content/uploads/2017/05/Proposed-Teletherapy-Guidelines-DRAFT-as-of-09.12.16.pdf

Association of Social Work Boards. (2015, March). *Model regulatory standards for technology and social work practice.* https://www.aswb.org/wp-content/uploads/2015/03/ASWB-Model-Regulatory-Standards-for-Technology-and-Social-Work-Practice.pdf

Association of State and Provincial Psychology Boards. (2013). *ASPBB telepsychology task force principles and standards.* https://www.asppb.net/page/Telepsych

Barglow, P. (2005). Self-disclosure in psychotherapy. *American Journal of Psychotherapy, 59*(2), 83–99. https://doi.org/10.1176/appi.psychotherapy.2005.59.2.83

Barsky, A. E. (2017). Social work practice and technology: Ethical issues and policy responses. *Journal of Technology in Human Services, 35*(1), 8–19. https://doi.org/10.1080/15228835.2017.1277906

Bograd, M. (1993). The duel over dual relationships. *Family Therapy Networker, 16*(6), 32–37.

Bridges, N. A. (2001). Therapist's self-disclosure: Expanding the comfort zone. *Psychotherapy: Theory, Research, Practice, Training, 38*(1), 21–30. https://doi.org/10.1037/0033-3204.38.1.21

Brodsky, A. M. (1986). The distressed psychologist: Sexual intimacies and exploitation. In R. R. Kilburg, P. E. Nathan, & R. W. Thoreson (Eds.), *Professionals in distress: Issues, syndromes, and solutions in psychology* (pp. 153–171). American Psychological Association. https://doi.org/10.1037/10056-008

Celenza, A. (2007). *Sexual boundary violations: Therapeutic, supervisory, and academic contexts.* Aronson.

Chester, A., & Glass, C. A. (2006). Online counselling: A descriptive analysis of therapy services on the internet. *British Journal of Guidance & Counselling, 34*(2), 145–160. https://doi.org/10.1080/03069880600583170

Cornell, W. F. (2007). The intricate intimacies of psychotherapy and questions of self-disclosure. *European Journal of Psychotherapy and Counselling, 9*(1), 51–61. https://doi.org/10.1080/13642530601164372

Drum, K. B., & Littleton, H. L. (2014). Therapeutic boundaries in telepsychology: Unique issues and best practice recommendations. *Professional Psychology: Research and Practice, 45*(5), 309–315. https://doi.org/10.1037/a0036127

Epstein, R. S. (1994). *Keeping boundaries: Maintaining safety and integrity in the psychotherapeutic process.* American Psychiatric Association.

Farber, B. A. (2006). *Self-disclosure in psychotherapy: Patient, therapist, and supervisory perspectives.* Guilford Press.

Federation of State Medical Boards. (2012). Model policy guidelines for the appropriate use of social media and social networking in medical practice. *Journal of Medical Regulation, 98*(2), 27–33. https://doi.org/10.30770/2572-1852-98.2.27

Federation of State Medical Boards. (2014). *Model policy for the appropriate use of telemedicine technologies in the practice of medicine.* https://www.fsmb.org/Media/Default/PDF/FSMB/Advocacy/FSMB_Telemedicine_Policy.pdf

Finn, J. (2006). An exploratory study of email use by direct service social workers. *Journal of Technology in Human Services*, *24*(4), 1–20. https://doi.org/10.1300/J017v24n04_01

Gabbard, G. O. (Ed.). (1989). *Sexual exploitation in professional relationships*. American Psychiatric Press.

Gabbard, G. O. (1996). Lessons to be learned from the study of sexual boundary violations. *American Journal of Psychotherapy*, *50*(3), 311–322. https://doi.org/10.1176/appi.psychotherapy.1996.50.3.311

Graffeo, I., & La Barbera, D. (2009). Cybertherapy meets Facebook, blogger, and second life: An Italian experience. In *Annual review of cybertherapy and telemedicine* (Vol. 144, pp. 108–112). https://doi.org/10.3233/978-1-60750-017-9-108

Greysen, S. R., Chretien, K. C., Kind, T., Young, A., & Gross, C. P. (2012). Physician violations of online professionalism and disciplinary actions: A national survey of state medical boards [Research Letter]. *Journal of the American Medical Association*, *307*(11), 1141–1142. https://doi.org/10.1001/jama.2012.330

Gutheil, T. G. (1989). Borderline personality disorder, boundary violations, and patient–therapist sex: Medicolegal pitfalls. *The American Journal of Psychiatry*, *146*(5), 597–602. https://doi.org/10.1176/ajp.146.5.597

Gutheil, T. G., & Brodsky, A. (2008). *Preventing boundary violations in clinical practice*. Guilford Press.

Gutheil, T. G., & Simon, R. I. (1995). Between the chair and the door: Boundary issues in the therapeutic "transition zone." *Harvard Review of Psychiatry*, *2*(6), 336–340. https://doi.org/10.3109/10673229509017154

Gutheil, T. G., & Simon, R. I. (2005). E-mails, extra-therapeutic contact, and early boundary problems: The internet as a "slippery slope." *Psychiatric Annals*, *35*(12), 952–961. https://doi.org/10.3928/00485713-20051201-02

Herlihy, B., & Corey, G. (2015). *Boundary issues in counseling: Multiple roles and responsibilities* (3rd ed.). American Counseling Association. https://doi.org/10.1002/9781119221586

Joint Task Force for the Development of Telepsychology Guidelines for Psychologists. (2013). Guidelines for the practice of telepsychology. *American Psychologist*, *68*(9), 791–800. https://doi.org/10.1037/a0035001

Kanani, K., & Regehr, C. (2003). Clinical, ethical, and legal issues in e-therapy. *Families in Society: The Journal of Contemporary Social Services*, *84*(2), 155–162. https://doi.org/10.1606/1044-3894.98

Kilburg, R. R., Kaslow, F. W., & VandenBos, G. R. (1988). Professionals in distress. *Hospital & Community Psychiatry*, *39*(7), 723–725.

Knox, S., & Hill, C. E. (2003). Therapist self-disclosure: Research-based suggestions for practitioners. *Journal of Clinical Psychology*, *59*(5), 529–539. https://doi.org/10.1002/jclp.10157

Kolmes, K. (2010, Summer). Developing my private practice social media policy. *Independent Practitioner*, *30*(3), 140–142.

Kolmes, K., & Taube, D. O. (2016). Client discovery of psychotherapist personal information online. *Professional Psychology: Research and Practice*, *47*(2), 147–154. https://doi.org/10.1037/pro0000065

Lannin, D. G., & Scott, N. A. (2013). Social networking ethics: Developing best practices for the new small world. *Professional Psychology: Research and Practice*, *44*(3), 135–141. https://doi.org/10.1037/a0031794

Lazarus, A. A., & Zur, O. (Eds.). (2002). *Dual relationships and psychotherapy*. Springer Publishing.

Menon, G. M., & Miller-Cribbs, J. (2002). Online social work practice: Issues and guidelines for the profession. *Advances in Social Work*, *3*(2), 104–116. https://doi.org/10.18060/34

Midkiff, D., & Wyatt, W. J. (2008). Ethical issues in the provision of online mental health services (etherapy). *Journal of Technology in Human Services*, *26*(2–4), 310–332. https://doi.org/10.1080/15228830802096994

Moleski, S. M., & Kiselica, M. S. (2005). Dual relationships: A continuum ranging from destructive to the therapeutic. *Journal of Counseling & Development*, *83*(1), 3–11. https://doi.org/10.1002/j.1556-6678.2005.tb00574.x

Mossman, D., & Farrell, H. M. (2012). Facebook: Social networking meets professional duty. *Current Psychiatry*, *11*(3), 34–37.

National Association of Social Workers. (2017). *NASW code of ethics*. https://www.socialworkers.org/About/Ethics/Code-of-Ethics/Code-of-Ethics-English

National Association of Social Workers, Association of Social Work Boards, Council on Social Work Education, and Clinical Social Work Association. (2017). *NASW, ASWB, CSWE, & CSWA standards for technology in social work practice*. https://www.socialworkers.org/LinkClick.aspx?fileticket=lcTcdsHUcng%3d&portalid=0

National Board for Certified Counselors. (2016). *National Board for Certified Counselors policy regarding the provision of distance professional services*. http://www.nbcc.org/Assets/Ethics/NBCCPolicyRegardingPracticeofDistanceCounselingBoard.pdf

Peterson, M. R. (1992). *At personal risk: Boundary violations in professional–client relationships*. W. W. Norton.

Pope, K. S. (1988). How clients are harmed by sexual contact with mental health professionals: The syndrome, and its prevalence. *Journal of Counseling & Development*, *67*(4), 222–226. https://doi.org/10.1002/j.1556-6676.1988.tb02587.x

Pope, K. S., & Bouhoutsos, J. (1986). *Sexual intimacy between therapists and patient*. Praeger.

Reamer, F. G. (2003). Boundary issues in social work: Managing dual relationships. *Social Work*, *48*(1), 121–133. https://doi.org/10.1093/sw/48.1.121

Reamer, F. G. (2015). *Risk management in social work: Preventing professional malpractice, liability, and disciplinary action*. Columbia University Press.

Reamer, F. G. (2017). Evolving ethical standards in the digital age. *Australian Social Work*, *70*(2), 148–159. https://doi.org/10.1080/0312407X.2016.1146314

Reamer, F. G. (2019, January). Boundary challenges in the digital age. *Social Work Today*. https://www.socialworktoday.com/news/eoe_0119.shtml

Reamer, F. G. (2020). *Boundary issues and dual relationships in the human services* (3rd ed.). Columbia University Press.

Reamer, F. G. (2021). *Ethics and risk management in online and distance behavioral health*. Cognella Academic Publishing.

Recupero, P. R., & Reamer, F. G. (2018). The internet and forensic ethics. In E. E. H. Griffith (Ed.), *Ethics challenges in forensic psychiatry and psychology practice* (pp. 208–222). Columbia University Press.

Roberts, J. (2005). Transparency and self-disclosure in family therapy: Dangers and possibilities. *Family Process*, *44*(1), 45–63. https://doi.org/10.1111/j.1545-5300.2005.00041.x

Schoener, G. R. (1995). Assessment of professionals who have engaged in boundary violations. *Psychiatric Annals, 25*(2), 95–99. https://doi.org/10.3928/0048-5713-19950201-08

Simon, R. I. (1992). Treatment boundary violations: Clinical, ethical, and legal considerations. *The Bulletin of the American Academy of Psychiatry and the Law, 20*(3), 269–288.

Simon, R. I. (1995). The natural history of therapist sexual misconduct: Identification and prevention. *Psychiatric Annals, 25*(2), 90–94. https://doi.org/10.3928/0048-5713-19950201-07

Simon, R. I. (1999). Therapist–patient sex. From boundary violations to sexual misconduct. *Psychiatric Clinics of North America, 22*(1), 31–47. https://doi.org/10.1016/S0193-953X(05)70057-5

Skinner, A., & Zack, J. S. (2004). Counseling and the internet. *American Behavioral Scientist, 48*(4), 434–446. https://doi.org/10.1177/0002764204270280

Sonnenstuhl, W. J. (1989). Reaching the impaired professional: Applying findings from organizational and occupational research. *Journal of Drug Issues, 19*(4), 533–539. https://doi.org/10.1177/002204268901900407

Stricker, G., & Fisher, M. (Eds.). (1990). *Self-disclosure in the therapeutic relationship.* Plenum Press. https://doi.org/10.1007/978-1-4899-3582-3

Syme, G. (2003). *Dual relationships in counselling and psychotherapy: Exploring the limits.* Sage. https://doi.org/10.4135/9781446218624

VandenBos, G. R., & Duthie, R. F. (1986). Confronting and supporting colleagues in distress. In R. R. Kilburg, P. E. Nathan, & R. W. Thoreson (Eds.), *Professionals in distress: Issues, syndromes, and solutions in psychology* (pp. 211–231). American Psychological Association. https://doi.org/10.1037/10056-011

Zur, O. (2007). *Boundaries in psychotherapy: Ethical and clinical explorations.* American Psychological Association. https://doi.org/10.1037/11563-000

Zur, O. (2012). TelePsychology or TeleMentalHealth in the digital age: The future is here. *California Psychologist, 45*(1), 13–15.

Zur, O. (Ed.). (2017). *Multiple relationships in psychotherapy and counseling: Unavoidable, common, and mandatory dual relations in therapy.* Routledge.

12
CONSIDERING RACIAL AND CULTURAL CONTEXT IN SEXUAL BOUNDARY VIOLATIONS

PRATYUSHA TUMMALA-NARRA

Attending to issues of race and culture, as well as to intersections of identities, is a critical ethical imperative in helping clients to cope with and heal from sexual boundary violations (SBVs). Power dynamics related to racism and other forms of social oppression can exacerbate the vulnerability of clients who are sexually exploited by their therapists. Yet, little attention is given in the psychological literature to SBVs in psychotherapy that affect racial and ethnic minorities. In fact, in my review of literature concerning SBVs faced by racial minority women, there was no scholarship focused on violations occurring in the context of psychotherapy. Questions of safety and protection in the therapeutic relationship are of utmost importance for all clients at any point in history. However, the current sociopolitical climate in the United States, characterized by heightened explicit racism and xenophobia, calls for closer attention to the experiences of violation that may be unique among racial minority clients.

This chapter explores the experiences of racial and ethnic minority clients with regard to disclosures concerning sex, sexuality, and violations in psychotherapy. Specifically, the client's conceptualizations of privacy around

https://doi.org/10.1037/0000247-012
Sexual Boundary Violations in Psychotherapy: Facing Therapist Indiscretions, Transgressions, and Misconduct, A. Steinberg, J. L. Alpert, and C. A. Courtois (Editors)
Copyright © 2021 by the American Psychological Association. All rights reserved.

sexuality, stigma against speaking openly about sexual violence, and racial-ized and sexualized stereotyping shape the client's experience of SBVs and decisions concerning disclosure. In the basic dynamic of psychotherapy, the therapist's role is to protect the client's privacy, and yet, the therapist asks to be allowed into the client's inner, private world. In this chapter, I explore how the meanings of this engagement vary with sociocultural experiences (including sociocultural trauma), with important implications for how racial and ethnic minority clients may approach SBVs. As literature addressing SBVs faced by racial and/or ethnic minority clients is virtually absent, this chapter draws primarily on literature focused on social, cultural, and contex-tual factors that should be considered in extending literature, dialogue, and training concerning SBVs in psychotherapy.

AN ETHIC OF CARE IN WHICH BOUNDARIES ARE MAINTAINED

Conceptualizations of ethics underlying the therapeutic relationship serve as critical frameworks through which SBVs are experienced and understood. Pope and Vasquez (2011) likened psychotherapy to surgery in that both rely on trust. They stated that surgery patients

> trust surgeons not to take advantage of their vulnerability to harm or exploit them. Therapy patients undergo a process of psychological opening up in the hope that their condition will improve. They trust us not to harm or exploit them. (p. 35)

Pope and Vasquez (2011) further pointed to Freud's observation that transference has the potential to harm in psychotherapy. Freud introduced the idea that the analysis of transference and countertransference is funda-mental to psychoanalysis, as it reveals unconscious fantasies of the other in the therapeutic relationship. He also noted that "psychoanalysis . . . is not afraid to handle the most dangerous forces in the mind and set them to work for the benefit of the patient" (Freud, 1963, p. 179). Freud under-stood that the analyst held considerable power when the patient trusted the analyst, and he believed that countertransference interfered with the patient's ability to explore unconscious material and with the therapist's interpreta-tion of the client's unconscious. There was an ethic of care underlying this notion, in that he recognized the importance of the client's experience and needs without the imposition of the therapist's unconscious needs and wishes. Interestingly, in recent decades, psychoanalytic theory has reconsidered the notion that views countertransference as only harmful to the client. Relational psychoanalysts, in particular, have drawn attention to the idea that countertransference is not only inevitable, but it is also something that can inform the dynamics within the therapeutic relationship (Dimen, 2017). Relational psychoanalysis has also extended the possibility that the therapist and client not only influenced each other based on personal life histories but also based on social location and position.

In parallel, multicultural and feminist psychologists, such as Comas-Díaz and Jacobsen (1991), have drawn attention to this phenomenon as well, coining the term *ethnocultural transference*. For example, the therapist and the client make assumptions about each other based on their sociocultural histories and identities as well as exposure or lack of exposure to specific sociocultural groups. Relatedly, the American Psychological Association's (APA; 2002) *Guidelines on Multicultural Education, Training, Research, Practice, and Organizational Change for Psychologists* (hereinafter, *Guidelines*; see also Clauss-Ehlers et al., 2019) detailed specific approaches in working with racial and ethnic minority clients in response to the neglect of sociocultural issues in traditional paradigms of psychotherapy. These *Guidelines* recognize that psychologists are cultural beings with attitudes and beliefs that influence perceptions of and interactions with others, and their conceptualizations.

The *Guidelines* raise important questions about the implication of unconscious processes in shaping perceptions of those whom we perceive as socioculturally different from or similar to ourselves. A psychoanalytic sensibility of ethics can help to expand our understanding of how sociocultural oppression is experienced intrapsychically and how its effects manifest interpersonally both within and outside of the therapeutic relationship. In psychoanalytic psychotherapy, an ethic of care requires that there is a respect for uncertainty and contradiction. There is a necessary mourning of loss, even that which occurs within the therapeutic dyad, where the therapist will never completely fulfill the unmet needs of the client. The therapist's conscious and unconscious desires interact with those of the client and, therefore, must be closely examined—this is an ethical position of psychoanalytic work (Kirshner, 2012).

When therapy itself poses a violation to the client's sense of safety and dignity, harm is experienced across multiple, interconnected layers that reflects betrayal at both interpersonal and systemic levels. The following case vignette illustrates the complex harm that is experienced by a client who faced SBVs interwoven with racism by a therapist, in addition to coping with sexual assault that occurred in adolescence. (Any information potentially identifying the client has been removed in order to protect the client's privacy, and permission to discuss this case material has been granted.)

SBVs WITHIN THE THERAPEUTIC RELATIONSHIP: CASE VIGNETTE

Celina is a 36-year-old straight-identified Dominican American cisgender woman with whom I worked in individual psychotherapy for 2 years. She was born and raised in an urban area of the United States, and her parents emigrated from the Dominican Republic to the United States as young adults. She sought psychotherapy after experiencing depressed mood related to loss and trauma early in her life. Celina was reluctant to seek the help of a therapist and specifically sought to work with a female therapist. Celina's mother died from an illness when she was 11 years old, and she and her brother were cared for thereafter by her father and a paternal aunt who lived with them. When she was 14 years old, she was sexually assaulted by a male stranger who broke into their home. For much of her adolescence and early adulthood, Celina experienced posttraumatic symptoms, such as nightmares, anxiety, and isolation. While a junior in college, she began working with a White female therapist with whom she developed a close connection. However, this relationship ended prematurely when her therapist abruptly stopped treatment after a few months in order to relocate to a different part of the country.

A few years after graduating college, after her feelings of anxiety, sadness, and loss escalated, Celina began working with a White male therapist. She had initially been reluctant to work with a White man, largely due to her experiences of racism that were heightened since college, and because of her traumatic experience of being sexually assaulted by a man. However, as this was a therapist who was available both to meet with her and accepted her health insurance plan, she decided to see him. Further, the therapist came highly recommended by her primary care physician. Celina worked with this therapist for approximately 6 months. Gradually, over the course of 3 months, she felt cared for by this therapist and began to openly share with him her longing for her mother, and the anxiety that she felt when around some men. She spoke of her feelings of being terrorized by the man who assaulted her. When the therapist asked her to describe the assault in more detail, she felt somewhat uncomfortable and explained to him that she wasn't used to talking about sex or the assault, especially with men. She told him that her father was not comfortable talking with her about the assault, even though he felt deeply saddened by what had happened to her. The therapist responded by asking her if her father's response was connected with being Dominican. Celina told the therapist that it is not typical for Dominican families to talk openly about sexual assault, after which the therapist told her that it must be difficult for her because she is American. Celina later recalled feeling ambivalently about the therapist's response, but she decided not to speak about this further.

Over the course of the next several weeks, she noticed that her therapist would make comments about her appearance, such as "You look good today," and "Did you change your hair? It looks nice." Initially, she perceived these comments to be affirming. In my work with Celina, she stated, "In these moments with him, I felt like he was probably trying to build up my self-esteem or something. So, I didn't think much of it." In one particularly difficult session a couple of months later, when Celina discussed her sadness about her mother's death and as she revealed more about her sense of being alone, the therapist asked if he could hug her. She gave permission for him to do so. The hugs continued in the next three sessions, and in the last of these sessions, she sensed that he wanted to kiss her. She decided to push him away from her and left the session. She later called the therapist and left a voicemail message to let him know that she would no longer be working with him. The therapist never followed up with her.

In our work, Celina was overwhelmed with shame as she described her experience with this therapist. She asked, "How could I have let him treat me this way? I really don't think I understood what he was doing. Maybe there is something wrong with me." Celina fluctuated between feeling angry toward the therapist and blaming herself for not detecting his negative intentions toward her. Above all, she felt betrayed by his abandonment of her, as he never called her back. She had hoped that he would call her and apologize for his behavior. In the course of our work together, she further discussed her fear of trusting White men, including therapists. When I asked her to share with me her fears of working with a therapist of any background, including me, she stated, "I don't know that I trust anyone really. I just know that I need help in feeling better. I just feel alone."

The importance of trust in the therapeutic relationship cannot be overstated, and gaining an understanding of the role of sociocultural context in the client's life is critical to establishing trust in psychotherapy. The APA (2017) *Ethical Principles of Psychologists and Code of Conduct* (APA Ethics Code), Principle E: Respect for People's Rights and Dignity, clearly notes that "psychologists respect the dignity and worth of all people" and that

> psychologists are aware of and respect cultural, individual, and role differences, including those based on age, gender, gender identity, race, ethnicity, culture, national origin, religion, sexual orientation, disability, language, and socioeconomic status, and consider these factors when working with members of such groups.

Principle E is only one of many standards and principles that were transgressed in Celina's case. Her previous therapist violated not only sexual boundaries but also the principle of securing her dignity based on race, ethnicity, and gender. The therapist also abandoned his responsibility to respond to her after she contacted him to terminate therapy. Although it may be obvious that Celina's previous therapist violated ethical practice of psychotherapy in a broader sense, it is important to consider how Celina's case illustrates the poignant ways in which sexual boundary violations are linked with social contexts. In particular, Celina's wish for a therapist to care for and help her stood in sharp contrast with the therapist's lack of understanding of her cultural background and experiences with racism; his inappropriate, unethical sexual behavior; and his abandonment of her. There was no recognition in this treatment of the destructive effects of their interaction and, as such, our work entailed mourning this trauma and loss.

Celina's case also highlights the ways in which clients may conceptualize privacy around issues of sexuality and sexual violence that differ from the therapist's conceptions in significant ways. The therapist's inquiry into these issues may itself be experienced as an intrusion over which the client may feel little control. It is critical that therapists attend to these differences in cultural worldviews and attend to the dynamics of power when considering whether or not to ask a client to reveal details of sex and sexual violence. Further, it is important that therapists attend to their own projections related to race, culture, and sexuality and how these projections impact the client's sense of safety and power in psychotherapy. This is especially problematic in a society where racial minority clients cope with racial injustice on an ongoing basis outside of the therapeutic space.

In cross-racial dyads, where the therapist is White and the client is a racial minority, special attention should be directed to power imbalances which, if left unexplored, could be detrimental to the client. Importantly, stereotypes of different racial and ethnic groups are infused with false narratives about sex and sexuality (Bryant-Davis & Tummala-Narra, 2017). The therapist who clearly holds a position of authority and power can use stereotypes to demean the client and those affiliated with the client's racial and/or ethnic group (e.g., family, friends, romantic and sexual partners). For Celina, the therapist's derogation of her racial and ethnic backgrounds is evident in the connection he draws between Celina's father's response to her sexual assault and Dominican ethnicity, as well as through the therapist's portrayal of himself as the more evolved, White American man. The therapist's behavior objectifies Celina by racializing and sexualizing her. As such, his betrayal is multilayered and mirrors broader societal dynamics and injustice concerning race and gender. It is also important to note that these dynamics were both implicit and explicit in their expression as, at times, the therapist made explicit stereotyped statements to the client and, at other moments, neither the therapist nor the client spoke directly about their racial and cultural differences. The silence around race and culture, coupled with stereotyping, impedes the possibility of an authentic, trusting space in which the client can safely explore her traumatic experiences.

PRIVACY, SEXUALITY, AND SOCIOCULTURAL CONTEXT

The ways in which individuals conceptualize and approach boundary violations both within and outside of a therapeutic relationship are influenced by sociocultural context. Specifically, interpersonal boundaries are shaped by cultural norms concerning expressions of intimacy. For example, in some cultural contexts (e.g., some South Asian countries), it is more common to see same-sex friends show affection toward each other physically than it is to see romantic partners show affection toward each other in public. In contrast, in mainstream U.S. context, it is widely accepted when heterosexual couples display physical affection toward each other. These types of cultural differences can have important implications for one's conceptualizations of privacy and sexual boundaries (Tummala-Narra, 2019). Relatedly, there may be taboos regarding open discussions about sex and sexual violence within families and ethnic and/or religious communities. Stigma attached to talking about sexuality may contribute to whether a client reveals details of sexual experiences with a therapist and potentially to whether or not the client feels as though he/she/they can reveal sexual and/or romantic feelings toward the therapist.

It is also worth considering that notions of privacy and sexual expression shift across contexts and time. This is evident in the experience of immigrants and refugees who are exposed to new cultural constructions concerning privacy and sexuality in an adopted country that contrast from those cultural constructions that exist in the country of origin. There are also differences in perceptions of acceptable norms regarding privacy across immigrant generations. For example, first generation immigrants (those who arrive to the United States as adults) tend to have perspectives on privacy and sexuality rooted in their cultures of origin that may diverge from those of their children and grandchildren who are raised in the United States. The second generation (those born and raised in the United States), on the other hand, contends with conflicting messages regarding privacy and sexual expression within families and ethnic communities and mainstream U.S. context (Tummala-Narra, 2019). These differences in conceptualizations of privacy can influence views of interpersonal boundaries and, at times, make it difficult to identify when the boundaries between therapist and client are crossed. Further, when the therapist and client are unfamiliar with each other's cultural perspectives regarding privacy and self-disclosure, the client may be even more vulnerable to boundary crossing by the therapist.

It is worth noting that there are also significant variations within and across sociocultural communities with regard to seeking help in coping with emotional distress, and the degree to which clients are comfortable sharing details of their personal lives in psychotherapy. Most often, racial and ethnic minorities seek help from informal sources, such as family, friends, clergy, and mentors. In some cases, there is stigma associated with seeking help from a mental health professional. There may be significant consequences for revealing details of family conflict or other painful experiences to people outside of one's family. Children may be socialized to refrain from sharing family matters with others, and the reasons for not disclosing these details may be based on an expectation that one remains loyal to one's family and/or ethnic community. For example, a client, Jasmine, who is a 30-year-old, second-generation Thai American woman, shared with me that telling me about her conflicted feelings about her sister made her feel as though she was betraying her sister and her Thai self. She stated, "I feel like I'm being less Thai, more American by talking about my sister." For Jasmine, her sense of loyalty to her family and to her cultural identity was threatened by disclosing her painful experiences to a therapist who is neither part of her family nor her ethnic community. Disclosing her experiences further posed a threat to her own identifications with Thai culture and community.

Revealing personal experiences in psychotherapy can be especially challenging when a client contends with conflicting sociocultural norms, especially when those in the home discourage seeking the help of mental health professionals, but in the mainstream, it is viewed in a more positive light. Revealing private information in psychotherapy can further contribute to a sense of shame and/or alienation from family and friends who have a negative view of or a lack of trust in mental health providers. Further, the client is even more isolated when a therapist causes harm by crossing sexual boundaries. Specifically, the client may feel more vulnerable to a therapist who crosses boundaries and attempts to "save" the client from disapproving loved ones.

In the case of sexual trauma, cultural constructions of privacy and sexuality influence how an individual experiences sexual violation and approaches disclosure of the violation. Specifically, gender norms across different cultural contexts impact the ways in which people learn about what is acceptable to discuss and disclose to others. It is worth noting the complexity of how sexual violence may be understood within families and ethnic and religious communities, and that individual meanings of cultural or religious practices may vary significantly.

Importantly, there is little empirical research or clinical literature that has examined the experiences of sexual violation faced by racial minority women outside of the context of domestic violence or intimate partner violence, or that faced by racial minority men. Yet, emerging empirical and clinical literature underscores the importance of attending to differences in how survivors across contexts conceptualize, experience, and respond to sexual violence (Tummala-Narra et al., 2019). These sociocultural differences can also have implications for sexual boundary violations within the therapeutic relationship. For example, in the case of Celina, her ambivalence about revealing the details of her sexual assault to her therapist was influenced by cultural norms regarding disclosure of violence. Additionally, her therapist's sexualization and violation of her compounded her sense of shame and betrayal. Although Celina took all measures to protect herself from further violation in therapy, she continued to wonder whether she should ever risk disclosing her assault to others, both because of the therapist's boundary violation and because of the implicit and explicit messages that she received while growing up warning her not to disclose abuse and violence to those outside of the family.

SOCIOCULTURAL OPPRESSION AND SEXUAL VIOLENCE

Conceptualizations of SBVs can be shaped by different forms of socio-cultural oppression and trauma. In particular, historical and ongoing racism, xenophobia, misogyny, homophobia, and other forms of discrimination contribute to fear and mistrust concerning disclosure of issues related to sexuality and violence among racial minorities in the United States. The contemporary U.S. climate is marked with an increase in hate-based crimes directed against racial and religious minorities, immigrants, LGBTQ+ people. On May 25, 2020, the murder of George Floyd by a White police officer once again underscored the devastating violence against Black and Brown people, and the COVID-19 pandemic has revealed the marked racial and economic disparities that place Black and Brown people at risk for contracting the virus, inadequate health care, and violence. The pandemic has certainly highlighted how racial minority communities are marginalized within health care systems, where their sociocultural contexts are either invisible or dismissed.

Additionally, with regard to perceptions of racial minorities in the United States and globally, racial stereotypes carry messages concerning sexuality such that men and women associated with certain racial and/or cultural groups are viewed as carrying nonstandard, non-White, Euro American forms of sexuality that are typically devalued (Bryant-Davis & Tummala-Narra, 2017). For example, in mainstream context (in person and in online spaces), Black men are often portrayed as dangerous predators and Black women are typically portrayed as hypersexual, while Asian men are portrayed as desexualized and Asian women are often seen as exotic, submissive objects. These stereotypes become internalized and shape attitudes regarding sexuality and sexual violation.

The therapeutic relationship can mirror broader social inequities and stereotyping such that the therapist and client enact dynamics related to race, gender, and social class, among other social locations (Holmes, 2016). A racial minority client who has experienced racism may have difficulty trusting that a White therapist will not devalue or dismiss the importance of sociocultural context. In a different case, a racial minority client who has experienced trauma within his/her/their family or community may wish to work with a White therapist, as this therapist may be associated with more acceptance in discussing sexuality and sexual violence (Tummala-Narra, 2016). Systemic and individual forms of racism and related power dynamics can contribute to imbalance in the therapeutic relationship, where the vulnerability of racial and ethnic minority clients is heightened. Amidst such dynamics, a transgressive therapist who takes advantage of the client's marginalized position contributes to further sociocultural oppression. For the client who experiences SBVs, the impact of multiple marginalization and traumatic experience can be profound and long-lasting.

DISCUSSION AND CONCLUDING THOUGHTS

The problem of shame and secrecy that characterizes sexual violations broadly and SBVs in psychotherapy is one that is pervasive across lines of race and culture. Psychoanalytic scholars (Grand, 2017; Pizer, 2017) have noted the ambivalence concerning sexuality within the history of psychoanalysis. Grand (2017), for instance, suggested that although sexual boundaries were initially conceptualized from the perspective of Judeo–Christian ethics, as a central aspect of the therapeutic relationship, nineteen century European patriarchal views of sexual desire contributed to an ambivalence regarding the violation of these boundaries. This "breakable taboo," in Grand's perspective, reflects a "sexual/moral/religious ambivalence" (p. 208). Certainly, the ways in which early analysts, including Freud, approached some of their female patients illustrates how patriarchy determined much of what was conceptualized as acceptable sexual behavior for the patient and the analyst. In the case of racial and ethnic minority clients, racist and xenophobic ideology can become intertwined with sexualization of the client, as well as unconscious and conscious beliefs of the inferiority of the client and the superiority of the therapist (and, therefore, the right to misuse power).

Recently, psychoanalysts have written about their own experiences of sexual violation by their therapists or analysts, marking an important turn in engaging with this problem. For example, Pizer (2017), in describing her experience of violation, called for a therapeutic culture that encourages clinicians to become actively aware of their affective life as it relates to love and sexual desire. She wrote, "experiences of intimacy, shared vulnerability, and transference are now embodied," referring to psychoanalytic process (Pizer, p. 164). She further suggested that the therapist and the client can misconstrue moments of embodiment, often reflecting early unmet needs. Pizer called on clinicians to make feelings of love and desire speakable in supervision and training, such that they can begin to own these feelings rather than project them onto others. Indeed, the lines between caring, affection, love, and sexuality can become blurred for both the therapist and the client. Relatedly, it would be important for clinicians to engage in more candid dialogue concerning race, ethnicity, and other aspects of sociocultural identity and context, such that clinicians can own a fuller range of feelings about these aspects of identity. It is critical for therapists to carefully attune to how a particular way of communicating affection is experienced uniquely by a client based on the client's sociocultural perspectives and on the client's experiences of being a racial minority within a particular context (e.g., U.S. society).

Dimen (2017) elucidated the dynamics of power in sexual boundary violations by noting that, in fact, there are two violations involved in sex between the analyst and patient. The first is "the analyst's abrogation of the tacit agreement, articulated by the Hippocratic oath, that doctors will not use those in their power, patients, for their own pleasure," and the second is "the rejection of the boundary between psychoanalysis and ordinary life" (Dimen, 2017 p. 170). Dimen further pointed out that SBVs in psychotherapy reflect social institutions and not only individual acts.

When considering cultural variations in how people approach sexual violence and experiences of stereotyping and marginalization, securing a safe space to talk openly about sexuality and sexual violation within and outside of one's family and community can be especially challenging for many racial and ethnic minority clients. For those who have suffered sexual violations, institutions facilitate silence and dismissal, making disclosure a shameful and precarious process. Violation itself can not only be sexualized but also racialized. Violation can also be experienced as colonizing, depending on the racial and ethnic background of the therapist and the client.

Too often, psychologists rely on limited training on issues of race and culture to guide their approaches to psychotherapy with racial and ethnic minority clients. At times, therapists overlook the impact that they and their lack of training or skills have on clients, and instead focus on their own experiences of having good intentions. These gaps in understanding have far-reaching consequences on clients who have been and continue to be socially and economically marginalized. They also served to reinforce White supremacist perspectives in psychotherapy that reflect distorted perceptions of sexuality among racial minorities (e.g., sexualization of Black and Brown women). As such, psychology training programs must move beyond general training on diversity issues and attend more specifically to how sociocultural oppression, such as racism and misogyny, contribute to perceptions of clients, dynamics of the therapeutic relationship (e.g., meaning of self-disclosure and boundaries), and to disparities in access to adequate mental health care.

REFERENCES

American Psychological Association. (2002). *Guidelines on multicultural education, training, research, practice, and organizational change for psychologists.* https://www.apa.org/about/policy/multicultural-guidelines-archived.pdf

American Psychological Association. (2017). *Ethical principles of psychologists and code of conduct* (2002, amended effective June 1, 2010, and January 1, 2017). https://www.apa.org/ethics/code/index.aspx

Bryant-Davis, T., & Tummala-Narra, P. (2017). Cultural oppression and human trafficking: Exploring the role of racism and ethnic bias. *Women & Therapy, 40*(1–2), 152–169. https://doi.org/10.1080/02703149.2016.1210964

Clauss-Ehlers, C. S., Chiriboga, D. A., Hunter, S. J., Roysircar, G., & Tummala-Narra, P. (2019). APA Multicultural Guidelines executive summary: Ecological approach to context, identity, and intersectionality. *American Psychologist, 74*(2), 232–244. https://doi.org/10.1037/amp0000382

Comas-Díaz, L., & Jacobsen, F. M. (1991). Ethnocultural transference and countertransference in the therapeutic dyad. *American Journal of Orthopsychiatry, 61*(3), 392–402. https://doi.org/10.1037/h0079267

Dimen, M. (2017). Eight topics: A conversation on sexual boundary violations between Charles Amrhein and Muriel Dimen. *Psychoanalytic Psychology, 34*(2), 169–174. https://doi.org/10.1037/pap0000110

Freud, S. (1963). Further recommendations in the technique of psychoanalysis: Observations on transference-love. In P. Rieff (Ed.), *Freud: Therapy and technique* (pp. 167–179). Collier Books.

Grand, S. (2017). Seductive excess: Erotic transformations, secret predations. *Psychoanalytic Psychology, 34*(2), 208–214. https://doi.org/10.1037/pap0000106

Holmes, D. E. (2016). Culturally imposed trauma: The sleeping dog has awakened. Will psychoanalysis take heed? *Psychoanalytic Dialogues, 26*(6), 641–654. https://doi.org/10.1080/10481885.2016.1235454

Kirshner, L. A. (2012). Toward an ethics of psychoanalysis: A critical reading of Lacan's ethics. *Journal of the American Psychoanalytic Association, 60*(6), 1223–1242. https://doi.org/10.1177/0003065112457876

Pizer, B. (2017). "Why can't we be lovers?" When the price of love is loss of love: Boundary violations in a clinical context. *Psychoanalytic Psychology, 34*(2), 163–168. https://doi.org/10.1037/pap0000126

Pope, K. S., & Vasquez, M. J. T. (2011). *Ethics in psychotherapy and counseling* (4th ed.). John Wiley & Sons. https://doi.org/10.1002/9781118001875

Tummala-Narra, P. (2016). *Psychoanalytic theory and cultural competence in psychotherapy.* American Psychological Association. https://doi.org/10.1037/14800-000

Tummala-Narra, P. (2019). Cross-cultural perspectives on privacy. In S. Akhtar & A. Abbasi (Eds.), *Privacy: Developmental, cultural, and clinical realms* (pp. 83–102). Routledge. https://doi.org/10.4324/9780429202278-6

Tummala-Narra, P., Gordon, J., Gonzalez, L. D., de Mello Barreto, L., Meerkins, T., Nguyen, M., Medzhitova, J., & Perazzo, P. (2019). Breaking the silence: Perspectives on sexual violence among Indian American women. *Asian American Journal of Psychology, 10*(4), 293–306. https://doi.org/10.1037/aap0000159

13

SEXUAL BOUNDARY VIOLATIONS OUTSIDE OF CISGENDER-HETEROSEXUAL DYADS

ELIZABETH CLARK AND KORI BENNETT

The most frequently reported sexual boundary violations (SBVs), the ones about which there is the most extant literature, involve a cisgender, heterosexual male therapist and a cisgender, (presumed) heterosexual female client. However, the possibility of SBVs exists in all therapy relationships, and all occurrences of such violations warrant attention and study in the service of protecting clients and clinicians from the destructive effects of such breaches. In this chapter, we provide an overview of the existing literature on SBVs within configurations outside of the often discussed "cishet" (cisgender and heterosexual) female-identified/cishet male-identified dyad. Examples of such dyads include but are not limited to the following:

- a cishet male client working with a cishet male therapist
- a straight, female and transgender (trans) therapist working with a cishet male client
- a cisgender bisexual female client working with a nonbinary queer therapist
- a nonbinary pansexual therapist working with a nonbinary queer client

https://doi.org/10.1037/0000247-013
Sexual Boundary Violations in Psychotherapy: Facing Therapist Indiscretions, Transgressions, and Misconduct, A. Steinberg, J. L. Alpert, and C. A. Courtois (Editors)
Copyright © 2021 by the American Psychological Association. All rights reserved.

Throughout, when we refer to the sexual orientation or gender identity of a person, it should be assumed that we mean the terms with which they self-identify. However, it should be noted that there is great variation in individual experience of sexuality and gender, both of which may be expressed or understood differently depending on each person's intersecting identities and contextual factors. In addition, two people who use the same descriptor (e.g., woman, nonbinary, bisexual, straight) may experience things quite differently from each other, and they may experience their own identities differently at different points in time.

Before we embark, we wish to acknowledge some tensions and difficulties of language that complicate the discussion. Some of the SBV examples we include are described in the literature as occurring within "same sex" dyads. However, this language is insufficient and misleading for several reasons. First, the use of the term "same sex" is confusing given that the word "sex" refers to a designation made by medical providers based on genital appearance, chromosomes, or secondary sex characteristics. In contrast, "gender" refers to an individual's subjective experience of self (i.e., gender identity) as well as the ways they present themselves through markers such as dress, behavior, or grooming (i.e., gender expression). Therefore, it is likely that examples in the literature, whether "same" or "opposite" sex, are referring to the gender (not the assigned sex) of the individuals in the dyad.

However, to speak of "same" and "opposite" gender is also problematic because these terms reify the inaccurate notion that sex and gender are binary and maleness and femaleness are "opposite" when, in fact, all are more accurately represented as spectra. Despite nearly all infants being assigned a female or male sex at birth, estimates suggest that up to 2% of the population is *intersex*, defined as the presence of genotypic (sex chromosomes) or phenotypic (internal and external genitals, hormones, and secondary sex characteristics) traits that differ from the "platonic ideal" of male or female development (Blackless et al., 2000, p. 151). Additionally, although most people do identify as male or female, many individuals experience themselves as neither or both and may use terms such as nonbinary, genderqueer, or agender to describe their gender identity. Therefore, continuing to use the language of "same" and "opposite" sex or gender excludes or misrepresents the experiences of intersex, nonbinary, and many gender expansive individuals.

We wish to acknowledge another tension present in any discussion of "same sex" SBVs: the term is all too easily used as shorthand for "gay" (or perhaps lesbian) SBVs, but this poses (at least) two problems. First, given the complexities of transference and countertransference in psychotherapy relationships, an erotic attraction can develop and be acted out between two people with the same gender identity, both of whom identify as cisgender and heterosexual; in other words, SBVs need not be identity-syntonic. Secondly, this labelling convention contains cissexist and mono-sexist assumptions, such that experiences of bisexual and/or transgender and nonbinary (TGNB) individuals are likely to be obscured or misrepresented. For example, in the case of a bisexual, trans female client who experiences a boundary violation with a cishet male therapist, the client's sexual orientation and lived experiences as a trans woman add nuances to the dynamics of the violation that would be missed by simply labeling it "opposite-sex." We elaborate further on some of these potential dynamics later in this chapter. Given that there is evidence that bisexual and trans individuals experience sexual abuse and assault at higher rates than their cisgender and gay, lesbian, or heterosexual peers (Stotzer, 2009; Walters et al., 2013), it is crucial to develop conceptual frameworks that describe SBVs without excluding or obscuring their experiences.

To summarize, what the term "same sex" offers in the way of alliteration and pithiness does not outweigh the conceptual minefields it contains. Therefore, we frame this chapter more broadly and inclusively, although recognizing that no discussion can cover all possible therapist–client dyads or all possible dynamics that might lead to SBVs within these dyads. Specifically, we examine therapist–client relational configurations that vary from the more often assumed or discussed cishet male therapist/cishet female client dyads. In this chapter, we use the language of "cishet dyads" to refer to cishet female therapist–cishet male client and cishet male therapist/cishet female client dyads and "non cishet dyads" to refer to other configurations. We do not discuss cishet female therapist and male client dyads; they are covered elsewhere in this text. Following the literature review herein, we offer an alternative framework through which to consider discussion of such dyads.

One final note on language: With the exception of initially including the terminology used by the authors we cite (which we will include in quotation marks), we use "LGBQ" (lesbian, gay, bisexual, queer) or "queer" to refer to nonheterosexual sexual identities; and TGNB (transgender/nonbinary), "gender expansive," or "trans" as umbrella terms to encompass those whose gender identities do not correspond with their assigned sex at birth. We recognize that we too are making choices about what should be kept and lost in the service of clarity and communication. Although we push against language predicated on the gender binary and biological essentialism, we own that the language we use continues to be limited in its ability to capture the diversity of human experience, and that this language will continue to evolve beyond what is currently available to us. As we transition to reviewing the existing literature, we ask that readers keep in mind the above caveats about language and join us in thinking critically about how these studies frame the issue and which experiences they capture and exclude.

OVERVIEW OF THE LITERATURE

Of the information on SBVs in psychotherapeutic settings, there is little that specifically addresses therapist–client configurations other than cishet dyads. A limited number of articles addressing or describing other dyadic configurations have appeared from the 1970s through the present. The lack of literature on SBVs impacting sexual and gender minority clients and therapists is perhaps not surprising given the degree of pathologizing perpetrated by psychiatrists and psychotherapists against LGBQ and gender expansive people. The 1973 removal of "homosexuality" from the *Diagnostic and Statistical Manual of Mental Disorders* was followed by the 1980 additions of "gender identity disorder of childhood" and "transsexualism," which, in turn, have been replaced by "gender dysphoria" (see American Psychiatric Association, 2013, p. 451; Drescher, 2014, 2015). Given the stigma that continues to surround identities and experiences deviating from cishet expectations, it also makes sense that shame and avoidance may have prevented cishet therapists from examining (much less writing about) erotic countertransferential feelings or behaviors toward clients to whom they might not expect to feel attraction.

The earliest studies that mention SBVs outside of cishet dyads typically do so in the context of discussions of the prevalence, correlates, and impacts of SBVs more generally, and they tend to focus on the reported genders of the participants, not their sexual orientations per se. Across multiple studies based on large surveys of providers, the most prevalent configuration of SBV is a male therapist and female patient, with studies reporting percentages ranging from 83% (Schoener & Milgrom, 1987) to 88% (Gartrell et al., 1987; Russell, 1984, as cited in Schoener et al., 1989) to 92.4% (Bouhoutsos et al., 1983) of all SBVs reported in the respective studies. However, these studies have produced divergent results regarding whether SBVs are equally common (Russell, 1984, as cited in Schoener et al., 1989), more common (Bouhoutsos et al., 1983; Gartrell et al., 1986), or less common (Schoener & Milgrom, 1987) in male–male than female–female dyads.

Holroyd and Brodsky (1977) explored psychologists' attitudes toward and experiences of erotic and nonerotic physical contact with patients, finding that roughly half of the respondents thought nonerotic physical contact such as hugging, kissing, or affectionate touching might be helpful to patients on occasion. In terms of "same sex" contact, more female therapist–client dyads reportedly engaged in nonerotic hugging, kissing, and affectionate touching at least occasionally than did male dyads. Although Holroyd and Brodsky did not explicitly state this, inquiry about nonerotic boundary crossings is relevant to the present discussion of SBVs in the context of the "slippery slope" noted by other authors (e.g., Alpert & Steinberg, 2017, p. 144; Celenza, 2007). When aggregating the responses for "same sex" and "opposite sex" therapy dyads, 10.9% of male and 1.9% of female respondents reported having engaged in erotic contact with clients. Holroyd and Brodsky noted that in the "same sex" therapy dyads, reports of erotic contact were rare and consisted mainly of erotic kissing and holding (as opposed to "intercourse"). However, given the heterosexist bias inherent in asking about "intercourse" (implying "real" sex), their findings should not be construed as meaning that the erotic contacts between "same sex" dyads were necessarily less serious or less harmful.

In their nationwide survey of U.S. psychiatrists, Gartrell et al. (1986) found that 7.1% ($N = 1,057$) of male and 3.1% ($N = 257$) of female respondents acknowledged sexual contact with their patients. Sexual contact was defined as "contact which was intended to arouse or satisfy sexual desire in the patient, therapist, or both" (Gartrell et al., p. 1127). Of all the reported sexual contacts in which gender was specified, 7.6% occurred between men and 1.4% occurred between women. However, because the sample was heavily skewed toward male respondents, these percentages may not reflect accurately the relative prevalence of SBVs in female/female versus male/male dyads. The same authors, in a follow-up article assessing psychiatrists' attitudes toward sexual contact with patients, reported that offending psychiatrists were significantly more likely to endorse certain "indications" or reasons that sexual contact might be acceptable (Herman et al., 1987). These included "to change the patient's sexual orientation," which is a chilling reminder of the complicity of some mental health providers in abusive sexual orientation change efforts disproportionately aimed at sexual minority individuals (Herman et al., 1987, p. 166).

Lyn (1995), the only researcher to date who has specifically surveyed gay, lesbian, and bisexual (GLB) therapists ($N = 234$) about SBVs, found that 3.4% (three women and five men) reported having engaged sexually with current clients, and 12.4% (13 women and 16 men) reported having engaged sexually with past clients. She noted that GLB therapists, due to the complexities that come with the tensions around seeking community support while maintaining appropriate boundaries with clients who may be a part of this community, may become more isolated. She also noted that most therapists in her study opposed sexual activity with both former and current clients.

Pope (1994) observed that studies show the overwhelming majority of perpetrators of SBVs are men and victims are women, and suggested that this fact alone might lead researchers to overlook other configurations. Addressing the lack of research on female perpetrators, Benowitz (1994) interviewed Caucasian female participants who had experienced SBVs while working with female therapists. She observed that "many of [the clients] were in the process of questioning and re-identifying their sexual orientation" and posits that this may have made them more vulnerable to SBVs (Benowitz, 1994, p. 71). Benowitz also noted that some of the offending therapists were perceived as heterosexual by participants, suggesting that therapists' own sexual identity exploration may be a contributor to SBVs in female dyads (see also Gartrell & Sanderson, 1994). Albrecht (2003) also researched female therapist–female client SBVs and suggested that stereotypes of women as nurturing and lacking in sexual initiative may contribute to the exclusion of such dyads from the SBV literature. Albrecht's and Benowitz's analyses highlight participants' feelings of betrayal, shame, and compromised capacity to trust, their powerful transferences to their therapists, and complicated feelings about the sexual part of their relationships with their therapists. Several other examples of female therapist–female client SBVs can be found in the new book produced by Therapy Exploitation Link Line (TELL, 2019).

Brown (1989) identified several dynamics that may contribute to boundary violations in lesbian communities, noting that women, perhaps especially those who also hold other marginalized identities (e.g., as sexual minorities, people of color, people with disabilities), may be more likely to deny or be unaware of their power. She wrote,

> The notion that a lesbian therapist is not particularly powerful because she, like her lesbian client, is oppressed in our culture is a dangerously seductive thought; and one very commonly used to rationalize the violation of boundaries by lesbian therapists who have become sexual. (Brown, 1989, p. 22)

Brown (1989) thus stressed the necessity of therapists' recognizing and owning the intrinsic power they have within their professional role and called on lesbian feminist therapists to engage in practices of self-reflection, self-care, and community care in order to address proactively vulnerabilities that might lead practitioners to violate boundaries. Additionally, both Brown (1989) and Gartrell and Sanderson (1994) suggested that feminist and lesbian practitioners may be reluctant to acknowledge SBVs perpetrated by women, noting that such practitioners' desire to escape from heterosexist, patriarchal structures might make it particularly painful to observe the way that abusive dynamics can be recreated in feminist and/or queer communities. They may also feel concern about hurting the larger community by association. Brown, Gantrell, and Sanderson noted, however, that failing to hold community leaders to a high standard of conduct carries greater risk for harm and may also reflect feminist and/or lesbian practitioners' own internalized sexism and homophobia.

Robinson (1993) and Gonsiorek (1995) noted that there is even less literature on SBVs in gay and bisexual male therapy–client dyads than there is on SBVs in female dyads. Robinson interviewed gay men reporting histories of sexual experiences with their male therapists and, comparing his findings to those of Benowitz (1991, as cited in Robinson, 1993), reported that male participants reported fewer posttraumatic symptoms than female participants, but the clients often described experiencing despair, negative self-image, and hopelessness at the end of the therapy relationship. In reflecting on the lack of data on SBVs in male therapist–client dyads, Gonsiorek noted that such dyads are rare in general, and that men are socialized to experience themselves as active rather than passive agents in sexual encounters, which may make it difficult for male clients to recognize the ways in which they have been exploited or violated.

Fickey and Grimm (1998) discussed considerations specific to gay and lesbian therapists with gay and lesbian clients, including clinicians' decision making around coming out in session and the challenges of working in a small community. They then described an experience in which one of the authors preemptively proposed termination to a client due to concerns about managing his own attraction to the client. Sharing this as an example of repair and reflection, Fickey and Grimm encouraged clinicians to draw on internal and external resources in responding to clinical situations in which "eros is present" (p. 87) and offered several suggestions as to how gay and lesbian therapists can prevent ethical transgressions when working with gay and lesbian clients.

COMMENTARY ON THE LITERATURE

Although the literature specifically addressing SBVs outside of cishet, male therapist–female patient dyads is spare, it does yield some convergent themes. Many authors recognize the role of both societal and internalized homophobia in maintaining silence around the issue. There is also considerable attention to the ethical complexities facing queer-identified therapists working with queer patients with whom they share community ties. An additional theme is the maintenance of awareness of the intrinsic power gradient between client and therapist, even when stripped of the gendered power differential of the male therapist–female patient dyad.

There is limited mention in the literature of the possibility that in male–female dyads, one or both people may be queer and/or trans. In one of the few articles to address sexual attraction between a cis male therapist and a cis female client where such attraction is identity-dystonic, Drescher (1996) described a "heterosexual" transference that emerged in his work with a lesbian-identified patient, challenging the assumption that an erotic dynamic cannot develop between gay men and lesbian-identified women or play out within treatment. Drawing on this analysis, Drescher argued that clinicians' attachment to their gender and sexual identities may impede their ability to identify and address erotic transferences and countertransferences that are incongruent with their identities.

Additionally, Morrow (2000) reported several instances of lesbian clients being sexually abused by straight male therapists under the guise of "curing" their sexuality. Additionally, Herman et al. (1987) reported that 7.1% of psychiatrists who had offended sexually endorsed the belief that trying to change the patient's sexual orientation was an acceptable reason for sexual contact with patients, compared to 0.7% of nonoffending psychiatrists. However, given that prevalence studies have generally not collected sexual orientation data nor asked about TGNB identity or experience, it seems likely that the absence of such dyads from the literature is more a result of erasure or invisibility of queer and trans identities than a reliable representation that such SBVs happen infrequently or not at all.

In literature that does specifically address SBVs involving dyads of the same gender or those that occur within queer communities, we found limited mention of sexual minority identities besides gay or lesbian, nor could we find any studies or articles that discussed SBVs in dyads that include a transgender client and/or therapist. These are significant limitations, given evidence that bisexual and transgender individuals have higher lifetime prevalence of sexual abuse and assault than cisgender gay men, lesbians, and heterosexuals (Stotzer, 2009; Walters et al., 2013), and that previous SBV literature has identified a past history of sexual abuse as a risk factor for victimization in treatment (Celenza, 2007). We suggest that other sexual minority communities, including those who identify on the asexual spectrum and those who practice BDSM/kink[1] and/or polyamory/consensual

---

[1]BDSM/kink = bondage, discipline, dominance and submission, sadomasochism/kink.

nonmonogamy, may also be at unique risk for SBVs in therapy. In the former case, given that some clinicians have attempted to "cure" nonheterosexuality through sexual contact (Morrow, 2000) and that biases regarding asexuality as pathological or intrinsically trauma-informed abound (Foster & Scherrer, 2014), it is reasonable to feel concern that individuals identifying on the "ace" spectrum (e.g., asexual, demisexual, gray ace) may be at risk for abusive therapy "interventions." In contrast, individuals involved in the kink and/or polyamory communities may be oversexualized by therapists, objectified both as sources of education about unfamiliar subcultures and as potential sexual partners because of mistaken stereotypes of having fewer or more lax boundaries around sexuality. They may also be encouraged to engage in extensive and detailed discussions of their sexual experiences to meet the prurient needs of voyeuristic therapists.

Finally, a very clear limitation in the literature is the pervasive absence of discussion of racial, cultural, socioeconomic, ability, and other identity factors that complicate both the power dynamics of the therapy relationship and perceptions of boundary violations within them. Bemak and Chung (2014) addressed the ways in which Euro American paradigms influence how clinicians understand boundaries and relationships in the United States, which they note continues to shift and evolve demographically regarding ethnicity and race. They emphasized the importance of avoiding reenacting historical traumas affecting clients of color through the application of culturally incongruent boundaries and encourage clinicians to consider community-based interventions, self-disclosure, gift giving, socializing with clients, touch, bartering, and the ways in which "different roles crease different boundaries" (Bemak & Chung, 2014, p. 87). Drawing on work by Barnett et al., they noted that "some boundaries are universal" including "engaging in inappropriate behaviors and sexual relationships" (as cited in Bemak & Chung, 2014, p. 86). The absence of cultural considerations from literature addressing SBVs involving cisgender queer/GLB and trans/gender expansive people is illustrative of how oppressive power structures can be reproduced in "LGBT" communities, privileging the experiences of upper- and middle-class White, able-bodied, cisgender and male U.S. citizens. Although we too are foregrounding sexual orientation and gender identity in the present discussion, we encourage ourselves and readers to consider critically how these identities interface with the cultural contexts and other identities of therapists and clients, adding specificity and complexity to the dynamics. Fors (2018) and Tummala-Narra (2016) each offered valuable frameworks for considering the interplay of power structures and intersections of identity in clinical work (although without a specific focus on SBVs, but see Chapter 12).

A NEW FRAMEWORK FOR DISCUSSING SBVs IN NONCISHET DYADIC CONFIGURATIONS

As noted previously, there are many problems with the ways in which SBVs that occur outside of cishet patient/clinician dyads are framed and discussed. Indeed, one of the challenges, as we noted in the introduction, is the grouping together of all such SBVs, a grouping that may include "opposite-" or different-gender dyads with one or more queer/trans members, as well as "same" gender dyads in which both parties identify as cisgender and straight. In order to facilitate our discussion of these many kinds of dyads, we propose the following descriptive language:

- "Identity-syntonic configurations" in which neither party's sense of sexual orientation or gender identity is threatened by SBV (e.g., a cis lesbian therapist and a cis female bisexual patient),

- "Identity-dystonic configurations" in which both parties' sense of sexual orientation or identity are threatened by SBV (e.g., a cishet male therapist experiencing attraction to a cishet male client),

- "Mixed-up configurations" in which the therapist (the party in the "up" or more powerful position) experiences the SBV as identity-syntonic, while the client experiences it as identity-dystonic (e.g., a cis gay male therapist with a cis straight male patient), and

- "Mixed-down configurations" in which the therapist (the party in the "up" or more powerful position) experiences the SBV as identity-dystonic, while the client experiences it as identity-syntonic (e.g., a cishet female therapist and a transgender, lesbian-identified patient).

We are not suggesting that identity-syntonic SBVs are necessarily *ego-syntonic* or experienced as acceptable, although there may be instances in which this is true. We also do not intend to suggest that identity is fixed and unchanging; rather, we refer to the individuals' sense of their identities at the time the SBV occurs, recognizing that both sexuality and gender identity can be fluid over time. Indeed, patients often use therapy to explore and clarify their identities, making it a space in which shifts in consciously held identity may be especially likely to emerge. (Therapists may do the same, however inappropriately; see, Gartrell, 2010, for one such example.) It may also be the case that identity-dystonic SBVs could play out relative to identities other than gender identity or sexual orientation.

In addition, there may be other elements of power (e.g., race, age, ability, citizenship status, religion) at play in the "up/down" dynamics. Even the example used below to illustrate a "mixed-up configuration" is one complicated by the heterosexual privilege held by the patient relative to his gay therapist. Despite these complexities, we use "up" and "down" to refer to power in the therapeutic relationship, underscoring the importance of holding in mind the power imbalance inherent in this relationship, even while considering other dimensions of privilege. In addition to avoiding the previously mentioned problems with "same" and "opposite" sex language, these terms serve to maintain a focus on (a) power, (b) identity, and (c) defensive processes blocking clinicians' awareness of erotic attractions and feelings that might contribute to SBVs.

VULNERABILITIES THAT MAY INCREASE THE LIKELIHOOD OF SBVs IN NONCISHET DYADS

Multiple Relationships in LGB/Queer and/or Gender Expansive Communities

Plaut (1997) noted, "Effective prevention [of SBVs] involves an understanding of the nature of trust-based relationships and the realization that the crossing of sexual boundaries reflects an extreme of a continuum of what are often called dual relationships" (p. 77). This clear, yet nuanced, understanding of clinicians enacting SBVs as exploiting the trust in one relationship (the therapeutic relationship) in order to create another (a romantic and/or sexual relationship) at the expense of the treatment and the client's well-being allows us to consider how "dual" or "multiple" relationships are connected to SBVs. Queer and/or trans clients often wish to work with someone in their communities. Each of the authors has worked with many clients who, at first contact, expressed an explicit preference to work with a gay, queer, and/or trans therapist (Bennett & Clark, in press). Because TGNB and/or queer/LGB communities are both diverse and small, multiple relationships are often unavoidable for queer/trans therapists working within community and, therefore, they must be negotiated carefully (Gartrell, 1992; Kessler & Waehler, 2005). To be clear, we have not come across any evidence suggesting that therapists identifying as part of the "LGBT" community are more likely to engage in SBVs than cishet therapists; to make such an unfounded assumption would enact an incredibly damaging stereotype of cisgender LGBQ and gender-expansive people as sexual predators. Rather, we name this stereotype both as a way to foster awareness around its potential activation as well as to discuss the special considerations important for queer/TGNB clinicians working with queer/TGNB patients.

Indeed, in their efforts to avoid even the appearance of boundary crossings and violations, queer and/or trans therapists risk reacting too rigidly when presented with boundary considerations relevant to multiple roles; for example, therapists sometimes mismanage these situations by opting out of meaningful activities as a means of avoiding clients, which can detrimentally impact the therapy and could, ironically, increase vulnerability to committing SBVs. This is consistent with other literature on SBVs, identifying them as resulting, in large part, from failures of self-care on the part of therapists, leaving the therapy narcissistically depleted and more likely to rely on their clients to meet emotional, social, and sexual needs (Celenza & Gabbard, 2003; Tylim, 2017). Recognizing this hazard, several authors encourage therapists to actively engage in such outside activities for their own well-being (Fickey & Grimm, 1998; Kessler & Waehler, 2005; Morrow, 2000). For example, Waehler, who identifies as lesbian, discussed a clinical situation in which a lesbian client expressed interest in becoming involved with a community group of which Waehler was a part. She shared her process of seeking supervision and utilizing Barret et al.'s (2001, as cited in Kessler & Waehler, 2005) eight-step ethical decision-making model in order to collaborate with her client on an appropriate approach to navigating multiple roles. Similarly, Morrow (2000) advocated for therapists discussing openly with clients the possibility of extratherapeutic encounters, offering reassurances about confidentiality, and inviting the processing of such encounters in session, if/when they occur.

Barriers to Recognizing, Preventing, and Addressing SBVs

Internalized homophobia, biphobia, and transphobia may make it difficult for cishet-identified therapists to recognize and address identity-dystonic attractions to clients with curiosity; rather, shame or discomfort may contribute to therapists avoiding or minimizing the situation. Queer and trans therapists may potentially experience hesitation around seeking consultation to address experiences of attraction, whether dystonic or syntonic, due to worries about perpetuating stereotypes of queer and trans people as predatory or abnormal. Therapists working in noncishet dyads may also be more vulnerable to SBVs due to actual or perceived lack of access to queer and trans-affirming supervision. We are also aware that many therapists are not comfortable, due to life experiences or lack of training, with discussing sexuality in general, thus making it difficult for them to bring any sexual subject matter (including erotic countertransference) into consultation spaces.

The disavowal of power is another potential barrier that may increase vulnerability to SBVs. Due to historical and personal experiences of disempowerment and marginalization, queer and trans therapists might have difficulty recognizing their own inherent power within the clinical dyad (as noted by Brown, 1989), which may be further compounded for those clinicians who also hold other oppressed identities (e.g., those who are disabled, Black, Indigenous, People of Color, economically disadvantaged). On the other hand, these experiences and others related to different kinds of oppression may make queer and TGNB therapists that much more sensitive to power dynamics. A similar paradox concerns queer and TGNB therapists' reactions to ethical guidelines. Some minority therapists may dismiss ethical standards as "oppressive" or "irrelevant" (Gonsiorek, 1995, p. 229) or see them as culturally incongruent (Bemak & Chung, 2014) or as antifeminist and reifying of patriarchal structures (Brown, 1989). On the other hand, due to an internalized sense of defect and the lived realities of oppression, queer, trans, and other minority therapists may feel more pressure to "follow the rules" in order to make up for perceived shortcomings and/or avoid evoking harmful stereotypes.

The following examples include vignettes containing different noncishet dyad configurations, as well as barriers to recognizing, preventing, and addressing SBVs.[2] We wish to emphasize that none of these dynamics, in and of themselves, constitute SBVs or are intrinsically high-risk or pathological, any more so than are erotic transference/countertransference dynamics present in cishet dyads. Rather, the dynamics we describe have the potential to become problematic and lead to SBVs only in combination with underlying and mismanaged vulnerabilities on the part of the therapist. As queer and/or trans clinicians ourselves, we also acknowledge feeling some of the same trepidation described by other authors about offering these examples and scenarios, wishing not to reinforce damaging stereotypes. However, we concur that the potential benefits to (queer and/or TGNB) clinicians, clients, supervisors, supervisees, students, and community members makes opening the space for reflections about these dynamics worthwhile.

Example 1: An Identity-Syntonic Configuration With Lack of Resources
S, a queer and trans female 34-year-old White therapist, is working with a lesbian-identified cisgender Filipinx 36-year-old patient, P. P has become increasingly flirtatious in their sessions. S recognizes that she will have to

---

[2]Any information potentially identifying the client has been removed in order to protect the client's privacy.

address and explore this with P in order to reinforce the frame and explore with P what might be playing out. As she reflects upon these dynamics outside of session, S acknowledges to herself that she is charmed by P, and that it feels good to have a cisgender queer woman, who is close in age, flirt with her in a way that affirms her gender and sexual orientation. S would like to talk about this with her supervisor, but she feels reluctant to do so after hearing her supervisor, a cis straight multiracial woman in her 50s, assume that S shares her attraction to men. Ultimately, after discussing her trepidation with a queer clinician friend for support, S decides to bring up her feelings and concerns in supervision.

Example 2: A Mixed-Down Shifting to Identity-Syntonic Configuration
R, a South Asian, cisgender, straight female 35-year-old therapist, is working with V, a 28-year-old White transmasculine straight patient who started hormone replacement therapy (HRT) a few months ago. During a peer consultation group in which she is discussing their work, R repeatedly misgenders V, with whom she has a strong therapeutic alliance. R experiences embarrassment due to thinking of herself as a trans-affirming ally and confusion in light of her genuine affection for V. She knows that aggression can play out through misgendering, but she does not sense that this dynamic is occurring in this instance. Through exploring the situation in supervision, R realizes that she has experienced increased discomfort in response to feeling more attracted to V as his physical appearance has shifted in response to HRT. R's supervisor, another cishet woman of color, also helps R explore how V's relative privilege as a White person may have been disrupting R's appropriate awareness of her power within the therapy dyad.

Example 3: A Mixed-Up Configuration With Stereotype Activation
P, a Black cisgender gay male therapist in his 40s, has been working for 1 year with J, a 21-year-old Korean American cis male patient who describes himself as "straight but not narrow." P felt paternal warmth toward J early in the treatment when J was experiencing distress related to a recent loss. More recently, he has noticed feelings of increased attraction to J, who has begun talking more about his relationship difficulties and taking longer to leave once the session has ended. P wishes to discuss his feelings with his peer supervision group, which is composed of mostly White straight and cis friends/colleagues who also live in his small town. P is worried that if he shares his feelings with the group, his peers will view him as a predatory older gay man "corrupting" a younger man, and he is also aware that stereotypes of Black men as hypersexual and Asian men as desexualized

could compound his peers' judgment. Ultimately, he decides to call his former supervisor, a gay cisgender man of Color who lives in a larger city several hours away.

RECOMMENDATIONS/FUTURE DIRECTIONS

The examples included in this chapter describe clinicians who are struggling to recognize, accept, and/or address their feelings and are challenged by internal and external barriers. The dynamics contained in these scenarios are both specific to queer and TGNB people and generalizable. For instance, S, the therapist in Example 1, is encountering the compelling experience of being seen accurately and desired. As we know from the work of Fraser (2005), Langer (2016), and others, trans people often grow up without feeling reflected accurately by those around them and society at large. In addition, they are often assumed to be straight and expected to adhere to White, misogynist standards imposed by dominant systems of power. S's experience of feeling seen by her client and not by her supervisor could be particularly challenging if S felt pressure to come out with regard to sexuality in order to get support.

The power of stereotype activation is another important consideration, as we see in Example 3. As P becomes aware of activated internalized stereotypes of older gay men as predatory and of Black men as hypersexual, he experiences shame and anxiety, which is amplified by the "mixed-up configuration" in which J, his cis, straight-identified patient is cast as a potential victim. P does not wish to act on his attraction to J, but he lacks local support in the form of gay-affirmative, culturally sensitive supervision. He thus deals with both internal and external barriers to seeking support and decides to reconnect to an older gay cis male supervisor who shares his experience as a person of color: a creative solution to a less than ideal, yet common, situation for queer and/or trans therapists working in rural areas and small towns.

We hope that our framework may be of help to those who are seeking new language to discuss the defenses, identities, and power dynamics that can impact therapists managing attraction or vulnerability to SBVs in non-cishet dyads. We also wish to note that although LGBQ and trans/gender expansive clinicians may experience vulnerabilities in their work that could contribute to sexual boundary violations, they may also have specific strengths. These include heightened sensitivity to boundaries and power dynamics which, in combination with self-care and community support, may lead to appropriate navigation of challenging dynamics and, in turn, to positive therapeutic outcomes. All clinicians and supervisors have a role to play in creating and maintaining a culture within our profession that makes space for the safe, supported exploration of challenging dynamics without relying on damaging stereotypes or lapsing into false dichotomies of "good/ethical" and "bad/unethical" practitioners.

REFERENCES

Albrecht, J. M. (2003). *Eros defiled: Sexual exploitation of female clients by their female therapists* (Publication No. 305470743) [Doctoral dissertation, Pacifica Graduate Institute]. ProQuest Dissertations and Theses Global.

Alpert, J. L., & Steinberg, A. (L.). (2017). Sexual boundary violations: A century of violations and a time to analyze. *Psychoanalytic Psychology, 34*(2), 144–150. https://doi.org/10.1037/pap0000094

American Psychiatric Association. (2013). *Diagnostic and statistical manual of mental disorders* (5th ed.). https://doi.org/10.1176/appi.books.9780890425596

Bemak, F., & Chung, R. C.-Y. (2014). Cultural boundaries, cultural norms: Multicultural and social justice perspectives on boundaries. In B. Herlihy & G. Corey (Eds.), *Boundary issues in counseling: Multiple roles and responsibilities* (3rd ed., pp. 84–91). American Counseling Association.

Bennett, K., & Clark, E. (in press). Crossing guardians: Signaling and safety in queer and trans therapist/patient dyads. *Psychoanalytic Psychology.*

Benowitz, M. (1994). Comparing the experiences of women clients sexually exploited by female versus male psychotherapists. *Women & Therapy, 15*(1), 69–83. https://doi.org/10.1300/J015v15n01_07

Blackless, M., Charuvastra, A., Derryck, A., Fausto-Sterling, A., Lauzanne, K., & Lee, E. (2000). How sexually dimorphic are we? Review and synthesis. *American Journal of Human Biology, 12*(2), 151–166. https://doi.org/10.1002/(SICI)1520-6300(200003/04)12:2<151::AID-AJHB1>3.0.CO;2-F

Bouhoutsos, J., Holroyd, J., Lerman, H., Forer, B. R., & Greenberg, M. (1983). Sexual intimacy between psychotherapists and patients. *Professional Psychology: Research and Practice, 14*(2), 185–196. https://doi.org/10.1037/0735-7028.14.2.185

Brown, L. S. (1989). Beyond thou shalt not: Thinking about ethics in the lesbian therapy community. *Women & Therapy, 8*(1–2), 13–25. https://doi.org/10.1300/J015v08n01_02

Celenza, A. (2007). *Sexual boundary violations: Therapeutic, supervisory, and academic contexts.* Jason Aronson.

Celenza, A., & Gabbard, G. O. (2003). Analysts who commit sexual boundary violations: A lost cause? *Journal of the American Psychoanalytic Association, 51*(2), 617–636. https://doi.org/10.1177/00030651030510020201

Drescher, J. (1996). Across the great divide: Gender panic in the psychoanalytic dyad. *Psychoanalysis and Psychotherapy, 13*(2), 174–186.

Drescher, J. (2014). Gender identity diagnoses: History and controversies. In B. P. C. Kreukels, T. D. Steensma, & A. L. C. de Vries (Eds.), *Gender dysphoria and disorders of sex development: Progress in care and knowledge* (pp. 137–150). Springer.

Drescher, J. (2015). Out of *DSM*: Depathologizing homosexuality. *Behavioral Sciences, 5*(4), 565–575. https://doi.org/10.3390/bs5040565

Fickey, J., & Grimm, G. (1998). Boundary issues in gay and lesbian psychotherapy relationships. *Journal of Gay & Lesbian Social Services, 8*(4), 77–93. https://doi.org/10.1300/J041v08n04_06

Fors, M. (2018). *A grammar of power in psychotherapy: Exploring the dynamics of privilege.* American Psychological Association. https://doi.org/10.1037/0000086-000

Foster, A. B., & Scherrer, K. S. (2014). Asexual-identified clients in clinical settings: Implications for culturally competent practice. *Psychology of Sexual Orientation and Gender Diversity, 1*(4), 422–430. https://doi.org/10.1037/sgd0000058

Fraser, L. (2005). Therapy with transgender people across the life-span. *American Psychological Association, Division 44 Newsletter, 21,* 14–16.

Gartrell, N. K. (1992). Boundaries in lesbian therapy relationships. *Women & Therapy, 12*(3), 29–50. https://doi.org/10.1300/J015V12N03_03

Gartrell, N. (2010). Boundaries for lesbian physicians. *Journal of Gay & Lesbian Mental Health, 14*(1), 19–27. https://doi.org/10.1080/19359700903368746

Gartrell, N., Herman, J., Olarte, S., Feldstein, M., & Localio, R. (1986). Psychiatrist-patient sexual contact: Results of a national survey. I. Prevalence. *The American Journal of Psychiatry, 143*(9), 1126–1131. https://doi.org/10.1176/ajp.143.9.1126

Gartrell, N., & Sanderson, B. E. (1994). Sexual abuse of women by women in psychotherapy: Counseling and advocacy. *Women & Therapy, 15*(1), 39–54. https://doi.org/10.1300/J015v15n01_05

Gonsiorek, J. C. (1995). Boundary challenges when both therapist and client are males. In J. C. Gonsiorek (Ed.), *Breach of trust: Sexual exploitation by health care professionals and clergy* (pp. 225–233). Sage Publications.

Herman, J. L., Gartrell, N., Olarte, S., Feldstein, M., & Localio, R. (1987). Psychiatrist-patient sexual contact: Results of a national survey: II. Psychiatrists' attitudes. *The American Journal of Psychiatry, 144*(2), 164–169. https://doi.org/10.1176/ajp.144.2.164

Holroyd, J. C., & Brodsky, A. M. (1977). Psychologists' attitudes and practices regarding erotic and nonerotic physical contact with patients. *American Psychologist, 32*(10), 843–849. https://doi.org/10.1037/0003-066X.32.10.843

Kessler, L. E., & Waehler, C. A. (2005). Addressing multiple relationships between clients and therapists in lesbian, gay, bisexual, transgender communities. *Professional Psychology: Research and Practice, 36*(1), 66–72. https://doi.org/10.1037/0735-7028.36.1.66

Langer, S. J. (2016). Trans bodies and the failure of mirrors. *Studies in Gender and Sexuality, 17*(4), 306–316. https://doi.org/10.1080/15240657.2016.1236553

Lyn, L. (1995). Lesbian, gay, and bisexual therapists' social and sexual interactions with clients. In J. C. Gonsiorek (Ed.), *Breach of trust: Sexual exploitation by health care professionals and clergy* (pp. 225–233). Sage Publications.

Morrow, S. L. (2000). First do no harm: Therapist issues in psychotherapy with lesbian, gay, and bisexual clients. In R. M. Perez, K. A. DeBord, & K. J. Bieschke (Eds.), *Handbook of counseling and psychotherapy with lesbian, gay, and bisexual clients* (pp. 137–156). American Psychological Association. https://doi.org/10.1037/10339-006

Plaut, S. M. (1997). Boundary violations in professional–client relationships: Overview and guidelines for prevention. *Sexual and Marital Therapy, 12*(1), 77–94. https://doi.org/10.1080/02674659708408203

Pope, K. S. (1994). *Sexual involvement with therapists: Patient assessment, subsequent therapy, forensics*. American Psychological Association. https://doi.org/10.1037/10154-000

Robinson, J. A. (1993). *Sexual contact between gay male clients and male therapists* (Publication No. 1627800048) [Doctoral dissertation, University of Southern California]. ProQuest Dissertations and Theses Global.

Schoener, G. R., & Milgrom, J. H. (1987). Helping clients who have been sexually abused by therapists. In P. A. Keller & S. R. Heyman (Eds.), *Innovations in clinical practice: A sourcebook* (Vol. 6, pp. 407–416). Professional Resource Exchange.

Schoener, G. R., Milgrom, J. H., Gonsiorek, J. C., Luepker, E. T., & Conroe, R. M. (Eds.). (1989). *Psychotherapists' sexual involvement with clients: Intervention and prevention*. Walk-In Counseling Center.

Stotzer, R. L. (2009). Violence against transgender people: A review of United States data. *Aggression and Violent Behavior, 14*(3), 170–179. https://doi.org/10.1016/j.avb.2009.01.006

Therapy Exploitation Link Line (TELL). (2019). *TELLing it like it is: When psychotherapists abuse and exploit* [Ebook]. https://www.therapyabuse.org/ebook-TELLing-It-Like-It-Is.pdf

Tummala-Narra, P. (2016). *Psychoanalytic theory and cultural competence in psychotherapy*. American Psychological Association. https://doi.org/10.1037/14800-000

Tylim, I. (2017). On transference, passion, and analysts' sexual boundary violations. *Psychoanalytic Psychology, 34*(2), 182–185. https://doi.org/10.1037/pap0000080

Walters, M. L., Chen, J., & Breiding, M. J. (2013). *The National Intimate Partner and Sexual Violence Survey (NISVS): 2010 findings on victimization by sexual orientation*. National Center for Injury Prevention and Control, Centers for Disease Control and Prevention. https://www.cdc.gov/violenceprevention/pdf/nisvs_sofindings.pdf

PART **IV** **DYNAMICS AND EFFECTS**

14 MIND F*CK

The Grooming Process in "Professional Incest"

CHRISTINE A. COURTOIS AND JUDITH L. ALPERT

This chapter describes and addresses the process of grooming and is a companion to Chapter 15 of this volume. "Grooming" usually connotes "intentional abuse," which may involve only one client or serial sexual contact with many clients, at times even concurrently. It is abuse which is more deliberate, premeditated and goal-focused, and more characterological than what is often known as "situational abuse," most often a one-time episode. It may also be the result of sexual addictions and compulsions or erotomania on the part of the therapist. At present, there is no absolute line of demarcation between the two, nor are there reliable data about which type is more common, although the two are often differentiated in the literature. In this chapter, the focus is on the more intentional and purposeful end of the spectrum. Situational abuse receives more focus in the interview with Dr. Celenza (see Chapter 4) as well as in the epilogue. We begin by considering grooming and then introduce related dynamics such as "gaslighting," betrayal trauma (individual and organizational) and resultant

The authors acknowledge Melise Mestayer and Holly Moy for their assistance with the literature search.

https://doi.org/10.1037/0000247-014
Sexual Boundary Violations in Psychotherapy: Facing Therapist Indiscretions, Transgressions, and Misconduct, A. Steinberg, J. L. Alpert, and C. A. Courtois (Editors)

attachment-based betrayal blindness and trauma bonding, as they are used by malignant or traumatic narcissistic or otherwise psychopathic predators/ therapists. We also discuss trauma dynamics and reenactments as different from transferential responses and the imperative of therapists to learn more about these dynamics to not get caught in them and to not act them out with the client.

Although our intent is to discuss sexual misconduct in psychotherapy, it must be recognized that such abuses also take place in other professional relationships, including supervision and consultation and in professional training programs and may involve similar dynamics. In fact, there is concern that some supervisors model an acceptability of boundary violations to their trainees when they engage in any type of dual relationships but especially those that are sexualized. In recent years, many states have extended prohibitions of sexual contact including sexual harassment by mental health and other professionals to all students/trainees, supervisees, employees, and even to the client's spouse/partner and other family members and related individuals.

Historically, the most typical dyad for sexual boundary violations (SBVs) involved the older cisgender heterosexual male therapist and the younger cisgender heterosexual female client (Gabbard & Lester, 1995; Schoener et al., 1989). Traditional sex roles, expectations, discrimination, sexism, and misguided theoretical formulations about women (see Chapter 9, this volume)—namely, the asymmetry of power and status between both parties— and the disparity between the greater number of male therapists and greater number of female clients were often cited as reasons for this scenario. More recently, J. Wohlberg (personal communication, March 2019) and her Therapy Exploitation Link Line (TELL) colleagues have noted that this typical dyad is no longer the only type that is recognized as reports of serious boundary violations perpetrated by female therapists have markedly increased and different pairings of all kinds (male to male, female to female and male, to and from individuals anywhere on the intersectionality spectrum) have been reported (for discussion, see Chapter 13). More female perpetration may be due to more women becoming psychotherapists, or it may suggest that it is the power and authority of the therapist role and the client's disproportionate lesser status, along with situational and characterological vulnerabilities—some of which are unique to the particular dyad—that are also at play. Given this, we will use male and female pronouns interchangeably in this contribution, as we refer to violating therapists and violated clients.

We deliberately chose a provocative title and subtitle to articulate the seriousness of the process and the consequences. In cases of grooming, a "mind fu*k" is involved, fueled by trickery and deception on the part of the therapist to achieve personal gratification of various needs through sexual means. We label SBVs in such circumstances *professional incest* because the behavior is highly taboo, perpetrated by an individual in a parentlike role who misuses the authority of the role to exploit rather than promote healthy growth, development, and individuation. Abusive therapists also fail in their responsibility to protect. Victims of incest are especially vulnerable to abuse of this sort due to the long-lasting impact of their original incestuous abuse and the fact that their histories are often fetishized by others, including some therapists (Courtois, 2010). Rather than being revictimized in another sexualized dual-role relationship, they require treatment that offers them conditions of safety from any type of exploitation so they can heal and develop new skills in self-protection along with a new sense of self.

INTENTIONAL ABUSE INVOLVING GROOMING

The grooming process is described in considerable detail in Chapter 15, so we provide only abbreviated information here. The following definition of adult sexual grooming by a therapist or other professional was offered by Sinnamon (2017, p. 484, italics added): "any situation in which an adult *is primed to permit themselves* to be abused and/or exploited for sexual gratification of another." The phrase "to permit themselves" may seem unfortunate and a misnomer but should not be taken to mean the victim is responsible for the abuse or to blame the victim. However, the phrase is accurate in describing what many client-victims have reported in hindsight as *a process* that produces in them great confusion, disorientation, personal disempowerment, psychological and behavioral passivity in many cases, and ongoing disconfirmation of their selfhood, reality, will, and perceptions. As noted by Van Dam (2001), for victims, grooming "orchestrates their participation" in their own abuse. Major goals of the grooming process are to create disorientation and self-doubt and loss of personal judgment and self-control in the client while developing increased dependence on and (over)valuation of the therapist. It is a chain of desensitization that results in the breakdown of the client's normal cautions, instincts and, in some cases, their ethics and morals, through subjugation to the therapist.

Sexual grooming cannot be easily and simply described because it does not follow a fixed set of rules and patterns other than involving emotional and psychological manipulation tactics and gradual encroachment on the client's life and reality over time. Abusers seem to have a keen ability to sense the needs and desires of each of their victims and to intuit how to manipulate and control them in ways that are carefully tailored. Moreover, they may use the client's transference responses or trauma and attachment-based dynamics including enactments and reenactments *against* her rather than *for* her due to mismanagement of their countertransference. Such scenarios are discussed extensively in the psychodynamic literature on transference and countertransference, especially when eroticized. Similar ploys can take place in contexts other than psychotherapy (e.g., cults, scams), and whatever the context, the motivation underlying each purposeful boundary crossing or violation is to enable the abuser to immediately or ultimately gain something from the vulnerable individual—in the case of the therapist, personal power and subjugation or expression of feelings or reactions, as well as gratification achieved via sexual contact. It is especially noteworthy that this goal is not immediately apparent because the abuser makes it seem as though it is he who is gratifying the needs of the victim (i.e., by providing special care and attention, providing unlimited approval, and so on). The grooming may be so subtle and gradual that it may go on for years, or even decades in some cases, before any sexual contact is introduced. Like more situational abuse, the usual course of grooming is to start with small verbal, physical, and behavioral boundary crossings; however, the point of differentiation between the two is that these are premeditated and deliberate rather than more inadvertent.

In other cases, however, the grooming might not follow this course and instead may escalate rapidly, a maneuver that might be calculated to shock, stun, disorient, and ultimately disarm the targeted individual. Whether the process is abrupt, relatively short term or more gradual, it generally involves the use of language designed to sow confusion, obfuscate and challenge the client's ability to think clearly and intentionally engage in behavior, and lower defenses and resistance. It may also involve verbalizations that meet the needs and longings of the client, paradoxically in the name of love, that is, what she "wants to hear" about how special, loveable, and wanted she is; how lucky she is to have the undivided attention and love of the therapist; the specialness and uniqueness of the relationship; and so on. From there, the typical course is a progression to seemingly innocent or accidental physical contacts and then on to relatively casual and low-level sexual ones, used to probe and test the client's gullibility, vulnerabilities, boundaries, and receptiveness. Moreover, the temptation of forbidden and taboo sex can be highly enticing and exciting to both parties.

It is this misinformation along with boundary crossings and violations that, taken together, create the context within which sexual abuse can occur. Grooming also works by mixing positive behavior and feedback with abusive elements, which can include blaming the victim and claims by the therapist–perpetrator that it is *he* who has been victimized ("You were so seductive and what we have is so special—see what *you* made me do?"). Traditional gender roles and expectations such as "boys will be boys" and tropes such as "males can't be expected to control their sexual urges when in the company of an available and seductive woman to whom they are attracted" and "females are not and cannot be sexually abusive" may be used as both rationalization for the behavior and projection of blame as well as intimidation.

With time, the behavior shifts, escalating to more serious sexual contacts, often accompanied by expressions of love for the victim, but sometimes followed by anger, blame, and contempt and then apology, setting up a repeat of the pattern (much like the "honeymoon" pattern or cycle that often accompanies spousal violence). The confusion and shame that usually ensue for the client-victim, partially the result of the silencing and secrecy that is insisted upon, sometimes involving threats of not being believed if they disclose or threats of harm to them or their loved ones, allow the behavior to continue, in the process entrapping her in subtle and not so subtle ways. Shame may be especially intense for those who are abused in relationships that they consider atypical to the norm (i.e., males abused by females, same-sex abuse) and may keep them from discussing or disclosing the abuse. In the typical scenario—whatever the configuration—the client takes on the responsibility and associated guilt and shame while missing the fact that it is the therapist who has the power and responsibility but who has off-loaded it. Most often, the victim keeps the secret and tells no one.

Sinnamon (2017) pointed out that grooming may extend beyond the intended victim to include colleagues and others, even family members of the client. Some abusive therapists are professionally successful, and some are at the height of their professions and careers. They usually present themselves and behave in ways that cause them to be valued as an ethical, credible, trustworthy, upstanding, and even distinguished mental health professional, or they use their power to provoke fear in others and maintain ironclad control. When abuse comes to light (if it does), it is this front of power, authority, rectitude, admiration, and fear that may cause colleagues and others to deny that the therapist could have done anything so egregious. This occurs even in communities and organizations where there has been gossip about the therapist and their laxity around sexual boundaries or around a tendency to dominate others and suppress any questioning of their behavior or authority, often over long periods of time. While denial is a common response among colleagues, it may also be affected by the gender of the perpetrator, with abuse by female therapists or same-gender abuse seen as less plausible or serious. In such scenarios, victims may be seen as less important than the alleged abuser and may have their reports dismissed due to knee-jerk denial and without adequate investigation. This is another misuse of power.

Dimen (2011), writing of her own abuse by a well-known analyst who slipped his tongue in her mouth during their initial session, described how her disclosure decades after the fact of this and other sexualized behavior was received by colleagues in her psychoanalytic institute. She wrote about the denial and even the complicity of colleagues who didn't know, didn't see, or didn't do anything—and didn't want to—at the time or later. Such dismissal and disregard added insult to injury and caused her additional distress, as she was made to feel "less than." Such personal betrayal is usually in the context of *institutional betrayal*, a dynamic described by Smith and Freyd (2014) that is contributory and reciprocal in therapist abuse and thus additionally damaging to the victim.

Although changes are taking place in a number of institutions, the typical response to disclosures or complaints of abuse in all types of organizations has been to mollify, placate, deny, or place the onus on the victim while protecting the alleged perpetrator (usually someone in power who holds special authority, prestige, and status or effectively intimidates others), who usually emphatically denies the allegations and blames the victim. In fact, intervention and reporting to outside authorities may be inverse to the degree of power and status of the alleged perpetrator in the organization. Freyd (2018) developed the acronym DARVO as shorthand for the most common institutional response: Defend–Avoid–Reverse Victim and Offender. Brown (2020) recently added another dimension when she described *institutional cowardice* as a powerful, often invisible manifestation of institutional betrayal.

There are now several models that describe the *adult grooming process* in therapist misconduct, with variation among them with respect to the description and labeling of behaviors and strategies and the number of stages involved; yet there is agreement that the process involves a (usually) gradual but calculated progression of behaviors and verbalizations designed to engage, mislead, and disempower the prospective victim with the goal of engaging them in sexual contact and a sexual relationship. The process resembles that found in child sexual abuse where a needy or otherwise vulnerable child is sought by a perpetrator and a relationship is cultivated that becomes the context for the abuse. A qualitative study of three disciplined therapists reported in "Neutralizing the Client: Therapist Accounts of Sexual Boundary Violations" by McNulty et al. (2011) found various ways these therapists equalized the power imbalance: minimizing the client's mental health problems, stressing the conventionality of the relationship and their own needs, and being unwilling to discuss with a supervisor what should have been a cause for concern. The victimized client's awareness that something is wrong may start early on, only to be challenged or assuaged by the therapist who uses her role and her power of persuasion and influence. This awareness and accompanying discomfort may continue, develop later, go underground for a period of time or resurface when secrecy is strongly suggested, insisted upon, or imposed by the therapist or if the client is threatened and made to feel unsafe.

On the basis of her advocacy work with TELL, the Boston-based website and helpline (see Chapter 15), Wohlberg (personal communication, March 2019) developed a three-phase model of grooming, each with its own characteristics.

Stage 1: Early Grooming Behaviors

Because most clients enter treatment with little or no understanding of therapy, even those who are highly mistrustful of authority figures tend to seek guidance from the therapist as the one who "knows the territory." In keeping with the preceding discussion, Simon (1999) noted that from the outset, most, but not all, therapies that become abusive look normal. Clues to something amiss are recognizable only in hindsight, if at all. According to Simon, there is violation when the primary source of the therapist's gratification is achieved from the client directly rather than from engagement in the therapeutic process with the client. Sources of gratification for the therapist are likely imperceptible to the client early on and may be less so even later in the process as enmeshment and gratification deepen and the client increasingly seeks the therapist's attention and approval. The unscrupulous and opportunistic therapist, for whom the client (especially one who was previously traumatized, as discussed subsequently) is a "sitting duck" (Kluft, 1990), implicitly—and ultimately explicitly—lets the client know what to do to gain and maintain that approval.

So the typical victim usually does not recognize, much less report, abusive behavior when it begins. It is now broadly recognized that something that is a memorable but not necessarily traumatic event can become traumatic through the prism of time, later experience, and a different perspective. When boundaries are crossed or violated from early on and gradually progress a little at a time, the client may think the question and timing are strange and even inappropriate but not necessary a sexual violation and may not be traumatized by it. In fact, clients may reassure themselves that such material is routinely brought up in psychotherapy and that the therapist knows best.

As the improper behavior continues and escalates, ever more seductive behavior is initiated, including repeated assurances that the client has come to not only the "right" place for help but to the "only" place. The therapist states or implies, "You are a special client, and I am the *only* therapist competent to understand and treat your issues." Increasingly, the therapist attends to the client's perceived "needs" and specialness by offering intensified care and attention in and out of the treatment setting. As this first stage continues, the therapist becomes increasingly familiar and casual in interactions. She compliments the client on her appearance and clothing and might gaze longingly in her eyes and stare at or make comments on her body.

During this stage, the victim may become increasingly dependent on the therapist's attention, getting a "fix" in the form of regular appointments during which they receive their "hit" of specialized attention. They may spend time between appointments anticipating and yearning for the next session and obsessing about the therapist. It is usually around this time that the therapist introduces the idea of more frequent and longer appointments, usually at the end of the day ostensibly "to have more time to be together" but also to evade detection. This additional consideration by the therapist may feel like "manna from heaven" to the client, providing more evidence of being special and wanted while countering feelings of not being loveable.

Stage 2: From Innuendo to Action

If one were to attempt to comprehend sexual boundary violations outside of the context in which they occur, it would be difficult to make sense of what has taken place because it seems illogical. During the two stages— which may take place over several weeks or months or over the course of years—client-victims are told repeatedly (but possibly intermittently in what is known to be a very potent form of learning reinforcement) that they are unique, desired by and irresistible to the therapist, who feels attracted to and seduced by them. There is repeated and ongoing misrepresentation; outright lying; denial; actions that do not match words; and positive, intermittent reinforcement to confuse and set expectations and projection of blame. The client's perception of what is happening becomes slowly and progressively manipulated over time, as the predatory therapist holds sway over reality and gains control and power. What takes place inside the therapy room may so greatly contrast with what takes place outside that the victim's reality and sense of self become challenged and discriminating between reality and fantasy compromised. The victim may doubt and question, but over time, her point of view is overtaken. She is increasing bewildered while simultaneously becoming "entranced," in the process losing her sense of identity, perception, and self-worth. She may also feel she is losing both her moral compass and her mind.

As the innuendo and suggestion continue to build, they lead to increasingly overt action. By the end of this stage, the therapist typically has (inappropriately) overdisclosed ever more personal life details, some of which might be "tall tales" of unavailable, chronically ill, and dying spouses; a meaningless marriage and an inadequate sex life; unruly or unappreciative children; an empty nest or other midlife crises; a painful separation or divorce that is in process or to come; illness; or professional and financial stress. This information has the effect of eliciting the client's concern and sympathy and, in the process, further engaging and ensnaring them. Being entrusted with such personal information can be especially seductive and gratifying for those clients who long to be helpful and who learned the role of caretaker in the family as a means of gaining approval or control. Caretaking often enhanced their sense of being personally selected and for being special and appreciated for having specialized abilities to respond to others. This in turn may lead to other dual roles, such as when a client's helpfulness extends to taking on clerical tasks like bookkeeping and billing services or cleaning the office and even providing housekeeping or child care in the therapist's home.

Although most of the grooming behavior occurs in the office setting, over time and as the relationship intensifies, it may move out of the office as it become less formal and professional and more relaxed, social, and romantic. An outside meeting for coffee may then become lunch and then an intimate dinner. A car ride or a walk in the woods or on a beach can lead to physical contact. The relationship looks more and more like courtship and dating rather than therapy. At some point, conversations become more sexualized. The therapist may confess her desire for more contact and begin to talk about her erotic fantasies about the client and encourage the same in turn. Some of this may be reinforced in late-night phone calls and by text or e-mail. If others in the client's and therapist's outside lives become aware of what seems like a growing obsession between the two, they may run up against a wall of anger, defensiveness, and denial if they attempt to point out, question, or stop it.

Stage 3: Now Clearly a Victim

This stage is when the relationship moves from the intensity and excitement of seduction and sexual innuendo to more explicit sexual behavior including undressing, mutual masturbation, oral sex (given and received), and intercourse. It is explicit and blatant and includes activities that may be observed, discovered, or reported to and by others, including spouses and confidantes, licensing boards or other authorities, subsequent therapists, or other survivors. In some cases, sexual activities are audio or video recorded by either party, ostensibly to provide a memento of the engagement; however, they can also be used as blackmail or as evidence in a lawsuit. By this stage, any semblance of "therapy" has long since passed, although "sessions" in which therapy issues are discussed may continue, ostensibly for sake of appearances should a spouse or office mate ask questions. Most abusers continue to bill for services and collect insurance and cash payments for their "sessions."

At this point, the client may be warned that should anyone find out about the relationship, it would have to end, and also that the therapist could lose his license, status, marriage and family, and possibly his freedom if he has to face charges, something he implies would be the client's fault. She is enjoined to secrecy and nondisclosure, with pleas ("Please don't do that to me, no one would understand what we have") or threats ("No one would believe you anyway. It would be your word as a client against mine— a well-regarded professional in my community who is being blackmailed by an unstable client"). The client has likely become increasingly and obsessively (or addictively or dissociatively) caught up in the relationship, isolated from his normal support systems, and conditioned or "programmed" into believing that he is responsible for the abuser's well-being, responsible for having seduced him into the relationship in the first place, and therefore also responsible for protecting him by keeping the secret. The victim may believe himself to be "in love," loved and unconditionally accepted by the therapist and believe that their lives will be forever entwined and they will have a life together. The therapist may actively encourage this expectation.

The sex itself can be highly stimulating and gratifying but can also be source of conflicted feelings and even disappointment. Many survivors describe the exhilaration and guilty pleasure associated with being engaged in and consumed by a taboo activity. Yet, especially if either party is married or in a committed relationship, they may feel guilty for their infidelity and ashamed. Some describe feeling hyperaroused or depersonalized (or both) during and after the sex, uncertain as to what is happening and how they are feeling. The addiction model may be a useful way of understanding the experience of victims who describe feeling alive when having sex with the therapist ("getting a dopamine hit") and empty and bereft between liaisons. A trauma history may also be implicated in that the client who spaces out during sex may do so because sexual contact is experienced as a trigger.

Paradoxically, many clients later say that they were not particularly physically attracted to the therapist (as many tend to be middle-aged or older and may not have "aged well"), but rather the excitement was provided by being seduced by what was provided and promised or how they were coerced. It is typically the nonsexual conditioning that creates the most psychological upheaval and damage for victims (Sinnamon, 2017). So clients are harmed not just by the sex, but more so by the grooming itself (see Chapters 6 and 15). However, in those cases when the sex is clearly aberrant and demeaning or violent, the sexual behavior may be the main source of trauma. And the ultimate loss of the relationship, whenever and however it ends, may be highly traumatic and experienced as a rupture rather than an ending.

Some therapists, often in the throes of their obsessive and compulsive behavior with the client, leave an indiscreet trail of evidence that might be discovered by significant others, employers, or colleagues and that might become important later on if the abuse is reported to a licensing board, to the police, or if a lawsuit is initiated. With so many means of communicating via text, email, and social media, the evidence may be overwhelming. In a case known to the first author, the abusing therapist kept an electronic diary that described in detail her growing involvement with a client, how she knew it was wrong and unethical (but didn't care), how she rationalized and hid it from others (including her husband and her employer and coworkers), and how she assumed they would react if they found out. She also blamed the client for having seduced her by offering to teach her about woman-to-woman sex after the therapist had inappropriately disclosed to her that she was conflicted about her sexuality and her marriage.

For this client, whose life was in total disarray and who was in a desperate state at the time, the involvement with the therapist became a lifeline that she quickly grabbed on to (sometimes referred to as the "love cure" or a flight into health). The therapist separated from her husband and moved in with the client, and they lived as a couple for a time, during which the therapist encouraged her to change her surname so she could not be identified as a former client. The "honeymoon" period ended when the client's symptoms began to reemerge, upsetting and angering the therapist, who believed them to have been resolved. The therapist responded by abruptly and without warning ending their relationship, causing the client to decompensate and be hospitalized after a serious suicide attempt. In subsequent therapy, the client learned of the unethical and illegal nature of the relationship. In response, she reported her former therapist–lover to her licensing board and additionally sued the therapist and her employer for damages.

Because the therapist's diary was known to the client, it was subject to discovery and subsequently introduced and admitted as evidence, along with other items, such as love letters, cards, and songs the therapist sang and recorded for the client. Unsurprisingly, the case settled before going to trial because the accumulated evidence was so damning.

GASLIGHTING

The term *gaslighting* comes from George Cukor's 1944 movie *Gaslight*, the story of a woman deliberately driven to the edge of sanity by her husband, who lies and questions her reality and perceptions for his own gain. In a similar vein, gaslighting in psychotherapy is a self-serving attempt by a therapist to take advantage of and misuse their position of power and influence to alter, modify, or distort a client's perception of reality for purposes of personal gratification. It is defined in the psychotherapy context as "the therapist's attack on the client's psychic reality, which results in the client believing that the reality that the therapist presents is the true one, regardless of the client's own perception to the contrary" (Caruth & Eber, 1996, p. 33). Gaslighting in the therapy hour has been referred to as the metaphoric rape of the client's mind or what has been more crudely termed a "mind f*ck" by the "the rapist" (Caruth & Eber, 1996). It has also been labeled "professional incest" by Courtois (2010) and others in recognition of the taboo nature of the sexual contact that involves a parental figure who is dominant and a less powerful child figure who is dependent. It thus involves a major betrayal. Many of the justifications and rationalizations used by abusive therapists and the resulting dynamics resemble those found in father–daughter as well as other forms of incest (Courtois, 2010).

In standard psychodynamic psychotherapy, therapists are trained to expect what is known as a *regressive transference*, a process in which clients project onto the therapist aspects of their relationship with important attachment figures from childhood, especially parents or other primary caregivers. The adult client who regresses in this way experiences himself as a child in relation to the parental authority figure who, in turn, is seen as all-knowing and all-powerful. In the throes of this regression, he is not able to independently assess his therapist (much like he was unable to assess his parents) and may come to believe father or mother can do no wrong and their viewpoint is always correct. Therapists who are so inclined can easily manipulate the transference to their advantage. When gaslighting is a component of the grooming process, the abusing therapist may further claim that sexual contact is good for both therapist and client, that it is good for her marriage, that it is in vivo sex education or sex therapy used to "teach her and loosen her up," that it is good for her mental health, or that it is due to her. After being gaslighted, the "gaslightee" surrenders independence and accepts rather than questions or rejects his viewpoint. In doing so, she seeks to avoid disappointing, angering, or losing him and their special bond (Gediman, 1991).

BETRAYAL TRAUMA, ATTACHMENT AND TRAUMA DYNAMICS, DISSOCIATION, AND TRAUMA BONDING

Betrayal has long been identified as a traumagenic dynamic of incest and child sexual abuse (Finkelhor & Browne, 1985) as well as other forms of victimization perpetrated by a parent or other relative, someone else in close relationship, or someone who holds a fiduciary relationship to the victim. Building on this background, Freyd (1996) developed betrayal trauma theory (BTT) to account for the unique traumatizing aspects of betrayal. Her theory, which has received extensive research support, posits that the closer the relationship between victim and perpetrator, the greater the betrayal and the more severe the consequences to the victim.

Freyd's theory was founded on attachment theory associated with such victimization. It is also used to better understand victim–perpetrator dynamics, as discussed by Gagnon, Lee, and DePrince (2017). When parents are impaired and abusive, absent, or unresponsive in significant ways early in a child's life, attachment or relational trauma occurs that then profoundly influences a child's psychophysiological development. The most serious attachment failures occur when parents and families are highly chaotic, violent or unsafe, inconsistent, and nonresponsive or unprotective (i.e., attentive and loving alternating unpredictably with all types of abuse, including negligence or nonresponse and separation, loss, and abandonment). These environments create insecurity in children and stunt their personal and relational development secondary to the damage done to their neurophysiology.

A particularly unfortunate consequence for the insecurely attached child (and later adult) is vulnerability to revictimization due, at least in part, to what Freyd (1996) labeled *betrayal blindness*. This term refers to the process by which those who have been betrayed by intimates may, as a result, be unable to recognize signs of danger or predation and thus become easy targets to be revictimized and retraumatized, often repeatedly. For example, victims of incest are more likely than those without such a history to serially engage with partners who are abusive and violent to them and to their children (Courtois, 2010). As Kluft (1990) noted, they may be "sitting ducks" to predatory others, including therapists, a susceptibility now extensively supported by research findings.

BTT offers another means of understanding the dynamics of therapist abuse. It is likely that many clients seek therapy due to the unresolved effects of childhood traumatic experiences of one sort or another, and most have an insecure or disorganized/dissociative attachment style. Those who are insecure/anxious may overrely on the therapist and continuously seek approval and attention, whereas those who are insecure/detached may goad the therapist into action and overinvolvement by being dismissive and even contemptuous toward them, causing them to feel helpless in response. These attachment styles and other dynamics, including the therapist's ability to stay emotionally regulated and to maintain boundaries in interactions with the client, are relevant in the discussion of therapist SBVs. Therapists may get caught up in their client's relational style and compromise the relationship in some way, including the violation of boundaries. Moreover, clients with "betrayal blindness" may be unaware of—and therefore susceptible to— a therapist's boundary incursions and involvement in dual relationships.

Freyd (1996) addressed another dimension of betrayal trauma: that children abused by a primary caretaker as someone on whom they are dependent are caught in an *attachment double bind*. Due to their survival-based dependence on that person, their accessibility and entrapment in the family, and for their own security and survival, *they had to stay attached to the very person who was doing them harm*. To do so, many temporarily or more permanently repress, sequester, or dissociate the abuse to maintain the needed relationship. This in turn results in lost memory and betrayal blindness.

A related dynamic is that of *trauma bonding*. This refers to the previously abused child's or client's seemingly inexplicable ability to continue under the influence of the abuser or to maintain love and other positive feelings, including loyalty and attachment. This puzzling bond must be understood by any subsequent therapist and not used to pathologize or further victimize the client (see Chapter 18). They must separate the abuser's behavior from the relationship between abuser and victim and understand that these dynamics relate to betrayal trauma where they usually have many other facets to their relationship besides exploitation and abuse (Middleton et al., 2017). The exploitation occurred in the context of the relationship, which was used to encourage and justify the sexual contact and to simultaneously trap the client-victim.

Messman and Long (1996) reviewed 18 studies and reported rates of therapist abuse in this population as similar to those found in a study by Pope and Vetter (1991), namely, that 32% of victims had a prior history of incest or other childhood sexual abuse. They also found such revictimization to be associated with greater mental health difficulties in later life. These individuals have been previously abused and are therefore vulnerable to reabuse because they often lack firm defenses and self-cohesion; moreover, they often experience dissociation, betrayal blindness, and trauma bonding when faced with a compromised or dangerous situation. As adults, they may repeat the past through compliance and submission to the will of the sexually abusive therapist who become endowed, via transference, with their father's (or other abuser's) power.

That many incest survivors are later exploited by their therapists speaks to their past conditioning into dual relationships and their ongoing vulnerability, which may be expressed in their traumatic transference and, not uncommonly, to their therapist's countertransference to them as they learn the details of their abusive histories. Some incest survivors are fetishized by their therapists (and others) as "damaged goods," sexually willing and available to any and all, and they may be subjected to fascination and voyeurism due to having been involved in such a taboo relationship. In contrast, some therapists become overinvolved in a misguided attempt to rescue, sexually educate (or reeducate) or compensate for the abuse, or "purify" the client. Others act out in anger, giving their client "what she deserves" and then abandoning her (Courtois, 2010).

Many abuse dynamics that are not strictly transferential but rather are trauma-based can enter the treatment relationship, including reenactment, repetition compulsion, attempts at mastery, and dissociation. Simply stated, as a child, the client had been treated as an object for purposes of the abuser's gratification. In treatment, they may be "easy" victims—easy to manipulate as they have been conditioned into expecting and accommodating dual relationships where trade-offs are the norm. Herman (1992), in her influential book *Trauma and Recovery*, noted alterations in relationship to the perpetrator (involving identification with or hatred of the aggressor as poles on a continuum, or alternation between the two) as a common response to childhood abuse, a dynamic that can play out with the therapist as well. When a therapist also has an abuse or trauma history, there may be a mutual trauma reenactment with the client with one or the other victim or victimizer.

These and additional transference–countertransference pressures can be quite strong, and it is solely the therapist's responsibility to identify and analyze them with the client. Although the client may hold the delusion of mastery in a sexual "conquest" of the therapist, in so doing, she has not overcome her past trauma; rather, she has repeated it. Nor has she conquered the therapist, but she has uncovered his venality. There is another side to the narrative at play here. The traumatic enactment makes clear to the client and reinforces her negative view of herself as a seductress, a slut, contaminated, "negatively special," harmful to others, and responsible for the therapist's aberrant sexual interest and interactions.

The client who was subjected to ongoing incest or other forms of chronic trauma likely used dissociation as a means of coping, a process that may continue into adulthood, particularly if the assaults by the primary abuser continue (believed to occur in as many as 15% of all cases) or if they are repeatedly abused by others. Dissociation may be prompted by triggers and reminders of the trauma in an intermittent or ongoing way. Dissociation involves a compartmentalizing or separation of information that should be connected, usually arising as a means of warding off knowledge of and coping with traumatization that is ongoing, entrapping, and not easily escaped. Many client-survivors will meet criteria for a dissociative disorder or the dissociative subtype of posttraumatic stress disorder.

Clients who are dissociative, particularly those with dissociative identity disorder, may have "part-selves" or alternate "states of mind" developed over the course of the abuse who may have different personal histories and motivations and who may take over executive control of the individual in response to various internal and external triggers. Some exploitive therapists have been known to use their client's dissociation against them. For example, if a sexualized part (often a child or young teen) emerges or is "called out" by the therapist, that part might be an "easy mark" who taunts or seeks to seduce the therapist because they are well-versed in dual or transactional modes of relating and do not understand being in a relationship that does not involve sexual contact or trade-offs. Alternatively, a teen part-self may be a protector and may engage defensively with the therapist. Kluft (2017) discussed these types of interactions in an article titled "Weaponized Sex: Defensive Pseudo-Erotic Aggression in the Service of Safety." Dynamics such as these are complicated and require a therapist to be cognizant of them and to know how to work with them without succumbing and acting them out with the client by engaging in sexual activity, even if the client "demands" it or engages in seductive behavior to solicit it. In fact, Putnam (1989) provided the following advice to therapists faced with such a challenge: It is far better to end a treatment than to "yield" to a client's entreaties and efforts because engaging in sexual contact will obviously retraumatize.

One other variation deserves mention: when a client crosses a sexual boundary and perpetrates an assault of some sort on the therapist (i.e., through exhibitionism or more direct action). This situation and its ethical, legal, and personal repercussions were recently discussed by Herbst (2015), who had the unfortunate experience as a therapist trainee of having a young male client with sexual behavior problems grab her breast at the end of a session. Her initial inclination was to protect her client; however, after a great deal of discussion with her supervisor, she ultimately made the decision to bring charges against him. She also chose to discontinue his treatment because it had been compromised, and they were now in dual roles with one another. These were not easy decisions for her, and she was assisted to reflect on her own reactions to the violation rather than on what the client needed. The client was referred to another therapist to continue his treatment for his sexual compulsivity and assaultive behavior.

Repeating what has been emphasized throughout this book, it is solely the therapist's responsibility to hold firmly to professional boundaries, even in the most pressured and enticing of situations. As we can see from this situation, this refers to the therapist's as well as the client's safety. Boundary violations are not tolerated no matter who initiates or perpetrates, and termination of treatment may be called for.

TRAUMATIC NARCISSISM

In his book *Traumatic Narcissism: Relational Systems of Subjugation*, Shaw (2014) described many types, contexts, and configurations of subjugating relationships that make emergence from submission difficult for the victim. Obviously, this is important information in understanding a type of abusive therapist, the dominating and traumatic narcissist. Shaw devoted a chapter to this topic and began with the following, quoted in its entirety due to its pertinence here:

> Traumatic narcissism . . . can be understood most simply as the action of subjugation. In the traumatizing narcissist's relational system, the narcissist fortifies himself by diminishing the other. The other is then conquered, controlled, or enslaved at worst—and exploited. Sadly, this happens often enough in relationships that are presented as therapeutic. I have heard story after story, from analysands, supervisees, colleagues, and friends of how a therapist, from any of the various schools of psychotherapy and psychoanalysis, was able to persuade her client of her infinite wisdom, and to go on to dictate and control all the significant choices and decisions in a client's life, sometimes for decades. I have learned of people told to marry or divorce certain people; to cut off all contact with family members, permanently; to assuage and comply with abusers; to dress differently, down to what kinds of earrings and bras to wear; to make donations and investments and expect never to see a return. . . . The list is quite long and horrible. I have heard these stories told

about therapists in remote rural and also in less remote suburban areas. I've heard hair-raising stories of control and exploitation about therapists in world-class cities, therapists who hold high academic or professional positions, or have well-known names through publications and media appearances. (p. 136)

He went on to discuss characteristics of these therapists:

The quality that so many of these controlling, subjugating therapists have in common, besides their charisma, is the ability to persuade themselves and others that all their words and deeds are offered out of selflessness, superior wisdom, and love. Those who fall under the spell of such a teacher, analyst, or guru, will feel elevated, renewed, redeemed—initially. The subjugation comes later. *What traumatizing narcissist therapists deeply deny to themselves is that their need of the client is as great or greater than the client's need of them* [emphasis added]. Holding on to the client means instilling in the client the fear that all will be lost if she leaves. It's a projection with which, all too often, the client identifies. What makes traumatizing narcissism so toxic and so confusing to those it traumatizes is that the narcissist delusionally believes his selfish, exploitative actions are the actions of love—and the narcissist is a great persuader. (p. 136)

Shaw also described the developmental history of the traumatic narcissist—and often of the client as well—as one of being repeatedly shamed and subjugated by their own traumatizing narcissistic parent(s), leading to a severely depleted sense of self and a sense of unlovability. This is described by others as the victim-to-victimizer process or the identification with the aggressor used as a means of attempting to work out the distress associated with past abuse. The narcissist often has ongoing problems with intimacy and sexuality and may view sexual contacts strictly as conquests and partners as objects to be used and discarded when they are no longer needed or complicit. Shaw further described the traumatizing narcissist's core as psychotic due to the self-delusion involved:

The child who becomes the traumatizing narcissist learns from these parents that whatever does not feel good inside is to be externalized—blamed on the actions of someone who is outside [emphasis in original]. Believing in one's own infallible righteousness and superiority, and believing that all the badness is outside, never inside, are delusions that are pathognomonic for traumatizing narcissism. (p. 138)

Some individuals with this history cope by reversing this position and becoming a therapist in the service of others. Yet these "wounded healers" whose own histories remain unacknowledged or unresolved can use their position to desperately seek from their clients and others the sense of lovability that is so elusive. This may result in their functioning as a traumatizing narcissist of their clients and others in their life. Clients may be susceptible to being dazzled by association with the traumatizing narcissistic and grandiose therapist, while not recognizing his controlling, needy, and even sadistic behaviors. It is no wonder that they take on responsibility while being duped and exploited.

THE ENDING OF THE RELATIONSHIP

How do such relationships end? In a wide variety of ways, but it should be recognized that some never do. In fact, many continue over many years and decades—intermittently or on an ongoing basis—at times due to the extent of any other dual affiliations, such as employment and business relationships, that have developed. In some circumstances, therapist and client even marry (and some may later divorce). Either party may bring the relationship to an end, or it may be ended as the result of observation and intervention by others such as the therapist's colleague(s) or employer or the spouses/partners and friends or family members of either party. A report to an employer, licensing board, or other outside authority such as the police or an ethics complaint may also put an end to the sexual involvement (although this is not guaranteed when sexual compulsivity or other issues are involved), even as the "therapy" might continue.

Many client-survivors report having experienced unanticipated endings that were announced unilaterally by their therapist with little or no notice, preparation, discussion, or explanation. This fits the definition of "traumatic ruptures" as described by Deutsch and colleagues in her edited 2014 book by the same title. Understandably, these sudden and unanticipated endings usually result in major devastation and despair and have potential for significant decompensation and increased suicidality, even homicidality. Endings of this sort are known to result from many causes and motivations, ranging from the therapist whose conscience or sense of ethics kick in (possibly under the influence of an outside consultation, an increased recognition of the conflicts and difficulties such a relationship creates in "real life" and to their spouse and children, or discovery and an ultimatum from a spouse or partner) to the therapist who can't handle the client's dependency or demands (and in some cases, their pathology and its symptoms, which might ebb and flow over time). It may be that the therapist tires of the client, possibly for not fulfilling the therapist's needs or fantasies, or ends the relationship to serially move on to other clients. Or a therapist might "come to his senses" after achieving sobriety or after other life transitions, both positive and negative. Effective personal treatment and the support from their own therapist or supervisor might help them to disentangle and end the relationship in a way that is less sudden and damaging to all parties.

Therapists who end the extra-therapeutic sexual relationship abruptly by "dumping" the client-victim with coldness and no evident consideration or who do so with anger and hostility create risk for themselves that, when their own self-interest is their sole focus, may not be obvious to them. Such endings can cause some clients to take action, involving one of all of the following: reporting the relationship to the therapist's spouse/partner, their employer or training organization, outside authorities, or a licensing board. Criminal charges might also be brought by authorities to whom the abuse was reported, and a trial may result. Or the aggrieved client might file a civil lawsuit for damages. These are not mutually exclusive actions. Tragically, such an abrupt ending and any media attention accorded to the case can result in self-injury and suicidality, up to and including completed suicide of either party and homicidal feelings, urges, and actions.

The client may need to "break the spell" before they are able to end the sexual contact. Disenchantment may begin when they are told or otherwise learn about the unethical nature of sexual interactions between therapist and client and understand that they have been and continue to be exploited and damaged by the involvement, even if they love the therapist. Some increasingly feel that their life and its trajectory have been hijacked and that if they stay in the relationship, their own values and morals will continue to be compromised and their goals and desires permanently sidelined. Some seek out a confidante or consultant to provide them with perspective and support. It may take many attempts with several starts and stops to fully disengage, especially when the therapist actively argues against ending due to their own high dependency, vulnerability to rejection/abandonment, or other needs (some of which may come as a surprise to the client), or when the therapist compulsively engages in retaliating or pleading with the client (up to an including stalking), or who threatens violence to self or others, including the client. Some client/victims have been driven to make a geographical escape by moving to a new location to elude the therapist.

The end of the relationship, however it occurs, does not end the emotional entanglements, repercussions, questions and musings. The ending can result in intense loss and mourning or what has been identified as *complicated bereavement* (prompted by the dynamics of trauma bonding and ambivalent attachment) and what Boss (2006) identified as *ambiguous loss* and Doka (1989) as *disenfranchised grief*, which can result when a relationship is taboo and has been kept hidden. Its loss subsequently tends to be hidden and therefore offers no public forum for acknowledgement and memorializing the relationship and its significance. This can leave the victim even further isolated and without support when they are bereaved and when it is most needed. Yet, the ending may result in a simultaneous sense of relief or freedom from both the confusion and the entrapment.

OUTCOME AND CONSEQUENCES

Victimized clients are often left to make sense of what happened to them as best they can. For many, the consequences and damages are extensive and long-lasting, affecting many aspects of their lives, including self-esteem and ability to trust their own perceptions, compromised mental and physical health, misuse of or addiction to drugs and various behaviors (gambling, eating, sex), ongoing and even increased dissociation, increased self-harm and suicidality, decreased ability to function, interrupted professional and career achievement, mistrust of others and their motivations and ability to be in healthy relationships, difficulty with intimacy, lowered ability to parent, and disturbances of spirituality and meaning-making, and so forth.

Many are left in anguish as they try to understand what happened and how they became so entangled. They struggle with issues of guilt and responsibility. It is obvious that many could benefit from a return to psychotherapy, something most resist due to their ongoing mistrust and shame. Yet, some do, in what can only be described as an act of courage and personal resilience (see Chapter 18). As well and despite the odds, many have a strength and determination to survive and to live highly meaningful and productive lives and go on to do so; however, they may always live "under the cloud" of what happened to them.

SUMMARY

The contemporary #MeToo movement has brought to light as never before how authority figures and powerful individuals use their influence over others who are less powerful to coerce and trick them into doing their bidding, including meeting their control, domination, and dependence needs through sexual means. Once they have been involved or compromised, they are trapped and it is ever more difficult for them to break out of the abuse. The coercive methods that are used are increasingly coming to light as more victims are breaking their silence and telling their stories and as more wide-scale serial abuse scandals by rich, powerful, and famous individuals (e.g., Harvey Weinstein, R. Kelly, Jeffrey Epstein, Larry Nasser) and involving organizations (e.g., the Catholic Church, Boy Scouts, Penn State), have been publicized and analyzed The public is more receptive to understanding how power and predatory dynamics within an ongoing relationship may be at play and how organizations and bystanders can play a contributory or complicit role. Psychotherapy is one such professional arena that is increasingly subjected to such scrutiny.

This chapter has considered various methods employed by psychotherapists in the process of intentionally conditioning and desensitizing adult clients for purposes of sexual exploitation and subjugation. Articulating these dynamics is important in helping victimized clients and their loved ones as well as subsequent therapists, licensing board members, and criminal justice professionals increase their understanding as they determine actions and outcomes associated with their respective positions.

REFERENCES

Boss, P. (2006). *Loss, trauma, and resilience: Therapeutic work with ambiguous loss.* W. W. Norton.

Brown, L. S. (2020). Institutional cowardice: A powerful, often invisible manifestation of institutional betrayal. *Journal of Trauma & Dissociation.* https://doi.org/10.1080/15299732.2020.1801307

Caruth, C., & Eber, M. (1996). Blurred boundaries in the therapeutic encounter: Some cinematic metaphors. *The Annual of Psychoanalysis, 24,* 175–185.

Courtois, C. A. (2010). *Healing the incest wound: Adult survivors in therapy* (2nd ed.). W. W. Norton.

Deutsch, R. A. (Ed). (2014). *Traumatic ruptures: Abandonment and betrayal in the analytic relationship.* Routledge, Taylor and Francis Group.

Dimen, M. (2011). Lapsus linguae, or a slip of the tongue?: A sexual violation in an analytic treatment and its personal and theoretical aftermath. *Contemporary Psychoanalysis, 47*(1), 35–79. https://doi.org/10.1080/00107530.2011.10746441

Doka, K. (1989). *Disenfranchised grief: Recognizing hidden sorrow.* Lexington Books.

Finkelhor, D., & Browne, A. (1985). The traumatic impact of child sexual abuse: A conceptualization. *American Journal of Orthopsychiatry, 55*(4), 530–541. https://doi.org/10.1111/j.1939-0025.1985.tb02703.x

Freyd, J. J. (1996). *Betrayal trauma: The logic of forgetting childhood abuse.* Harvard University Press.

Freyd, J. J. (2018, January 11). When sexual assault victims speak out, their institutions often betray them. *The Conversation.* https://theconversation.com/when-sexual-assault-victims-speak-out-their-institutions-often-betray-them-87050

Gabbard, G. O., & Lester, E. (1995). *Boundaries and boundary violations in psychoanalysis.* Basic Books.

Gagnon, K. L., Lee, M. S., & DePrince, A. P. (2017). Victim–perpetrator dynamics through the lens of betrayal trauma theory. *Journal of Trauma & Dissociation, 18*(3), 373–382. https://doi.org/10.1080/15299732.2017.1295421

Gediman, H. (1991). Seduction trauma: Complemental intrapsychic and interpersonal perspectives on fantasy and reality. *Psychoanalytic Psychology, 8*(4), 381–401. https://doi.org/10.1037/h0079299

Herbst, A. (2015). Ethical considerations when a client crosses sexual boundaries: My experience as a student therapist. *Psychotherapy Bulletin, 50*(1), 33–36. https://societyforpsychotherapy.org/ethical-considerations-when-a-client-crosses-sexual-boundaries-my-experience-as-a-student-therapist/

Herman, J. L. (1992). *Trauma and recovery*. Basic Books.

Kluft, R. P. (1990). Incest and subsequent re-victimization: The case of therapist–client sexual exploitation with a description of "sitting-duck" syndrome. In R. P. Kluft (Ed.), *Incest-related syndromes of adult psychopathology* (pp. 263–288). American Psychiatric Press.

Kluft, R. P. (2017). Weaponized sex: Defensive pseudo-erotic aggression in the service of safety. *Journal of Trauma & Dissociation, 18*(3), 259–283. https://doi.org/10.1080/15299732.2017.1295376

McNulty, N., Ogden, J., & Warren, F. (2011). 'Neutralizing the patient': Therapists' accounts of sexual boundary violations. *Clinical Psychology & Psychotherapy, 20*(3), 189–198. https://doi.org/10.1002/cpp.799

Messman, T. L., & Long, P. J. (1996). Child sexual abuse and its relationship to revictimization in adult women: A review. *Clinical Psychology Review, 16*(5), 397–420. https://doi.org/10.1016/0272-7358(96)00019-0

Middleton, W., Sachs, A., & Dorahy, M. J. (2017). The abused and the abuser: Victim-perpetrator dynamics. *Journal of Trauma & Dissociation, 18*(3), 249–258. https://doi.org/10.1080/15299732.2017.1295373

Pope, K. S. & Vetter, V. A. (1991). Prior therapist–patient sexual involvement among patients seen by psychologists. *Psychotherapy, 28*(3), 429–438.

Putnam, F. W. (1989). *Diagnosis and treatment of multiple personality disorder*. Guilford Press.

Schoener, G. R., Milgrom, J. H., Gonsiorek, J. C., Luepker, E. T., & Conroe, R. M. (Eds.). (1989). *Psychotherapists' sexual involvement with clients: Intervention and prevention*. Walk-In Counseling Center.

Shaw, D. (2014). *Traumatic narcissism: Relational systems of subjugation*. Routledge, Taylor & Francis Group.

Simon, R. I. (1999, March). Therapist–patient sex. From boundary violations to sexual misconduct. *The Psychiatric Clinics of North America, 22*(1), 31–47. https://doi.org/10.1016/S0193-953X(05)70057-5

Sinnamon, G. (2017). The psychology of adult sexual grooming: Sinnamon's seven-stage model of adult sexual grooming. *The psychology of criminal and antisocial behavior*. Elsevier. https://doi.org/10.1016/B978-0-12-809287-3.00016-X

Smith, C. P., & Freyd, J. J. (2014). Institutional betrayal. *American Psychologist, 69*(6), 575–587. https://doi.org/10.1037/a0037564

Van Dam, C. (2001). *Identifying child molesters: Preventing sexual abuse by recognizing the patterns of the offenders*. Haworth.

15

GROOMING AND THE DYNAMICS OF ABUSE AS EXPERIENCED AND VIEWED THROUGH THE EYES OF VICTIMS AND PEER ADVOCATES

Cases from TELL

JANET WOHLBERG

The Therapy Exploitation Link Line (TELL) is the largest and oldest-known all-volunteer entity in the world (I rejected the word "entirely" because TELL also serves as a tool for educating professionals about the nature of such abuse and treatment issues, and also serving as a resource for media, etc.) dedicated to the support of individuals who have been abused and exploited emotionally, psychologically, physically, and financially by rogue members of the mental health professions. The vignettes in this chapter are real stories of real people, selected from the thousands of stories told by victims to TELL volunteers over the past nearly 4 decades of TELL's existence. These vignettes are by no means meant to provide an exhaustive description of the range of grooming methods used by abusers, nor do they illustrate the seemingly infinite range of variables and nuances in these destructive relationships. But while every story that comes to TELL is unique, there are certain themes and styles that emerge repeatedly. The vignettes that follow are meant to describe some of these common themes. Names and identifying details have been altered to protect confidentiality in all vignettes except for Wanda, who prefers that we use her real name.

https://doi.org/10.1037/0000247-015
Sexual Boundary Violations in Psychotherapy: Facing Therapist Indiscretions, Transgressions, and Misconduct, A. Steinberg, J. L. Alpert, and C. A. Courtois (Editors)

GROOMING: DEFINITION AND OVERVIEW

Grooming is the term used to describe a set of behaviors that enable a therapist to manipulate and control a patient to achieve an outcome desired by the therapist for their own gratification rather than for the benefit of the patient. It is an ongoing process that continuously reinforces the patient's belief that the nontherapeutic relationship is what they desire and need while sustaining the therapist's dominance and power over the patient. Unlike transference, a naturally occurring part of many therapies, grooming is purposefully instigated by the therapist. Whether this process begins as a conscious act by the therapist, whether the therapist simply sees opportunity, or both, is unclear.

A question that regularly arises is whether a patient can also "groom" a therapist, methodically luring the unsuspecting therapist into an otherwise untherapeutic and harmful relationship. This question misses the requirement for all therapists to set and maintain safe and therapeutic boundaries even for the most manipulative and seductive of patients. No amount of personal drama or lack of fulfillment in a therapist's life allows for the use of patients to fill those gaps, nor does provocative patient behavior. As noted by Boston attorney Linda Jorgenson, even if the patient is a prostitute naked and begging for sex, the therapist is absolutely precluded from acting on temptation.

Any detailed description of the grooming processes used by rogue psychotherapists to abuse and exploit those in their care presents at least two potential dangers: (a) providing a how-to for would-be abusers and (b) encouraging the victim's nearly universal question, "How could I have been so stupid?" The latter is especially problematic as most discussions of grooming focus on the obvious, most tangible, and most easily understood aspects of the process: the red flags. These may include but are not limited to moving a victim to the last appointment of the day, making suggestive comments about the victim's appearance, offering to see the victim for free or at a greatly reduced fee, making pointed self-revelations, giving and taking gifts, allowing the victim to run up a bill, involving the victim in the therapist's social life, and asking the victim to do personal tasks such as babysitting or office work.

When red flags are perceived only as singular events and not as parts of patterns of perhaps hundreds of micro and macro boundary incursions, victims feel foolish for having missed "the obvious" and blame themselves for their "stupidity." Focusing on individual red flags obscures the many insidious grooming behaviors that we have found to be far more damaging.

These include the careful cultivation of dependence on the therapist as not just *a* source but *the* source of healing and support, shifting the attention of treatment away from the patient's needs to those of the therapist's, increasing the victim's financial and emotional investment in the relationship, and assuring the victim that he or she is "different" and special.

WHEN DOES ABUSE BEGIN?

Emma (Canada)

A victim of incest and lifelong sexual exploitation, including being sex trafficked beginning at age 6 with the cooperation and for the profit of her family, Emma sought therapy from a prominent British Columbia feminist therapist, Pamela Sleeth, to deal with her dissociative identity disorder (DID) and other issues. It took Emma well more than a decade before she was able to recognize not just the constant stream of red flags but that from her initial appointment, when Sleeth spent more than an hour telling Emma of her expertise, brilliant work, outstanding training, and revered position that Sleeth was systematically establishing her dominance over Emma and instilling in her a believe that she, Sleeth, was Emma's "savior come at last."

In the community of feminist therapists, the "therapy" was set up to meet Sleeth's needs and not those of her patient. Over the course of their "relationship," the therapy extended to multihour sessions on the pillow-lined floor of Sleeth's office, to multiday sessions at Sleeth's remote country cottage in which there was a single bed. Their first overt sexual act took place 8 years after the "therapy" had begun, after which Sleeth declared that they were now "partners."

Sleeth made Emma her medical proxy, required her to work in the house that Sleeth demanded they buy together, and required Emma to run her personal errands. Throughout, Sleeth made clear that Emma was to keep the true nature of their "relationship" secret. When Emma was finally able to end the relationship, Sleeth sued her, claiming that Emma had no financial right to their jointly purchased property. Sleeth increasingly flaunted her exploitative relationships with other clients and verbally abused Emma publicly and privately. Emma's determination to end the relationship was costly both emotionally and financially.[1]

---

[1] For a complete description of how this relationship evolved and how Emma has healed, see: Fox, B. (2018). *Coming to voice: Surviving an abusive therapist.* https://www.amazon.com/Coming-Voice-Surviving-Unethical-Therapist-ebook/dp/B07K5XR5HX

Rarely is a patient abused by a psychotherapist quickly or in the absence of psychological manipulation and foreplay. If a patient walked into a psychotherapist's office on day 1 or 2 of treatment, or even on days 5 or 10, and the therapist and patient engaged in a sexual act, most laypeople and professionals would quickly recognize the therapist's behavior to be unethical and unprofessional. They might even deem the act criminal assault or rape. As one TELL founder suggested, if there was a sign on the therapist's door that read "Should you choose to enter here, you risk losing your family and friends, becoming your therapist's emotional and possibly sexual servant, losing your sense of self and soul, and ultimately being betrayed and abandoned," most patients would know to flee.

Lacking such an early warning system, therapist–patient relationships are able to evolve over prolonged periods during which abusive therapists nurture victims' dependence, encourage adoration, and systematically separate victims from as many relationships external to the therapist–patient dyad as possible, doing so slowly and methodically so as to be imperceptible to victims both while it is happening and in retrospect. It is a phenomenon akin to watching the grass grow. So gradual may the evolution of the abusive relationship be that few victims can pinpoint where and when "therapy" ended and abuse began.

It is unlikely that the change occurred simply when the victim's appointment time was moved to the end of the day, when therapist and patient took their first walk in the woods, when they shared their first hug, or even when they first had sexual intercourse. Rather, it is likely that there were not just dozens but hundreds of boundary incursions, some beginning as early as day 1, that, in the victim's desperation to hold on to what appeared to be a lifeline, went unseen or denied as well as justified by the therapist as part of the therapeutic process.

The elements of grooming are designed, consciously or not, to fit the unique set of factors each victim brings to the treatment room. We can discern no predictable patterns of form, timing, and intensity. Ultimate termination of the formal treatment relationship does not necessarily end the hold abusers have over those they have groomed.

Marva (Middle East)

Marva, a highly educated professional woman, related the following story of how her belief that she had been "saved" by her psychiatrist slowly evolved into a relationship that was both confusing and emotionally threatening. Said Marva:

> "Differently special" was the term my psychiatrist used for me after terminating therapy. It was his way of reassuring me that I was not an ordinary client,

a claim he made consistently throughout the course of our 1-year "therapeutic" relationship. I went to him because I was in an abusive marriage, engaged in self-harm, had low self-esteem, and was suicidal. He was an acclaimed military psychiatrist known for using "unorthodox" approaches. He diagnosed me with borderline personality disorder. Initially he served as a witness to my abuse and made me feel visible and significant. He was the first to acknowledge that I was the victim of spousal rape and that I had an obligation to myself to leave the marriage. After an unwanted pregnancy, I left my husband, had an abortion, and filed for divorce. I went back to school, my self-harm episodes decreased significantly, and I was no longer suicidal. I started liking myself. After many months, my psychiatrist started hugging me at the end of sessions, something I found comforting and safe. I told him I loved him. He said he loved me too and that he no longer considered me a client. He shared intimate details of his relations with his partner and encouraged me to express and explore my romantic fantasies since we were "in a safe space." He gave me marijuana. He discussed other clients with me. I interpreted his methods as innovative rather than unethical. I felt I was the chosen one. Despite knowing for months that he would be transferring, when "therapy" ended, I felt abandoned and lost. We stayed in touch. After a year, he told me I was a "desirable woman" and that he wanted to sleep with me. I was afraid of the emotional aftermath of a sexual relationship and turned him down, but it has taken me 5 years to end contact with him, forgive him, and make peace with what happened. I still struggle with self-forgiveness and have a constant sense of loss, grief, indescribable numbness, and an unnamable something that keeps eating at me. (Used with permission of the anonymous author)

Grooming does not stop when abusers succeed in being embraced as the longed-for partner and lover, the only one who can truly understand the victim, and the ultimate savior. Instead, the manipulations continue to move the abuse into darker places, further deepen the hold abusers have over their victims, and ensure the secret. Increasingly, abusers justify the abuse, convincing victims that they are getting what *they* want and need. (In cases of therapists being abused by other therapists, abusers may explain away the relationships as "We can do this because we are colleagues, and we understand each other.")

While the most overt parts of Marva's grooming took place after her formal treatment ended, in the following case, Mary's began well before.

Mary (New York, United States)

Mary's relationship with her abuser began when he served as backup coverage for her regular therapist. She describes the evolution of the relationship as follows:

I was 34 when my phone calls with AH began: I left his office for the last time shortly before my 61st birthday. I guess I fell "in love" with him before I actually met him. I was in treatment with a female therapist, an ordained minister who named neither my sexual assault by a female counselor at an evangelical college nor my being molested by the wife of my church pastor as abuse. Instead, she followed her own agenda: She diagnosed me as having DID, convinced me my father had molested me, and eventually diagnosed me as a survivor of Satanic cult abuse. I was dependent on her and needed backup whenever she was away; thus began a phone relationship with her colleague, AH. I looked forward to her vacations to be able to talk to him. He quickly refuted her diagnosis and description of me. In time, he declared her incompetent.

Our phone conversations were like talking to a man I might have met through a dating ad, and the calls became more frequent and personal. We joked a lot. I begged him once to meet me for a drink: He refused. Later he would often bring this up as a sign that I had no boundaries. Finally, during the therapist's vacation, I went to a real session with AH, meeting him in a tiny room on the top floor of his institute. Despite his being older, slightly over-weight, and balding, in my eyes he was a movie star. After a 2-year buildup of telephone flirtation, the transference was incredibly intense. At the end of the session, when he took my hand and held it, I felt like I would never wash my hand again. A short time later, when he went away for a week, he sent me a postcard from San Francisco. While I was hurt that he didn't sign it "Love, AH," I was mesmerized by receiving something he had touched. When I early on reverted to self-harm, he would stroke the cuts, a sign to me that he loved me. He never told me he did.

The treatment plan he proposed was to address my "unhealthy boundaries" with women, not by exploring the violence and sexual abuse by a schizophrenic mother and subsequent female abusers but by "internalizing him" to enable intimacy with men. For many years, he hugged me at the end of each session. It was when he had a reaction to my bringing in vacation photos, one show-ing me in a bathing suit, that I realized I had an effect on him: He acted both offended and, at the same time, stimulated. I think now that his reaction was calculated. He encouraged me to share nude and increasingly more explicit photos of myself to "get in touch with my body." I had a desperate longing for connection, and he was offering that.

I did not enjoy what became constant sexual banter during sessions, especially when he would get an erection and sit with his legs open. If I looked in his direction and lowered my eyes an inch or two, he would ask, "Are you checking me out?"

Gradually, the man I had fantasized about was revealed to be different than the not-so-attractive man sitting across from me. Yet I was still enthralled and longed for the hugs he no longer gave at the door but were meted out as he saw fit. And, as I left each session, he would remind me not to "forget your assignment," which was to enact masturbatory fantasies about him to be discussed in detail, often with accompanying photos, when we next met.

When I became involved with another man, AH insisted that we have a joint session during which he badgered my boyfriend with questions he couldn't answer. By the time the session was over, the relationship with my boyfriend had ended. It didn't occur to me to go against AH's decision, but the sexual fantasies about him were gone for good.

The next 13 years had its own extreme and bizarre abuse until I finally left. There was never any treatment of the trauma that brought me to therapy in the first place except for AH's insistence that I no longer have contact with anyone in my family. When AH raised his fee, I found another therapist but didn't bring up the abuse for months because it didn't occur to me that he had done anything wrong. Comparing AH's treatment of me with legitimate therapy has been an integral part of recognizing how abusive his behaviors were and that I am not to blame for what happened. I know the truth now, and while I can never get back those lost years, I have finally begun to heal, and I am slowly learning to trust.

VICTIMS AS NURTURERS

Many abusers, recognizing opportunities presented by the natural and socialized tendencies of their prey to be nurturers, make their victims responsible for their well-being and professional standing, as well as that of their spouses, children, parents, and even grandparents, as part of the "bargain" to maintain the "relationship." Abusers have been widely reported to play on victims' nurturing instincts by claiming, for example, personal illness, ill children, and difficult marriages. Dozens of victims have reported that their abusers "made them promise" never to do anything to hurt them—and even years after the abusive relationships end, many victims still feel bound by that promise.

While escalating the roles of victims as caretakers, abusers also decrease the likelihood of exposure by: increasing their victims' isolation; keeping them off balance, sometimes with Stockholm syndromelike behaviors; promising ever-higher levels of connection and healing; and by reinforcing the fear that there is nothing for the victim outside of the therapy relationship.

Grace (Missouri, United States)

Raised in a severely dysfunctional family, Grace was neglected and abused by her parents and two of her siblings. She was sexually abused at age 4 by a teenaged neighbor, later by three of her brother's friends, and was a victim of date rape at age 20. When she sought therapy with Dr. Miles, Grace was single, 32, in a high-pressure profession, distressed, drinking to excess, and deeply scratching and cutting herself. Early in the treatment, Dr. Miles recorded children's stories for Grace to listen to between sessions. Comforting and soothing, they created an unbroken connection to Dr. Miles and became Grace's "safe place." Quickly her feelings for him became that of a young child for a loving parent. Over the next several years, with his encouragement and reassurance, Grace disclosed her sexual fantasies about Dr. Miles. In response, he explained transference. Slowly and increasingly, he also shared his own sexual fantasies, details of past experiences, and his attraction to her. Grace described her subsequent experience as follows:

> After 4 years, we began having sex, after which he would cycle between saying how wonderful it felt to how wrong it was. He would say it was damaging to me and then that it was okay—and we would do it again. I didn't pay for sessions when we had sex but did pay for the sessions when we discussed having had sex. I was confused by the relationship and asked him about talking to another therapist. He said that he and I were the best people to work on the situation. I took this to be another thing that was special between us. At no time was giving him up an option. I believed I would die without him.

Dr. Miles assured Grace that their relationship was not in jeopardy and that they were, instead, in a unique place in which they could do "deeper therapy." The cycle of erotic talk and sex and apologies continued. Eighteen months after the first sexual intercourse, Dr. Miles abruptly terminated the "therapy." (Used with the permission of the anonymous author.)

Abusive therapists make no attempt either to rein in or to remediate boundary crossings so long as the relationships are meeting their needs. Each purposeful boundary crossing enables the abusing therapist to derive personal gratification. Abusive therapists are seemingly unconstrained by ethical or professional concerns or concerns about the well-being of their patients. As described by former Massachusetts psychotherapist Amy L. Johnson, "There are too many choice points before therapists carry out abuse and exploitation . . . too many times for a therapist to stop and consult with other professionals. . . . This is not an impulsive embrace at the end of a session; there is a lot that needs to happen prior to sexual contact. It generally involves many small boundary violations over time that disarm and confuse the client in subtle ways."[2] In our experience, the grooming process almost always includes carefully calculated tests of the depths of the patient's susceptibility that then proceeds to purposeful plans to control and exploit the patient.

Wanda (Texas, United States)

As a candidate at the Boston Psychoanalytic Society and Institute, Wanda felt honored to be assigned to "Ed" Daniels for her training analysis and by his apparent interest in her. She wrote,

---

[2]See "The hardest thing I've ever had to do." In *Telling it like it is: When psychotherapists abuse and exploit.* http://www.therapyabuse.org

Instead of talking to me about why I was sad and crying, he would say we should meet more often. Since this was a so-called training analysis, I began with four appointments a week in October. By late spring, I was meeting with him 7 days a week. All this was well before he approached me with a sexual hug. He must have felt when he did that I was totally hooked. In January, after he said that I never looked at him as I was leaving, I looked at him on the way out. He had some sort of deep-eyed look. At the end of the next appointment, he was standing by the door for the first time ever as I was leaving. He hugged me, pressing his crotch into me. I left in a daze. I am amnesic as to what happened in the next unknown number of appointments, but later that month I found myself telling an analytic colleague that I was "head over heels in love" with Ed. She assumed I was talking about transference. In that time of total amnesia apparently I split in half, and sex began. I had had a number of sexual relationships before getting married. I am not amnesic to any of those first sexual encounters—only with Ed.

Mostly, as he was increasing my appointments, he sat behind me and shuffled papers and answered the phone while I did my duty and said whatever came to mind. He said very little. Once he said if he were Winnicott, he would come hold my hand. In retrospect I realize that he was testing to see if I was ready for him. At the time, I rationalized that he was teaching me as my training analyst.

In the face of his relative silence and my desire to be a good patient, saying whatever came to mind, I regressed to a state of intense nonsexual longing. This longing was only relieved by being in an appointment. He was very specific in how he groomed me. If he had rushed things, and if he had been physical sooner, it is very likely I would not have fallen victim to him. The right approach with me was silence and intellectual deprivation. He never gave an interpretation of anything I said or felt in that year of grooming. Instead by increasing appointments, he presented his presence as the answer to what was bothering me, and I deeply regressed.

The "relationship" lasted more than 9 years, ending when I left, telling him I no longer knew who I was and that my marriage was beginning to suffer. I had no idea I had been abused until almost 2 years later when I became mesmerized by the Anita Hill hearings and said to myself, "She is telling the truth, and he is a dirty old man." After that I got dangerously depressed and finally sought subsequent treatment. The psychoanalyst I saw did not name as abuse what had happened to me at the hands of his colleague. I had to discover that later after finding TELL and beginning to read about the topic.[3]

Boundary violations that include sex must be seen in the context of a systematic process that begs the question of when "sex" begins. Does sex begin when the therapist tells an off-color joke? Tells her that she is attractive? Engages in intimate, late-night phone calls? Hugs her goodbye? Kisses her? Discloses his own sexual fantasies? When patient and therapist take off their clothing? Not until penetration? Can it be sexual abuse if penetration has not occurred?

---

[3]For more on Daniels, see http://www.psychsearch.net/edward-daniels-2

The degree of fragility and vulnerability of a patient may determine the length of time it takes for the patient–therapist relationship to devolve to the sexual. This may be many years, but in some situations, the process may be greatly shortened by the use of prescription and nonprescription drugs and alcohol.

Kent (Massachusetts, United States)

A strikingly handsome and highly intelligent 29-year-old, Kent turned to a psychiatric nurse practitioner, Karen L, for help with problems completing his graduate school studies, alienation from his mother, and confusion over his relationship with his abusive father who had died when Kent was 15. Recommended by his primary care provider, Karen had recently arrived in Kent's small rural town with an agenda unknown to either the provider or Kent. After the second appointment, Karen prescribed antianxiety medication, which Kent initially found helpful. Within weeks, Karen added myriad other medications, told Kent repeatedly that he was special and unlike any patient she had ever worked with, and increasingly commented on his good looks. As Karen added more drugs, Kent became unable to get out of bed. He described this as being in a "zombielike trance." Karen assured him that this indicated "progress" in the therapy and that Kent was "finally" breaking through the denial that had been holding him back. Karen then had Kent move into her house so she could "closely monitor and care for him" because, she said, he was "special." Within days of moving him into her house, she moved him into her bed with professions of love and promises of a beautiful life together.

For 4 months, while they had sexual intercourse, Karen regularly woke him to have sex in the middle of the night. While Kent observed that Karen took her temperature, he did not know until several years later that she was doing so to track her ovulatory cycles. At the end of the 4 months, Karen disappeared as quickly as she had come. Less than a year later, she called Kent to tell him that he had a son, that he would never see him, and that if ever tried to make contact she would "have him committed." While Kent went on to free himself from the drugs, complete graduate school, and begin a challenging career, on the 10th anniversary of his son's birth, he committed suicide. The letter he left made clear that his experience with Karen and his longing for his son were major factors in his decision to end his life. Karen is still a practicing nurse practitioner.[4]

---

[4]Kent's story was written, with the help of his mother, by his TELL advocate.

While more than two thirds of those who turn to TELL report some level of suicidal thinking, in TELL's nearly 40 years, Kent is only one of two known to have followed through.

HOW DO ABUSIVE RELATIONSHIPS END?

Most therapist–patient abusive relationships end when abusers tire of victims and their demands for more attention and greater personal commitment—and often when victims threaten to "out" the relationship to spouses or colleagues. Abusers have made promises that they never intended to keep and see decreasing reasons for doing so. Abusers may begin to insult and belittle their victims, cancel appointments, claim that a spouse or other has become suspicious, blame the victim for what took place, and position themselves as the victimized. Some end the relationships abruptly, leaving victims all the more confused and bereft. We estimate that abusers end abusive relationships more than 80% of the time but may attempt to reassert control over victims who begin civil or licensing board actions by claiming to their victims that what they "shared" was true love, offering sincere-sounding apologies, claiming that the abusive behavior has been a source of great pain and guilt for them, and that the two should get together to talk about their relationship.

VICTIMS AND SUBSEQUENT TREATERS

It is with these raw and traumatized patients, self-blaming, feeling guilty, unable to trust either themselves or others, and still protecting their abusers, that subsequent treaters are confronted. The issues that brought these patients to therapy in the first place have not only gone untreated, they have been exacerbated. Long programmed to be the caretakers of their abusers, victims may give only highly edited narratives of what took place. Dozens of victims report guarding their abusers' identities for months and even years of subsequent treatment and concealing much of what they experienced as the most shameful and embarrassing parts of the abuse. Many continue to long for their abusers and believe that they drew the abusers into the relationships despite knowing, intellectually, that they have been exploited and betrayed.

While some mental health professionals appear to believe that TELL is "antitherapy," this is directly counter to TELL's mission and practices. As stated at TELL's website, TELL does not provide therapy but instead strongly urges victims to seek competent subsequent treatment. Because most victims of therapy abuse have difficulty trusting, especially therapists, TELL volunteers serve as "sounding boards," urging victims to be open and honest with their subsequent treaters and guiding them through the process. From time to time, TELL volunteers find themselves having to urge a victim to seek a new subsequent treater when the treater they are seeing significantly replicates the behavior of the abuser; fails to acknowledge that what took place was harmful, unethical, and unprofessional; assigns the blame for the abuse to the victim's desires and defects; or exhibits other behaviors that minimize the experience.

Subsequent treatment of those abused and exploited by psychotherapists is covered elsewhere in this book, but TELL's observations, based on thousands of reports from victims, suggest general trends that may predict why some subsequent treatments succeed while others are doomed from the outset or early on. On this basis, TELL offers a few suggestions:

- From the point at which a patient reveals what took place, validate that the experience is real and meaningful and that the perpetrator's behavior was unethical, unprofessional, and unacceptable, but do so without exhibiting *overt* anger. Recognize that the victim may still feel he or she "loves" the abuser or is, at best, ambivalent.

- Never tell a victim that they have to trust you. Not only is that likely to be what the perpetrator claimed, a victim has many valid reasons not to trust you.

- Do not push a victim for details of what took place before the victim is ready and willing to reveal them. Remember that those details are likely heavily shrouded in shame and self-blame.

- In states where there is mandated reporting of abuse, let victims know that if they share the name of the perpetrator, you will be required to report.

- Because victims struggle to gain or regain power and control over their lives, do not report or otherwise take action against an abuser or offer to do so for the victim. It is up to the victim to decide when and how to take action: Doing so is an important step in the healing process.

- When a victim decides to take action, suggest that they seek out resources such as those available at TELL to help assess what avenues of action might be available and what is involved.

Be aware that you can do everything right but still not succeed in your attempts to work with a victim because the victim is not ready to address what took place or make the "leap of faith" necessary to open themself to the perceived dangers of doing so.

TAKING ACTION

Given the victim's confusion, the nature of the abusive relationship, shame, social pressures and judgments, concern for families and marriages, and promises to never betray their abusers, few victims pursue civil suits or other legal actions. Those who do are often silenced with nondisclosure settlement agreements that keep them from speaking out about the abusive events or following up with reports to licensing boards.

Abusers who have early-on diagnosed their victims with pathologies that suggest, for example, lack of ability to differentiate between truth and fantasy and even psychosis, are often quick to use these diagnoses to discredit victims who report.

In the past, it was the rare abuser who paid a price (e.g., anything out-of-pocket or loss of license) for having severely violated a patient's boundaries and inflicted serious harm. Although that is changing and today more abusers are being held accountable, the majority of those sued by their victims still go on their way, free to abuse again. Those who do lose licenses frequently change venues and reinvent themselves in roles such as life coaches, counselors, and spiritual guides. Some request and achieve reinstatement of their licenses. Public education and movements such as #MeToo have begun to bring about visible change.

Those in the helping professions who want to accept assertions by abusing colleagues that what took place was a mistake, that it will never happen again, that it was based on true love, that they have been rehabilitated, and that they should be allowed to continue to practice, perhaps after a refresher course in ethics or a packaged or online "rehabilitation" program, are misguided and undermine the reputation of their professions. Integrity requires professionals to ask themselves: "Would I send someone I care about, my parent, my spouse, my child, my best friend to this person? And if the answer is no, then why send anyone else?"

TELL

TELL (http://www.therapyabuse.org) was founded in Boston in the 1980s when a client, "D," told Boston social worker Nancy Avery that she felt she could only move ahead in her healing if she could talk to others who had had similar experiences.

"D" had been sexually exploited by a psychiatrist, Richard Ingrasci, to whom she had turned after having been given a difficult medical diagnosis. Ingrasci, who claimed to specialize in holistic medicine and treating women with chronic, disfiguring, and fatal diagnoses, practiced what he called "vaginal rolfing." He often stood his naked clients in front of mirrors and required them to watch as he stroked their bodies. He had intercourse with many. According to the testimonies of some who filed charges against him with the Massachusetts Board of Registration in Medicine, he told patients that they had become ill because they had failed to love their bodies. He was going to teach them how to remedy that. In the face of multiple complaints, Ingrasci ultimately resigned his license.[5]

Recognizing the healing benefits of helping victims network with one another, Avery sought out colleagues who were treating women who had been exploited in therapy settings. Avery was able to bring together four women for the first known therapy group specifically dedicated to this problem. Says Avery, "There is nothing that any therapist can do for a victim that comes close to what meeting another victim can do." The wisdom of Avery's statement has been borne out time and again by the connections victims make through TELL.

At the conclusion of the Avery's multiweek group therapy, the four women decided they needed something more. Seeing my name and story in *The Boston Globe*, they invited me to meet with them: The five of us founded TELL.[6] Within 6 months, and with the help of additional *Boston Globe* publicity, monthly meeting attendance grew from five to nearly 50. Today, TELL is Internet only and is supported by a small group of volunteers on three continents who give peer support to victims from around the world. In addition to other resources and readings, TELL offers a free e-book at its website that includes first-person accounts of abuse and commentaries and history by experts.

Because TELL is not engaged in research and keeps no databases, it does not collect statistics on just how often sexual abuse of patients takes place. However, judging from the steady 40,000 to 45,000 visitors who access the TELL website each year, it is clear that the number is significant.

In our earliest communications with victims, TELL Responders validate victims' stories and suggest that it is not the person but the dream that has

[5]See https://www.upi.com/Archives/1989/05/25/Editors-Note-nature-Another-psychiatrist-target-of-Massachusetts-sex-probe/5539612072000/ and https://www.psychsearch.net/robert-ferrell
[6]See https://www.psychsearch.net/lionel-schwartz

been lost and must be mourned when the abusive relationship ends. This is an idea, along with pointing out that what took place was abuse and not an "affair," that must be reinforced continuously as we work to educate victims about what therapy and therapists should and should not be.

Victims of abuse that did not culminate in sexual intercourse often question whether they have actually been abused. Nonsexual abusive treatment may be dismissed by family, friends, and even subsequent treaters as "What's the big deal? Nothing really happened." In our experience, however, it is the nonsexual grooming processes that create the most psychological upheaval and damage. The exceptions occur when sex has been demeaning, such as when abusers have required victims to crawl naked on their hands and knees and beg to be allowed to perform oral sex, be urinated or defecated upon, taken to S&M parlors, masturbated while being photographed, and so on.

Many victims who find TELL are too untrusting to talk to professionals about what took place and fearful of being pathologized rather than believed. Instead, victims who turn to TELL report being more comfortable with peer support and the relative anonymity of the internet.

Our hope is that TELL can be seen as an adjunct to therapy and a partner to reputable and informed therapy and therapists.

CONCLUSION

What is clear from considering the sadly true stories of Marva, Emma, Grace, Mary, Kent, Wanda, and many thousands of others who have been groomed and exploited by abusive psychotherapists is that grooming cannot be easily and simply described. Although abusers appear to be universally calculating and opportunistic, the process of grooming does not follow a fixed set of rules and patterns. Abusers appear to understand the needs and desires of each of their victims and have a keen sense of how to manipulate and control them. Although it is possible that abusers simply "ring many doorbells before someone finally answers," the intimate nature of therapy, generally undertaken in private rooms and out of sight, affords extreme levels of opportunity for those who choose to draw on it.

The bad news is that grooming and abuse appear to be inevitable in a species that is hierarchical by nurture and nature. In the words of psychoanalyst Wanda Needleman: "While many victims have backgrounds that make them clearly vulnerable, I had experienced neither abuse nor neglect. If I can be groomed by someone like Ed Daniels, then anyone can be groomed."

The good news is that with support, knowledgeable subsequent treatment, and validation that what happened to them was abuse, that it is not their fault, and that they are not alone, healing is not only possible for victims but probable. With the exception of Kent and one other known to us, whose pain became intolerable, those who volunteered their stories for this chapter should be embraced as testaments to the strength and resilience of the human spirit and to their own inner strength and determination to survive and lead productive lives.

16

THREE SURVIVORS SPEAK

Stories of Confusion, Shame, Anguish, and Resilience

CHRISTINE A. COURTOIS, JUDITH L. ALPERT, AND GOLDIE EDER

Our intent in this chapter is for the reader to hear the personal narratives of people who experience sexual boundary violations (SBVs) in treatment. For this purpose, we sought out three survivors to interview, two of whom had been identified by colleagues by means of purposive sampling and one who was a former patient of one of the authors who had volunteered when she learned about the book and its topic. All three candidates agreed to be interviewed about their experience because doing so provided them with both an opportunity to tell their story and, in the process, to understand more about it and to educate others. As noted throughout this book and in other publications on the topic, survivors of therapist abuse rarely have a forum in which they can discuss their experience in any detail and with a knowledgeable respondent. On the basis of our clinical experience and review of relevant literature on SBVs in therapy and its aftermath, the three authors developed a standardized set of questions used in all interviews, with each interviewing one survivor volunteer. Before the interview, each was sent informed consent and publication permission forms to sign, as well as a copy of the interview questions they would be asked. Interviews were

https://doi.org/10.1037/0000247-016
Sexual Boundary Violations in Psychotherapy: Facing Therapist Indiscretions, Transgressions, and Misconduct, A. Steinberg, J. L. Alpert, and C. A. Courtois (Editors)

conducted by phone after the individual reviewed the questions and then indicated readiness to be interviewed. The interviews took place in one to three 90-minute sessions. In summarizing the experiences of these survivors, we have changed their names and any other identifying information that would compromise their anonymity, but all other information is unaltered. A draft of this chapter was sent to them before submission for publication. They were asked to review the chapter for accuracy and to give their final approval.

We begin by providing a brief introduction to each of the three survivors, written by the corresponding interviewer, followed by discussion of some common and individual themes that emerged from the three interviews with commentary. Of note: The abuse of each of three survivors began at different ages, ranging from childhood to adulthood, offering a different window into some of the age-related dynamics. It is also clear that each survivor was emotionally vulnerable due to previous experiences of abuse and neglect or because of felt isolation and loneliness at the time they started the therapies reported here, and that the offending therapist capitalized on these experiences or feelings. In the final section, we review relevant literature on characteristics of survivors and aftereffects and relate it to the material provided by these individuals.

KEN: ABUSED BY HIS MALE THERAPIST AS A CHILD

Being maltreated was familiar to Ken, who reported abuse beginning at age 6 months. His parents, also abused as children, were his first tormentors. They abused him physically, verbally, emotionally, and by means of neglect and abandonment. They kicked him out of the house at age 17. As a result, as a child, Ken thought people could do whatever they wanted to him and that he had no right to say anything, try to stop it, or fight back. Tellingly, Ken was an angry kid who got into a lot of trouble in school. His principal threatened expulsion if he did not receive therapy, so his parents complied with the referral they were given. Ken was 9 when he began treatment and reports being abused in the very first session by his male therapist, a psychiatrist. Ken met with this therapist once a week for 2 years, with abuse occurring in almost every session. The "treatment" ended when Ken's family moved. Nudity of Ken and his therapist during sessions was standard, as were physical exams during which the therapist wore a doctor's coat and stethoscope and played with Ken's genitals to arouse him and then mastur-bate him to orgasm. Although Ken recalls less about the acts he was made to perform on the therapist, he remembers what the therapist's genitals looked like and that he had difficulty swallowing during one session and vomited afterward. Ken thinks porn may have also been involved.

Ken had no understanding of what was supposed to happen in therapy or how it was supposed to help him. His parents were disengaged and never inquired about his treatment, so he never felt he could go to them for help. As far as he knew and according to what the therapist told him, the behaviors during the session were normal; however, as they proceeded, Ken came to believe they were wrong, but he also felt that everything in his life was like that—wrong. He felt ashamed, humiliated, and embarrassed. He was also very confused because he sometimes looked forward to the sessions as he was given attention, listened to, and allowed to do such things as smoke the therapist's cigarettes and put his feet on the therapist's desk, and he received candy and gifts. At age 12, he told his older brother what had happened with the therapist, but he received no reaction or response. He disclosed the abuse to his mother as an adult, and she said his father knew about the abuse but did not indicate how he knew or why he never intervened or protected him.

Ken is now a bisexual man in his early 60s. Although the abuse occurred 52 years ago, he reports that he has been haunted by it. He is dissociative, especially when having sex, and knows his self-esteem and ability to trust others were severely compromised by being treated as an object. He made unsuccessful attempts to locate his previous psychiatrist with the goal of protecting other children from what he went through. This has been very confusing as he now wonders who this man was and whether he was even a psychiatrist. How is it that he can't be located and that there is no record of him or his practice? Ken was suicidal as a child and adolescent and homeless several times as a young adult. He describes himself currently as a happy and successful person with a stable job. He has worked hard to be healthier and to feel less shame and attributes his stability to his extensive spiritual work, psychotherapy, and ongoing participation in men's sexual abuse groups.

JOANNE: ABUSED BY HER THERAPIST AS AN ADOLESCENT

Joanne describes having had a relatively happy early childhood and family life, but she may not have received enough validation from her parents as she developed an engaging and pseudomature style with adults in the community in attempts to get special attention and approval. When she was a young teen, her success and high potential as an athlete resulted in her parents engaging a private male coach for her. She and the coach developed a close friendship but "My specialness ended one night on the way home from practice in an isolated, dark parking lot—a scene that would be repeated many times. It spread to abuse in the family room of my own home while my parents were upstairs. My . . . [athletic] practices turned to dread, and my interest in the sport plummeted." She was in shock when he began to fondle her and tried to get her to masturbate him—she had been raised Catholic, had not received any sex education, and did not have any context to understand what he was doing.

Subsequently, Joanne changed dramatically from "good girl" to "good delinquent." She began to drink beer and found that alcohol brought her great comfort. Drinking took over all aspects of her life. She became deliberately sloppy in her clothing and appearance in order not to bring attention to her body. She was increasingly rebellious and uncooperative at school and in the community and attracted attention from authorities several times. Her parents were appalled and teachers confused and concerned, but no one asked whether anything adverse had happened to her. When the coach left town suddenly, reportedly due to his sexual abuse of another female athlete, her mother asked if he had ever done anything to her. The question unnerved her. She didn't trust adults to be able to help so she said no.

In desperation as her alcohol-fueled behavior spiraled out of control, Joanne's parents put her in therapy with an addiction specialist. Joanne initially resisted their sessions. Over time, she experienced the therapist as kind and caring. They first worked on her alcoholism, and she describes her early efforts at sobriety as rocky with many relapses. They began to meet more frequently and for longer sessions, something Joanne did not question because she knew she needed help. But she did resent Friday afternoon sessions that stretched on for hours, with no advance notice, and seemingly at the whim of her therapist. Joanne believed her therapist was avoiding going home and was using her as an excuse not to. During that same period, the therapist began to touch her during breath training and ostensibly to check her liver and began to end sessions with a long hug. They had increasingly frequent phone contact and began to meet outside the office to talk and take walks together. One Friday night, Joanne got drunk and told her therapist about the relapse on their regular Saturday morning phone call. The therapist told Joanne to come over to her house so they could talk about it. Joanne ended up staying overnight. The therapist's husband opposed this plan and reacted by directing his anger at Joanne. That night, she reports she awakened briefly to find her therapist trying to unbutton her jeans, supposedly to make her more comfortable.

With support and coaching, Joanne was finally able to stop drinking, something her parents were proud of and attributed to her "shining star" therapist. Around that time, on one of their "therapeutic walks," the therapist spontaneously kissed Joanne on the lips, and Joanne kissed her back. This was the beginning of "an intense, secret, emotional and physically driven relationship" that took over both their lives. There was never any discussion about what was happening, that it was same-gender and sexual, and that it was compulsive and all-consuming. The amount of time they spent together increased significantly, something no one questioned. Quoting Joanne: "To the outside world, she was still my therapist. My in-office appointments were time locked in a room to have sex. Our time together outside the office was any opening we could figure out to rendezvous. We even took vacations together." It is not clear when, if, or how her therapy ended. Her therapist left her husband. He blamed Joanne and although he threatened to call her parents, he never did. Meanwhile, Joanne's long-term relationship with her high school boyfriend ended abruptly after she casually and rather flippantly told him about having had a sexual relationship with the therapist during the time that they were dating. She describes him as shocked and devastated, and he broke up with her shortly after her disclosure.

Following her separation, the therapist moved into her own apartment, which provided them a standing location to meet; it caused Joanne new anxiety about being "outed" and their being perceived as a lesbian couple. Joanne had become increasingly conflicted about their sexual contact as her sexual identity was firmly and exclusively heterosexual; she could not understand or reconcile how she became sexually involved with a woman. She was very relieved when the therapist called for a 3-month hiatus so she could engage in her own therapy. After the 3 months, the therapist contacted Joanne to resume their relationship, but they never again had sex, something that was not discussed. The therapist resumed dating men, which Joanne encouraged, and their contact lessened and eventually became very sporadic.

Joanne started a career, married, and had children. While this was happening, she occasionally thought about her abusive therapist, but she did not think about the sexual aspect of their relationship. Joanne felt warmly toward her and thought of her as a family member whom she might someday introduce to her family. It was only after 20 years, when she found the Therapist Exploitation and Link Line (TELL; see Chapter 15), that she understood she had been used. At first it was difficult for her to take this in, but slowly she came to understand that she was, indeed, groomed, and she came to understand the impact of the abuse on her internal world. Despite this understanding, she continued to feel connected to her and miss her and what they had. Her husband who was in treatment for service-related posttraumatic stress disorder, disclosed Joanne's history to his psychiatrist who was the first to label what happened as abuse and as unethical. Over time, her husband and his psychiatrist's perspectives helped to break through her denial and resulted in her seeking help and finding TELL.

CAROL: ABUSED BY HER MALE PSYCHIATRIST AS AN ADULT

Carol was in her 40s when she was sexually abused by a male psychiatrist. She was married with two adolescent daughters and worked outside the home during the 5 years of her treatment and abuse. Carol sought treatment after reading about borderline personality disorder (BPD) in a self-help book and considering that it might apply to her. She sought consultation from a national expert who worked at a local renowned psychiatric treatment center. Specifically, she sought treatment for symptoms of anxiety, depression, and insomnia that selective serotonin reuptake inhibitor medication only partially treated. The BPD expert referred Carol to a local psychiatrist in his center's network, and she started treatment with him once a week, soon increasing to twice a week.

Before long, the therapist offered to be available by phone or pager 24/7 between sessions, which initially surprised but also impressed Carol. She soon became increasingly dependent on the between-session contact, craving ever more communication and reassurance. About 6 months into treatment, Carol started having "feelings" for the therapist, which she disclosed in a letter as she felt too discomfited to tell him in person. Initially, he reacted by telling her these feelings were natural and they "would work through them," but before long he was giving mixed messages about what their involvement could be. He complimented her on her appearance and made suggestive comments about her body, and noted their special connections around topics related to philosophy, religion, and so on. He began to hug her at the end and, eventually, at the beginning of sessions. Over time, he expressed sexual fantasies about her. During one phone call, he told her he loved her. It took her awhile for her to tell him she loved him, but when she did, he told her he already knew. Both became increasingly flirtatious, trading fantasies, but acknowledging they "couldn't have what they want." Her need for contact escalated, and she obsessively called or paged him until he called her back with reassurances that he cared about her. Over time, Carol became more emotionally and behaviorally dysregulated, and on more than one occasion went into his medicine closet and grabbed handfuls of medication, threatening to commit suicide. She would also grab other patient's medical records which were left on furniture in the office, an action that resulted in his wrestling with her for them. He did little to manage the escalating situation or to develop a new treatment plan. It is not known if he sought consultation although at one point, he suggested she seek a consultant. She refused because she thought she would be told to stop seeing him.

Toward the end of the treatment, the therapist disclosed that he and his wife had not been intimate for about 10 years. Although he had originally said that sex between therapist and patient was prohibited by professional ethics, he responded to her flirting with him by saying, "See, isn't this fun?" and because Carol thought he was getting ready to kiss her, she kissed him. The contact between them then intensified and became sexual during the last month of treatment. Although they never had intercourse, therapy sessions continued during this last month with "extra time on the couch" for physical and sexual contact. She was billed for these sessions. They agreed to keep the behavior secret. Although Carol fantasized about marrying him, she knew this was unlikely. He told her he would never leave his wife. She began to feel he was using her, and she confronted him and demanded he turn himself into the Board of Registration of Medicine. The therapist instead disclosed to a colleague that he had been intimate with a client. This led to a violation report to the Board of Medicine. Therapy came to an abrupt and traumatic halt as he voluntarily agreed to stop practicing medicine and never responded to Carol's attempts to reach him afterward, even though he initially had told her he hoped to be able to continue to prescribe her medications or at least continue as a nonprescribing physician to be her psychotherapist "after all this dies down."

Carol subsequently became obsessed with the therapist and unsuccessfully attempted to see him at his home and in other settings. She had contacted the Board of Medicine and rescinded her report in a misguided attempt to protect him, something she now regrets. She researched options such as a lawsuit or criminal charges and decided not to file either one. Carol eventually lost her job and went on disability due to her ongoing decompensation and inability to function. She is now remorseful about her neglectful and detached behavior with her husband and daughters during the treatment period and afterward.

At some point, she learned about TELL. They referred her to a therapist who helped her understand that what her previous therapist did was wrong and constituted abuse and that he was solely responsible. After that therapist retired, Carol continued with a new male therapist whom she feels is supportive and has appropriate boundaries. She continues to have difficulty finding and keeping a psychiatrist who can prescribe medication for her. Carol ended the interview by stating,

> I can feel very frustrated. The abuse left me feeling hopeless. He seemed like the most caring and selfless person. I thought if he wasn't who I thought he was, then there are not good people and nothing worth living for. Every time I get an ounce of hope it dwindles. I need to find a reason or purpose for what I went through. I've had a couple of opportunities where I thought I could share my story, but they fell through. I thought your project had fallen through too [due to some of the delays involved].

Despite her eagerness to participate, Carol delayed the interview until her current therapist returned from his vacation to have his emotional support. She anticipated discussing the abuse and her misguided former therapist might revive her emotional turmoil and pain.

COMMON AND INDIVIDUAL THEMES IN THESE PERSONAL DESCRIPTIONS

Common and individual themes are interwoven in these personal descriptions, many of which match those found in the extant research literature on the aftereffects of therapist abuse and in the personal descriptions that have been published in survivor memoirs (see Bates & Brodsky, 1989; Freeman & Roy, 1976; Shepherd, 2017) and clinician and responder descriptions.

Abuse Is Highly Variable, as Are Aftereffects and Symptoms and Their Presentation

Although there are commonalities, we emphasize here that there is no "one size fits all" abuse scenario. There is a tendency to categorize therapist abuse as being on either the "slippery slope" pole or the "psychopathic therapist" pole, but the reality is that therapist abuse falls all along the continuum. Nor are aftereffects all the same, experienced to the same degree in each case or manifest in the same way. As is illustrated by Joanne's case, victims can appear asymptomatic for years and even decades. They may be highly functional during periods of denial, minimization, and knowledge sequestration due to dissociation and due to the distractions provided by the demands of family and career. In such cases of delayed expression of posttraumatic stress disorder, initial posttraumatic responses go dormant or remit for some time, making the victim susceptible to their later spontaneous emergence, usually in response to trigger events or experiences that are highly idiosyncratic and unpredictable. Assessment of each individual's experience is needed because dynamics and many other factors, including severity of occurrence, duration, and aftereffects; means of engaging, grooming, or silencing the victim; and consequences vary; they can also manifest at different points in time, as illustrated by these three cases.

Age at Onset

The age at onset of these abusive therapies differs. The victim's personal history and age and stage of development at the time of the abuse influenced aftereffects and their expression. For example, Ken's previous and ongoing maltreatment by his parents had already caused him to feel somehow deserving of abuse and powerless to protest, feelings that were unfortunately intensified rather than ameliorated by his "therapy." Due to his age at onset and his previous history, dissociation would likely be a primary coping mechanism for him at that time and possibly later. In his interview, he reported discontinuous memory of the abuse and being generally dissociative as an adult, especially during sexual experiences.

Joanne's experience with her coach, occurring suddenly in early adolescence, had profoundly negative effects. These most likely contributed to her use of alcohol to cope and self-soothe. Her later abuse by her therapist caused more extreme disconnection and led to the development of what she described as "a dual life." When she connected the two (i.e., by facing that her therapist used and abused her), it resulted in intense emotional pain and self-hatred. In Carol's adult-onset therapy, proper boundaries were mishandled from the start and resulted in the reinforcement of gross overdependence on her therapist and resultant personal insecurity. She "fell in love" with him, which was followed by mutual seduction and the later sexualization of their relationship. This, in turn, set her up for decompensation rather than the amelioration of her presenting symptoms. She reported less dissociation than Ken and Joanne, possibly because her abuse occurred during adulthood.

History of Previous Abuse

A history of previous abuse increases vulnerability and often results in more serious consequences. Two of the three respondents (Ken and Joanne) had previous histories of abuse, Ken from his parents and Joanne from her coach. Carol's history is less defined but individuals with her symptoms and possible BPD diagnosis usually have histories of invalidation in childhood.

Therefore, all of them had symptoms that brought them to treatment and were expressed in different ways: Ken, due to anger and acting-out behavior; Joanne, due to addiction and negative changes in behavior, motivation, and self-presentation; and Carol, in unremitting depression, anxiety, and emotional dysregulation. All three entered treatment in highly vulnerable conditions— conditions used against them by their therapist. Their abuse was replete with betrayal of them as individuals and of their trust and need; the abuse constituted betrayal trauma.

Therapist–Abusers

The violators and referral sources varied. Ken saw a male psychiatrist who was married with children and was recommended by the school principal. Currently, he questions the identity of his therapist. Was he really a psychiatrist, or was he a pedophile or pornographer? Why has he been unable to locate information about him despite an extensive search? Joanne's abuser, a licensed "addiction therapist of sorts" was married and ostensibly heterosexual. However, she was unhappy in her marriage and sought to leave it, seems to have been conflicted about her sexual orientation, and may have been in the throes of a manic/compulsive episode of some sort. Carol's therapist was also a psychiatrist who was married, and her referral to him came from an acknowledged expert in BPD. Her therapist was well regarded, and she approached him from a position of trust. She was surprised but delighted by his offer of boundless availability that resulted in her overreliance and intensifying need for his reassurance. He appeared to have a high need to be needed and to be perceived as an all-giving therapist. Over time, he disclosed being in an unhappy marriage that lacked sexual intimacy. After the relationship with Carol became sexual, he disclosed that he had no intention of leaving his wife. These three professionals represent a range of credentials but, more importantly, a range of personality types and characteristics that match those identified by Gabbard (1994): those who are predatory psychopaths with paraphilias (Ken's), lovesickness and mania (Joanne's), and masochistic surrender (Carol's).

Means of Engagement and Escalation of Contact

In two of these three cases, the therapist was described as helpful early on. Joanne and Carol describe getting and appreciating needed attention and care. Ultimately, their needs were used against them, and both were subjected to increasingly serious boundary crossings that led to sexual boundary violation. Joanne's therapist progressively engaged her by complimenting her on her "niceness and gentleness" and by relying on her learned deference to adults. She broke standard boundaries, however, regarding length, timing, and location of sessions; phone calls; and physical contact during sessions. She was also inappropriate in her interventions when Joanne relapsed, including when she had her stay overnight at her home. Carol's therapist offered her 24/7 availability, which reinforced overdependence on her part. She also "fell in love with him" during this time, leading to later sexualized conversations and shared fantasies, increased hugging and other physical contact, and then to sexual activity (but not intercourse) over the course of several weeks, before she "came to her senses" and confronted him.

Ken's abuse began much more immediately and blatantly with an inappropriate physical exam involving genital inspection and manipulation in the first session. Mutual nudity and masturbation occurred in almost every weekly session for 2 years. Ken reported that none of what went on in treatment was therapeutic. He felt used as an object and never considered that he could complain or refuse the contact because he was bad and deserved mistreatment. Ken described being groomed by the therapist's attention to him and bribed and rewarded with candy, cigarettes, and special privileges. He was enjoined to secrecy around the nudity because "people wouldn't understand."

Feelings and Thoughts During Abuse Period

Ken did not know how to understand or to process what was happening in sessions, made all the worse by his lack of understanding about therapy. He initially thought that the behavior was normal; however, over time he came to feel it was wrong. Yet he maintained the belief that it was his fault and he could not refuse, beliefs that benefited his abuser. He experienced shame, humiliation, and embarrassment, feelings that further trapped him as they interfered with his telling anyone. Ken also described having conflicted feelings about the sessions because he liked the attention and gifts and being able to engage in other "special" activities.

Joanne described compulsive, risky, furtive, and escalating sexual interactions with her therapist in a wide variety of settings. She did not question much (e.g., that it was same-gender interaction with her then-married and ostensibly heterosexual therapist) but instead went along in a way that sounds robotic or dissociative. Although she enjoyed some of the sexual contact and described learning how to be sexual, her wish was to have their special relationship without the sex. No one around them inquired about their

290 • *Courtois, Alpert, and Eder*

relationship. In fact, when the relationship was disclosed to two professional colleagues, they enabled it. When the therapist separated and got an apartment, they no longer needed to be furtive in their meetings and began to look more like a "normal" couple. This was a wake-up call for Joanne, who saw herself only as heterosexual, wanted a traditional marriage and a family, and did not want to be in a same-sex relationship. To Joanne's relief, after the therapist's 3-month break, the friendship resumed but not the sexual contact. Perhaps the therapist had been treated for her compulsive and hypersexual behavior, both signs of bipolar disorder. We can only speculate. There was little discussion between them about what had happened, except that they spoke often about their special friendship and developed a joint fantasy of being together in their later years. The therapist wanted Joanne to care for her in her old age. Over time, the therapist began to date men, which Joanne supported. Contact between them gradually decreased with Joanne unsure how or when it ended. Joanne continued to imagine resuming some sort of relationship with her therapist in the future, even to the point of having the therapist meet her husband and children. It is only in the last decade that Joanne has begun to put the pieces of her dual life together and acknowledge the misconduct and its extent. She has been able to do this because of many factors, primary among them her husband's ongoing outrage about the misconduct and its toll on her and his challenges to her ongoing denial and idealization of the therapist.

Carol, in contrast, began to have feelings for her therapist early in her 5-year treatment, due to his active encouragement of her dependence through over-availability and infantilizing. He initially maintained proper personal boundaries, but these eroded over time when the boundary violation escalated. When this led to sexual contact, it had the paradoxical effect of breaking through Carol's fantasy, causing her to suspect he was using her. She then confronted him and urged him to report his unethical conduct to his licensing board. He later relinquished his license to practice. She testified to the abuse to the Board of Medicine where she felt she was interrogated. Later she recanted due to her conflicted feelings about the therapist, an action she now regrets. She was unsuccessful in her attempts to contact her therapist afterward and later stalked him in her attempts to resume contact. She also sought information about taking civil action against him, but the lawyer she consulted discouraged her due to her perceived fragility.

Short- and Long-Term Effects of Abuse

All three respondents reported significant and long-lasting interruption of their lives and negative impact in a variety of life domains. They were forced to expend great effort on maintaining emotional equilibrium and on recovery efforts, including subsequent therapy and self-help, and all three demonstrated perseverance and personal resilience in these efforts. At the end of treatment, each of them was more vulnerable than when they started, and their problems had compounded. Notably, whatever age at onset, all were confused, both during and afterward, and questioned their involvement. Each felt manipulated but also responsible, feelings that began to change during their recovery efforts. Some of these feelings intensified at different points in their lives, leading them to feeling helpless, hopeless and suicidal. All maintained suicide as a possible "out" if things got too bad and as a way to "do away with" the self they had come to hate.

All three respondents had posttraumatic reactions and symptoms. They reported different degrees of dissociation, with Ken's emerging episodically and especially during sexual activity and Joanne's being the most ongoing and dense. Dissociation allowed Joanne to separate from the abuse, maintain a highly positive memory of her therapist as a "good mother figure," have a successful marriage and family, and a thriving career. As her dual life began to merge, facing the reality has resulted in great anguish and increased suicidal urges, and she again returned to alcohol as a means of chemical dissociation. She continues to question how she could have engaged in homosexual behavior and is fearful of what others would think of her were they to know.

Carol and Joanne expressed ambivalence toward their former therapists, and all three interviewees reported unfinished business. Each would like to locate their therapists. They seek to prevent what happened to them from happening to others. Joanne initiated a phone call, which led to the therapist wanting to get together. They subsequently met a couple of times for lunch. She reported the therapist's expressed delight in seeing her again; however, during one of their meetings, the therapist told her that a colleague had lost her license due to sexual involvement with a patient. Although this did not lead to a discussion of their relationship, Joanne believes her therapist was communicating that she knew their interactions were wrong and unethical but was also seeking reassurance that Joanne would not report her causing her to undergo the same fate as her colleague. She was relying on what she knew about Joanne's character and again used their special relationship to ensure secrecy. Maintaining silence is another way that abused clients can remain special to the therapist, and thus is another way they can be manipulated (for detailed accounts, see memoirs by Penfold, 2006; Russell, 2020; and Shepherd, 2017). Joanne recently researched her former therapist and found some pictures of her on the Internet to which she had an unexpected highly aversive physical and emotional response, including rage about what had happened and all that she had lost. Despite this, she continues to struggle with feelings of ambivalence and even love for the therapist.

Joanne has prospered in her career as a medical professional but questions whether she would have entered a helping profession had she not been abused and reinforced for her caretaking. She would like her transgressive therapist to know of her success because "she would be proud of all I have accomplished," the type of affirmation she rarely received from her own mother. However, due to continuing to feel like an imposter and sometimes a hypocrite, she struggles with accepting her colleagues' accolades regarding her management and clinical abilities. Joanne has had difficulties finding a subsequent therapist. Two of them, even though they knew of her history and claimed expertise in treating survivors of therapist abuse, inexplicably crossed nonsexual boundaries, causing her enormous consternation, shock, and mistrust that resulted in her ending the treatments. She was terrified to enter treatment again but with the encouragement of her husband and his psychiatrist, she did. Throughout her treatment and since then, she has continued to rely on the ongoing support and perspective of her TELL respondent and has continued to stabilize and separate from the past, something she reported with pride in her interview.

Carol, in contrast, lost her job and ability to work and ended up on disability. Several times she was hospitalized or admitted to partial hospitalization programs. She has had difficulty finding outpatient therapists but eventually was referred to a female therapist with whom she worked successfully for 5 years, until the therapist's retirement. She is now working with a male therapist whom she trusts. She emphasizes the need for survivors to have a context in which to discuss abuse and to break the secrecy because the topic is difficult to admit to and discuss with family and friends who may not understand or know how to respond. She describes ongoing ambivalence toward her abusive therapist, on the one hand wanting him to think she is completely recovered and, on the other, to know how much he hurt her and the continuing negative impact of his actions.

Bystanders

In terms of family members and others, all three survivors wonder why no one questioned what was happening or intervened, especially when they suspected or knew about the abuse. Ken later learned that his father knew but did nothing. Joanne's family was "blinded" by gratitude toward the therapist who had helped her curb her addiction and return to functioning. They never questioned the excessive time the two spent together. Carol's husband and daughters endured her obsession, absences, inconsistencies, and hospitalizations. She was surprised to get a supportive and nonblaming response from one of her daughters when she disclosed why she was no longer seeing her therapist. That one of her daughters had announced her "boyfriend" was on the phone when he returned a call, indicates some suspicion regarding their overinvolvement. Both Joanne and Carole feel guilty about how their husbands and children were impacted by their reactions in the aftermath of the abuse.

LITERATURE ON AFTEREFFECTS

How do the feelings and effects reported by these three survivors compare with those in the literature? Studies of the aftereffects of therapist abuse began in the late 1970s consisting mostly of surveys of random samples of therapists who were asked if they had ever been sexually involved with a patient and of patients who were asked to describe the circumstances and the consequences of their reported abusive experiences. After reviewing both the historical and newly available literature and research and extending it to clergy and other professionals, Pope (1989, 1994) concluded that although the behavior was rather frequently reported and well known in professional circles, its acknowledgment and the publication of the early findings were actively disavowed and suppressed in these same circles, leading him to call it "the problem that had no name." In a series of papers, presentations, and books, he reported on the findings and identified patient–therapist sex as unethical, abusive, and highly damaging and called on psychology (and other professions) to actively confront its occurrence, prohibit it as always unethical, and develop methods for intervention for both parties on the part of professions and licensing boards, and possible remediation or retraining for the perpetrator-therapist.

Pope (1989, 1994) challenged the then-prevalent patient-blaming and the subsequent disbelief and questioning of the victim's veracity as being due to sexism and a gross misunderstanding of the dynamics of sexual abuse. He identified what he described as a *patient–therapist sex syndrome* consisting of the following effects on the victim: (a) ambivalence, (b) guilt, (c) feelings of isolation, (d) emptiness, (e) cognitive dysfunction, (f) identity disturbance, (g) inability to trust, (h) sexual confusion, (i) mood lability, (j) suppressed rage, and (k) increased suicide risk. As can be seen, these are closely aligned to effects reported by our three interviewees.

Since then, this list has been supplemented by additional research and clinical findings. As an example, in 1989, two Boston therapists, Estelle Disch and Nancy Avery, investigated reports of SBVs in therapy and founded Boston Associates to Stop Treatment Abuse (BASTA). This group joined with Jan Wohlberg to form Therapist Exploitation Link Line (TELL) and provided groups, workshops, and a mechanism of support to and from other survivors of sexually transgressive therapists, including referrals to subsequent therapists who understood the specialized needs and issues involved. They learned from survivors that the validation received from participating in a group or peer-mentoring process was invaluable in learning about sexual abuse in psychotherapy and that they were not alone ("the only one this ever happened to"), nor were they an outlier ("it wasn't just me"). These processes provided a place where they could clarify and redefine their often-confusing experiences and feelings, especially their ambivalence toward those who had hurt them, and a place to grieve what had been lost. Some participants were moved to action such as filing complaints to licensing boards, filing civil lawsuits, issuing demand letters to perpetrators, and reporting their abuse to the police.

The results of Disch and Avery's (2001) questionnaire study of 149 women and men who had been sexually exploited as adults by medical/mental health professionals and clergy members reported a common theme: the therapist's deliberate attempts to foster emotional dependence in the counselee. Many reported that survivor clients had both positive and negative feelings about the practitioner. Some of the feelings included feeling special, cared for, excited, loved, in love, and as if they had found the love of their life. Some, however, reported feeling confused, and others felt pressured or coerced to sexually engage. Two thirds of the respondents took the initiative to end the relationship, with the last contact being a negative one. Almost none reported a planned or orderly termination process.

The researchers assessed the impact of the abuse and found that respondents were particularly high on the following: loss, overwhelming emotions, isolation, and shame with those with a history of childhood sexual abuse describing a more negative response (Disch, 2006). About half of respondents reported experiencing both nightmares and panic attacks. Many reported existential and actual losses due to the abuse—loss of a part of self, missing out on important parts of family or other life events, loss of close family or friend relationships, loss of hope in having a future healthy intimate relationship, and damage to ability to function competently or to work.

Difficulty in trusting other helping professionals is common. Even entering a private office and being alone with a therapist or other helper was experienced as anxiety-provoking and prohibitive. Many who do return to therapy begin with traumatic transference reactions toward the new therapist and are fearful of once again being manipulated and used. Many also have difficulty getting past what is usually the lack of closure caused by sudden, unanticipated, and unexplained ending by the former therapist, which creates an additional trauma of rupture and abandonment (Deutsch, 2014). Disch and Avery (2001) provided recommendations for how subsequent therapists should work with patients who have been abused and the interested reader is referred to their work (see Chapter 14 of this volume for a discussion of subsequent treatment).

CONCLUSION

We are grateful to these three survivors for giving us the opportunity to interview them and to discuss their experiences of abusive therapy in this text. Their stories are deeply touching. Each story, unique to the individual and his or her life circumstance, illustrates different ways that sexual transgressions take place. Their stories share many themes with others reported in the research and clinical literature. Their aftereffects are also consistent and reinforce what is known about the damaging consequences that result when professional standards and boundaries are not maintained. Along with those consequences, however, these survivors also demonstrate tenacity and resilience in their lives and their attempts to recoup what they have lost and ultimately recover. They remind us of the ongoing need for self-knowledge and self-reflection on the part of therapists and the importance of the physician's oath to "do no harm."

REFERENCES

Bates, C. M., & Brodsky, A. M. (1989). *Sex in the therapy hour: A case of professional incest.* Guilford Press.

Deutsch, R. A. (2014). *Traumatic ruptures: Abandonment and betrayal in the analytic relationship.* Routledge.

Disch, E. (2006). Sexual victimization and revictimization of women by professionals: Client experiences and implications for subsequent treatment. *Women & Therapy, 29*(1–2), 41–61. https://doi.org/10.1300/J015v29n01_03

Disch, E., & Avery, N. (2001). Sex in the consulting room, the examining room, and the sacristy: Survivors of sexual abuse by professionals. *American Journal of Orthopsychiatry, 71*(2), 204–217. https://doi.org/10.1037/0002-9432.71.2.204

Freeman, L., & Roy, J. (1976). *Betrayal: The true story of the first woman to successfully sue her psychiatrist for using sex in the guise of therapy.* Stein & Day.

Gabbard, G. O. (1994). On love and lust in erotic transference. *Journal of the American Psychoanalytic Association, 42*(2), 385–403. https://doi.org/10.1177/000306519404200203

Penfold, P. S. (2006). *Why did you keep going for so long? Issues for survivors of long-term sexually abusive "healing" relationships.* Therapist Exploitation Link Line.

Pope, K. S. (1989). Dual relationships between therapist and client: A national study of psychologists, psychiatrists, and social workers. *Professional Psychology: Research and Practice, 20*(5), 283–293.

Pope, K. S. (1994). *Sexual involvement with therapists: Patient assessment, subsequent therapy, forensics.* American Psychological Association. https://doi.org/10.1037/10154-000

Russell, K. E. (2020). *My dark Vanessa: A novel.* William Morrow.

Shepherd, A. (2017). *Mending the shattered mirror: A journey of recovery from abusive therapy.* Words on the Wing.

17 WHEN COLLEAGUES BETRAY

*The Harm of Sexual Boundary
Violations in Psychotherapy Extends
Beyond the Victim*

JENNIFER M. GÓMEZ, LAURA K. NOLL,
ALEXIS A. ADAMS-CLARK, AND
CHRISTINE A. COURTOIS

Sexual boundary violations (SBVs) perpetrated by clinicians in psycho-therapy are a long-standing problem (Pope et al., 1979), indicative both of a fundamental abuse of power and mismanagement within the therapeutic relationship and complex harms that often extend beyond the primary victim to family members, colleagues, institutions, and the field at large. As a feminist explanatory framework, *betrayal trauma theory* (BTT; Freyd, 1996) refers to abuse and exploitation that occurs within close relationships that should be trustworthy and sacrosanct (e.g., familial, romantic, fiduciary). Research to date has substantiated the additive effect of this *interpersonal betrayal* to other elements and sequelae of the trauma. Betrayal trauma theory has been extended to institutions (e.g., institutional betrayal; Smith & Freyd, 2014). Societal power further affects the incidence of betrayal, with harm and violence within cultural minority groups (e.g., racial minorities; women) conferring a cultural betrayal (e.g., Gómez, 2019b) that further exacerbates outcomes. Another form of betrayal trauma perpetrated by colleagues (i.e., colleague betrayal trauma) was identified by Courtois (2017). SBVs in psychotherapy often involve all four types of betrayal: (a) the

https://doi.org/10.1037/0000247-017
*Sexual Boundary Violations in Psychotherapy: Facing Therapist Indiscretions,
Transgressions, and Misconduct*, A. Steinberg, J. L. Alpert, and C. A. Courtois (Editors)

client is the primary victim, (b) families and peer/colleagues are secondary, (c) institutions are tertiary, and (d) the entire field of psychotherapy is further impacted. These violations and betrayals occur within, and are affected by, differences in power dynamics at the personal, role, institutional, professional, and societal levels.

We begin this chapter with a vignette that illustrates SBVs and various betrayals. We then briefly highlight the relevant ethics codes from the American Psychological Association (APA; e.g., 2017). Next, we provide overviews of the literature on betrayal trauma theory (e.g., Freyd, 1996), institutional betrayal (Smith & Freyd, 2014), and colleague betrayal (Courtois, 2017), with a brief introduction to cultural betrayal (Gómez, 2019a). We then detail the implications of this problem for clinicians, organizations, and professional training programs, with an emphasis on suggestions that both reduce the likelihood of SBVs and mitigate harm when they do occur.

A SEXUAL BOUNDARY VIOLATION VIGNETTE

Dr. P is a 60-year-old White man, a clinical psychologist who has been practicing for 30 years at the Eastside Clinic. As the clinic director, he is responsible for overseeing operations, carrying an individual therapy caseload, running clinic team meanings, managing therapists and student clinicians, supervising psychology doctoral students, writing letters of recommendation, and generally serving as a role model. He is well regarded in the community and has a reputation as an ethical and responsible psychologist.

Eighteen months ago, Dr. P began treating Jae, an African American, heterosexual woman in her late 20s. She presented with a long history of abusive relationships, and she was seeking to better understand herself to end this pattern. She reported that, beginning in childhood, she had been sexually and psychologically abused by her father. The incest lasted until age 16 when she ran away from home. Her then-boyfriend initially offered her shelter and solace, yet ended up physically, sexually, and psychologically abusing her for the next 5 years until Jae was able to leave him for good at age 21. Despite her success as a professional pianist, Jae battled with depression, anxiety, shame, very low self-esteem, self-blame, suicidal ideation, and occasional nonsuicidal self-injury. Moreover, her involvement in abusive romantic relationships continued. Her latest bad relationship and its breakup provided the impetus for Jae to begin therapy. She hoped to learn skills for dealing better with her emotions and learning ways to develop healthy friendships and romantic relationships.

From virtually the first session, Dr. P felt a connection to Jae, which he presumed was a good predictor of a strong therapeutic alliance. Simultaneously, Dr. P's long-term marriage began to unravel, leaving him feeling bereft, incompetent, and ashamed. He started noticing a strong emotional and physical attraction to Jae and rationalized that it was harmless, and even potentially helpful. Instead of self-monitoring this response and using it to understand himself and Jae, he instead began to disclose his unhappiness and discuss his life circumstances with her. She responded by being sympathetic. He then began to find ways to extend Jae's therapy sessions, including scheduling them in the evening and at outside settings (e.g., coffee, dinners). She was initially flattered by his attention and slowly became his confidante. He behaved in an increasingly seductive way with Jae, and over time, he initiated sexual contact. She did not feel comfortable with this part of their relationship but felt powerless to stop it given both Dr. P's role as her therapist and his significance as the closest, most supportive person in her life. Jae was also concerned that if she tried to stop their relationship, he would do something to harm her or himself, as he had confided the depth of his depression and despair to her.

One night, after staying late to finish clinical case notes, Dr. P's supervisee, Dee, a queer Latina doctoral student, witnessed Dr. P romantically kissing Jae in the hallway following an evening session. She checked the master schedule and learned that Jae was Dr. P's client. Since Dr. P was her direct clinical supervisor and director of the clinic, Dee did not feel comfortable going to him to report this transgression, even though she was well aware of the ethical and moral implications of his behavior. Instead, she disclosed what she had observed to Dr. F, a White female staff psychologist who, despite being fairly new to the clinic, had been vocal in supporting ethical and professional standards in the clinic team meetings. Unfortunately, Dr. F initially dismissed and downplayed Dee's disclosure until she herself witnessed an inappropriate interaction between Dr. P and Jae. Dee felt betrayed by Dr. F's disbelief. Both Dee and Dr. F felt betrayed by Dr. P's misbehavior.

Although Dr. F recognized her responsibility to intervene per the APA's (2017) *Ethical Principles of Psychologists and Code of Conduct* (hereinafter, Ethics Code) and report this major ethical violation to the state licensing board, she was worried for her professional reputation if she "tattled" on well-respected Dr. P, who, after all, was her boss. She rationalized that even in the era of #MeToo (https://metoomvmt.org), those who dared to disclose sexual mistreatment of any sort in the workplace were still being publicly shamed and blamed. Due to this concern, Dr. F did not confront Dr. P about his behavior or report Dr. P's unethical behavior within the clinic or to the Board. Moreover, despite her own verification of the misconduct, Dr. F told Dee that she must have been mistaken and that her lack of ethics in disclosing something so far-fetched and damaging would be reflected in her clinical trainee evaluation. Dee was devastated and subsequently did nothing to further report Dr. P. She continued in supervision with him where she was cognizant of her contempt toward him.

RELEVANT ETHICAL STANDARDS

This vignette demonstrates several serious violations of APA's (2002, 2010, 2017) Ethics Code. A primary mandate involves establishing and maintaining appropriate and health-promoting professional boundaries in work with clients, students, and colleagues. Any type of sexual behavior (e.g., suggestive comments, writings, and harassment) or sexual contact between therapists and clients is explicitly forbidden, a proscription that has been more recently extended to relatives of clients, students/trainees, and employees (see Chapter 2).

Importantly, psychologists are obliged not only to maintain proper and professional interactions with others but also to act if they observe or otherwise learn of misbehavior on the part of a colleague(s) by bringing the ethical issue to the involved colleague if possible and reporting the ethics violation to the appropriate authorities or licensing board. Psychologists should also seek to create environments that allow others to report ethics violations without fear of punishment or retribution.

BETRAYAL TRAUMA THEORY

Betrayal trauma theory (Freyd, 1996) is a framework within which to conceptualize therapists' (and other authority figures') sexual and other forms of boundary violation. BTT asserts that high betrayal traumas, such as sexual and other traumatic violations committed by individuals who are in relationships of trust and power with the victim, carry a harm above and beyond that of the abuse itself (Freyd, 1996). Consequently, high betrayal traumas are associated with costly mental health outcomes (Edwards et al., 2012; Freyd, 1996; Freyd et al., 2001, 2007).

BTT created a new paradigm for traumatic interpersonal injury and avenue for researching the dynamics of exploitive and abusive relationships, particularly the impact of betrayal by a person of significance in the victim's life. As such, it applies to therapists who abuse their power and betray their roles, responsibilities, and ethical and professional standards through SBVs. For instance, Courtois (2010) and others have referred to SBVs as *professional incest* due to the violation of the power differential, authority role, and fiduciary responsibilities inherent in the relationship, the violation of a taboo relationship, and the imperative of the therapist to work in the client's best interest.

Moreover, in perpetrating SBVs, therapists may prepare their victim in some way, often by increasing their dependency and making them feel special, a process known as *grooming* (see Chapters 14 and 15). Like other abusers, therapists may misrepresent and rationalize their motives and behavior to themselves and to the victim, a process known as *gaslighting*. This misrepresentation betrays, confuses, and wounds victims. Therapists can further harm their clients by blaming them for the abuse that the therapists themselves perpetrated. As noted in other chapters, Freyd (1997) posited that by denying abuse, attacking the victim, and by "playing the victim" (a behavior repertoire captured by the acronym DARVO—deny, attack, reverse victim and offender), perpetrators of interpersonal violence are often able to escape culpability. Since its initial conceptualization, the elements of DARVO, as perpetrator responses to confrontation by the victim, have been linked to victim self-blame (Harsey et al., 2017) and, by extension, nondisclosure. However, recent experimental work suggests that education about DARVO could mitigate its effects on individuals' perceptions of perpetrators and victims (Harsey & Freyd, 2020).

INSTITUTIONAL BETRAYAL

Expanding the concept of BTT beyond the interpersonal level, Smith and Freyd (2013, 2014) developed the concept of *institutional betrayal* to describe trust violations committed by agents and representatives of larger organizations and institutions. Institutional betrayal occurs when an organization does not intervene or protect members who are mistreated by others within or affiliated with the organization (Smith & Freyd, 2013, 2014). In other words, institutions have an obligation—often unstated but generally understood by members—to create and maintain a healthy environment, including safety and security for all. Along with the responsibility to protect members from danger, organizations are responsible for responding when a dangerous situation is identified or a member reports being hurt in some way. However, much in the same way that incestuous families can coalesce to protect the family and its reputation by repudiating and even shunning the victim member while supporting the abuser (e.g., Delker et al., 2018), organizations can do the same. Thus, institutional betrayal is an additional harm above and beyond the initial traumatic event that compounds the negative effects of the original violation (Smith & Freyd, 2013, 2014).

There are multiple ways that institutions can betray individuals. Generally, such incidences of institutional betrayal exist at the intersection of two key dimensions: omission/commission and apparently isolated/systemic (Smith & Freyd, 2014). Institutional agents commit acts of omission by, for instance, failing to offer appropriate belief, evaluation, follow-up, intervention, or assistance for people who report sexual victimization. Moreover, acts of commission include actively covering up reports of misconduct to maintain the institution's status and reputation (Smith & Freyd, 2014). Although an institutional betrayal could be perceived as a one-time, isolated occurrence, it may instead be a systemic issue, such as routinely covering up abuses and lacking procedures for responsive organizational interventions (Smith & Freyd, 2014). Other common examples of institutional betrayal include discriminatory and oppressive behavior, normalizing abusive contexts, retaliation (including public shaming or ridicule, harassment, stalking, shunning, loss of employment or status), and other punitive acts (Smith & Freyd, 2014).

Research has indicated that institutional betrayal has deleterious effects on people who are victimized in universities (mental health outcomes; Smith & Freyd, 2013; Wright et al., 2017) and the military (posttraumatic stress disorder, depression, suicidality; Monteith et al., 2016). In this way, institutional betrayal can be additive to the original experience of betrayal trauma, often with dire consequences for the victims. Moreover, multiple institutions, including governments (Smidt & Freyd, 2018), law enforcement agencies (Gómez & Freyd, 2014), religious organizations (Smith & Freyd, 2014), athletic organizations (Smith & Freyd, 2014), health care systems (Smith & Freyd, 2017), professional organizations (Gómez et al., 2016), and judicial systems (Smith et al., 2014), have engaged in institutional betrayal. Smith and Freyd (2014) identified several organizational characteristics that make institutional betrayal more likely: prestigious standing in the community, strict standards and requirements for membership, and the prioritization of achievement and status (Smith & Freyd, 2014)

INSTITUTIONAL BETRAYAL, POWER, AND CULTURAL BETRAYAL

A feminist tenet is that power plays an important role in the dynamics of all forms of betrayal trauma across interpersonal and institutional levels. Power can be due to societal privilege (e.g., White, male, heteronormative, cisgendered, upper class) as well as hierarchical status within an institution (e.g., being the boss, administrator, commander, director, owner). Perhaps because of interpersonal, structural, and societal power, the effect of institutional betrayal may be particularly damaging for individuals who are already marginalized by society and of lesser power (e.g., racial/ethnic, sexual, and gender minorities; Freyd & Birrell, 2013; Smith et al., 2016).

Additionally, some marginalized populations are at increased risk for violence and other victimization due to minority race (Native American, American Indian, and other Indigenous populations, Black/African American, Latinx American, Multiracial), sexual orientation (lesbian, gay, bisexual), gender identity (transgender, gender-fluid, or intersex), age, or ability (physically disabled or mentally handicapped; National Center for Victims of Crime, 2012). Therefore, systemic oppression and trauma are more regularly experienced in these populations due to their lower status, power, and vulnerability (Burstow, 2003, 2005). Compounding marginalization (e.g., racial and gender minority; intersectionality, Crenshaw, 1991; multiplicity, Hames-García, 2011) can contribute to both the incidence and meaning-making of trauma, which in turn can negatively influence identity (Gómez, 2019a).

Moreover, traumatic harm that occurs within cultural minority groups, such as between women and People of Color, is also affected by lower societal status and economic inequalities. Implicit in within-group harm among individuals who are marginalized in society, cultural betrayal exists as a violation of the (intra)cultural trust (e.g., in-group connection) that serves as a buffer against societal inequality (Gómez & Gobin, 2019). As a unique traumatic dimension of harm, cultural betrayal in trauma results in deleterious mental, behavioral, and cultural outcomes (e.g., Gómez, 2019a, 2019b; Gómez & Freyd, 2018; Gómez & Gobin, 2019).

COLLEAGUE BETRAYAL

Colleague betrayal was introduced as another manifestation of betrayal trauma (Courtois, 2017) and has also been identified in psychoanalytic writings about collateral damage to colleagues and training institutes when a colleague transgresses sexually (Goren, 2017; Slochower, 2015). *Colleague betrayal* refers to behavior on the part of a teammate, associate, or colleague— including students, trainees, and supervisees—that violates ethical and professional standards regarding the maintenance of boundaries, the creation of dual relationships, the welfare of the client, the welfare of colleagues, the reputation of organizations, and the reputation of the profession or other entity as trustworthy and moral. Colleague betrayal can take many forms, including sexual malfeasance and assault, and can be perpetrated without regard to the consequences and the potential for harm. In some cases, it occurs because organizational representatives are ordered to take an action or a position to protect the organization (in other words, to dismiss, deny, or otherwise cover up) under threat of losing their jobs. It is often the case in therapist sexual abuse that the violating therapists are aware that they are doing something out of bounds but minimize the consequences to others and rationalize their misbehavior to themselves. As with other forms of perpetration, sexual abuse can be intentional, premeditated, and occur serially, or it can be situational, resulting from ignorance, inexperience, insufficient training, naivete, or carelessness. When an organization charged with protecting its members and monitoring adherence to ethical, legal, and moral codes, denying, minimizing, disregarding, or even punishing the victimized individual may be additionally damaging. The aforementioned institutional betrayal (e.g., Smith & Freyd, 2014) can be conceptualized as encompassing colleague betrayal.

BETRAYALS AND IMPLICATIONS OF THE SEXUAL BOUNDARY VIOLATIONS VIGNETTE

In revisiting and analyzing the vignette at the start of this chapter, we see SBVs—even those that occur in a "slippery slope" fashion, as opposed to intentionally sadistic and extreme—can be intertwined with and compounded by interpersonal, colleague, institutional, and cultural betrayal. Dr. P engaged in direct interpersonal betrayal of his client, Jae, as well as institutional betrayal in his role as therapist. In doing so, Dr. P revictimized Jae, who sought therapy as a survivor of previous sexual, physical, and psychological violence. Dr. P additionally betrayed his colleagues, clinic, and profession, including his supervisee, Dee, and fellow therapist, Dr. F, who are both of lower institutional and societal power due to their professional status at the clinic and their gender or sexual identities. Dee and Dr. F are victims of Dr. P's colleague betrayal. Dr. F then perpetrates cultural and institutional betrayal against Jae and Dee (whom she gaslights and threatens with punishment), as well as colleague betrayal against the clinic and profession by not reporting the violation, in some states a violation of the law.

Taken together, this vignette shows the complicated landscape of betrayal trauma. The direct and collateral damage can be profound. Jae, the primary victim, is betrayed not only by the sexual abuse that takes place in what should be a protected relationship where she is of lesser power and status (and of marginalized race and gender), but further by the failure of witnesses to intervene. Dr. P goes unconfronted and unstopped in his behavior.

IMPLICATIONS FOR CLINICIANS, INSTITUTIONS, AND PROFESSIONAL TRAINING PROGRAMS

As Hook and Devereux (2018a, 2018b) argued, widespread ignorance about both the prevalence of boundary violations in mental health professions together with inadequate training can exacerbate the harm of sexual transgressions in psychotherapy. Within this context, we argue that BTT (Freyd, 1994, 1996) offers a useful framework that can guide the ethical decision-making of licensed practitioners, foster institutional change (including revisions to initial and continuing education requirements for licensure), encourage training program development, and catalyze much-needed cultural change within the field of psychotherapy. Because the implications of colleague betrayal for clinicians, institutions, and professional training programs are vast, programmatic changes that foster institutional courage and healing among individuals (clients and colleague therapists alike) who have been harmed by SBVs in psychotherapy may be particularly impactful and perhaps necessary for laying a solid foundation onto which new policies and institutional norms may emerge. In this section, we discuss the implications of BTT (and more recent conceptualizations of colleague betrayal) for institutions (including licensing boards) and professional training programs with particular attention to actions that not only prevent the occurrence of such violations but ensure that when such abuse occurs, mitigates additional harm to the client and other parties (e.g., colleagues, institutions).

Implications for Clinicians

Although awareness of the problem of SBVs within the field of psychotherapy appears to be growing, cultural change within the profession, such as shifts that will impact policies, licensing requirements, and training, will take time. In the meantime, in their roles as practicing therapists, colleagues, and leaders within institutions and training programs, licensed clinicians have a key role to play in addressing the ongoing problem of SBVs within the field. Given the difficulties of speaking up when observing a colleague engaging in SBVs, we recommend that all licensed clinicians actively seek out support and continuing education and consultation opportunities that will help them address these violations and colleague betrayals effectively when they occur. Such efforts can empower clinicians to become advocates for cultural change within the profession. There are additional recommendations for clinicians in positions of power within institutions, including professional training programs specifically.

Implications for Institutions

Colleague and institutional betrayals following sexual transgressions by a colleague are not inevitable. To foster healthy and equitable environments and prevent institutional betrayal, researchers recommend several steps. In terms of prevention, institutions should provide training to its members at the beginning and throughout employment regarding definitions of boundary violations, reasons for and prohibitions against them, their potential negative consequences and wide range of primary and secondary victims, and steps to be taken if and when they occur. Despite these efforts, violations can still occur and call for vigilance and response on the part of all who observe something that seems problematic (Gabbard, 2017). This training can include education on *institutional cowardice*, a type of institutional betrayal that includes a "knowing or consciously motivated act, an intentional decision to go in a particular direction and allow a vulnerable person or persons to be harmed" (Brown, 2021, p. 2). Common acts of institutional cowardice include absence of an apology, ceasing all contact and support for a victim who reports abuse while offering support to the alleged perpetrator, and doing nothing while knowingly witnessing institutional betrayal under the guise of simply following the rules (Brown, 2021).

Importantly, steps toward institutional change should be taken, such as the establishment of simple and clear policies for investigating and addressing reports of misconduct and discrimination (Freyd & Birrell, 2013), including multiple avenues for reporting; educating institutional members about existing policies and procedures, including how they are operationalized in response to a report (Freyd & Birrell, 2013); encouraging and promoting transparency in organizational operations (Gómez & Freyd, 2014; Smith & Freyd, 2014); conducting self-studies to identify areas of the institution that may pose potential harm to members (Gómez et al., 2014, 2016; Smith & Freyd, 2014); and praising rather than punishing complainants and whistle-blowers (Freyd & Birrell, 2013; Gómez et al., 2014; Smith & Freyd, 2014; Smith et al., 2014). Perhaps most important, if an institutional betrayal does occur, institutions should acknowledge it, apologize to the primary victim as well as to affected others, and reach out to the organizational community, which may also be shocked and traumatized by the transgression, whether by an older, influential, and esteemed colleague or by a trainee or novice therapist (Freyd & Birrell, 2013; Smith et al., 2014). By taking and implementing these actions, institutions can not only uphold clear professional and moral standards and avoid committing acts of betrayal through indifference, cowardice, and inaction, but can open pathways for communication (Smith et al., 2014) and environments that foster personal and professional security that help members thrive.

Implications for Professional Training Programs

In addition to institutional change, increased emphasis on prevention throughout professional training is urgently needed because many practitioners know little about SBVs (Hook & Devereux, 2018a, 2018b), much less about sexuality, erotic transference, and what to do if a situation of risk develops. To be effective, we believe such a shift must be incentivized and backed by professional licensing boards that regulate initial and continuing education requirements for licensure. The following suggestions are by no means comprehensive; however, members of professional training programs, such as doctoral clinical and counseling psychology programs and internships, psychoanalytic institutes, counseling and social work programs, and psychiatry residencies can consider the following recommendations for increasing knowledge in this domain and reducing the prevalence of SBVs and colleague betrayal in their organizations and the field at large.

1. Acknowledge the realities of sexual misconduct among psychotherapists today.
   a. Actively seek out up-to-date information about the prevalence of sexual misconduct by therapists and work to keep this knowledge current.
   b. Recognize the inadequacy of current professional training approaches to prevent and address SBVs. Acknowledge that providing therapists with an ethics code, instructing them about what boundaries not to cross, discussing cases, and supervising therapists until they are licensed are necessary components of ethics training but insufficient for preventing SBVs in psychotherapy.
   c. Acknowledge that some institutions may have a high tolerance for SBVs in training environments and that this constitutes a risk to all, primarily to the victim but also to other members (Peltz & Gabbard, 2001). Conduct regular self- and external-assessment designed to identify and address such risk.

    d. Attend to group- and institutional-level dynamics that may make SBVs and colleague betrayal more likely (e.g., inequality in hiring and promotion, tolerance of ongoing discrimination and harassment).

2. Evaluate and improve training curriculum as it relates to SBVs.

    a. Consider how different theoretical orientations account for boundary violations (including but not limited to sexual misconduct; see the chapters in Part II, this volume) and critically evaluate the evidence base for the current model of teaching trainees about SBVs.

    b. Modify curriculum to avoid framing the potential for boundary violations in terms of "discontinuity models" that separate therapists into "good–bad" or "ethical–unethical" (Gabbard, 1996).

    c. Where appropriate, normalize the existence of strong countertransference responses to clients (including the pull to engage in boundary violations) that need to be monitored and managed with support rather than hidden.

    d. Lower the stakes of disclosure of therapist countertransference to supervisors by actively encouraging ongoing self-reflection and disclosure of countertransference reactions in supervision. Provide support for therapists in working through countertransference reactions and make referrals for additional support (e.g., counseling for the therapist) as needed.

3. Teach trainees about power as it relates to interpersonal and institutional dynamics and model transparent conversation about power differentials that exist within psychotherapy.

    a. Explicitly name power differentials throughout all aspects of training and model open discussions of power.

    b. Support trainees in developing a deep understanding of differences in power that exist between therapist and client. Emphasize that with regard to power, therapist and client are never peers within the context of psychotherapy.

4. Integrate trauma-informed psychoeducation about institutional, colleague, and cultural betrayal into professional training to help provide training and supervising therapists with conceptual frameworks for understanding experiences of colleague betrayal when they occur.

    a. Actively foster opportunities within the training program for discussion of betrayal trauma and help the group understand its responsibility to members and members' responsibility to the group and profession.

   b. Educate seasoned therapists and support staff responsible for training new psychotherapists about the harm of SBVs via formal and informal continuing education opportunities about institutional, colleague, and cultural betrayal within the field of psychotherapy.

5. Increase dialogue about colleague betrayal by encouraging intra- and inter-organizational conversations about institutional dynamics that impact professional training.

   a. Create nonevaluative, safe spaces for trainees and supervisors to engage in conversation about institutional, colleague, and cultural betrayal.

   b. Note that a "slippery slope" of comparatively small boundary violations may lead to sexual misconduct (Strasburger et al., 1992); encourage dialogue about institutional dynamics that allow, foster, or reinforce comparatively small boundary violations.

6. Include deliberate practice and experiential learning activities (e.g., Rousmaniere, 2019) throughout all phases of therapist training to help trainees recognize and respond to countertransference reactions with the potential to lead to SBVs.

   a. Create opportunities for trainee therapists to practice responding to adverse idealizing transference, which is client responses that idealize the therapist (and may lead them to romanticize the therapist), as such responses are often cited as an important factor in many boundary violations, especially for therapists with a strong need to be liked, approved of, or who are prone to overengagement with clients (Hook & Devereux, 2018a).

7. Encourage all trainee therapists to engage in their own individual psychotherapy or other culturally congruent forms of healing throughout training.

   a. Emphasize the importance of therapists seeking outside help for personal problems known to increases risk for SBVs (e.g., long-standing or unresolved problems with self-esteem, experiences of boundary violations by a parental figure, personality disorders, relationship problems and losses; Celenza, 1998, 2007; Hook & Devereux, 2018b).

8. Provide trainees and supervising therapists with effective strategies for whistleblowing.

   a. Take proactive steps to ensure that whistleblowers are not neglected or maligned when they raise concerns; this includes modeling healthy responses to disclosure.

    b. Create opportunities for trainees and supervising therapists to practice responding to potential colleague boundary violations and betrayals *before* SBVs occur.

9. Solicit frequent anonymous feedback from clients, trainee, and supervising therapists about the general atmosphere of the professional training program.

    a. Evaluate this feedback against the recommendations for preventing institutional betrayal (as described earlier).

    b. Celebrate progress in cultivating an environment that values institutional courage. Consider regularly recognizing courageous actions and individuals through internal awards.

10. Actively look for examples of institutional courage and reward individuals who speak up about their own and others' boundary violations.

    a. Highlight comparatively "small" instances of appreciating those who point out problems in the training environment to cultivate a culture where

        i. colleague betrayal is less likely to occur and

        ii. when it does occur, institutional courage and healing are possible.

Need for Further Research About Colleague Betrayal in Psychotherapy and Effective Training Practices

Although the history of SBVs in psychotherapy is long, open discussion of this phenomenon in psychotherapy has proven challenging, and systematic research in this area is still relatively new (Celenza, 2011). On one hand, significant attention has been given to the prevalence and harm of SBVs in psychotherapy (e.g., Gabbard, 1994, 1996, 2017; Lamb & Catanzaro, 1998; Norris et al., 2003; Sarkar, 2004; Simon, 1999; Strasburger et al., 1992), with most training programs including at least one formal course in ethics that provides psychoeducation about SBVs. Nevertheless, relatively little empirical research has been conducted to assess the prevalence of colleague betrayals or the implications SBVs have for institutions. Moreover, disproportionate attention has been given to the intraindividual and personality characteristics of transgressing therapists with comparatively little attention given to group and institutional dynamics that can make SBVs more likely to occur (e.g., inadequate, inattentive, or dismissive or punitive supervision; disbelief that SBVs could occur). Given the dearth of information about such betrayals, therapists of all levels (trainees, newly licensed clinicians, and experienced practitioners alike) may have difficulty contextualizing, framing, or responding to their experience of colleague betrayal.

Consequently, there is an urgent need for empirical research that (a) documents the prevalence of colleague betrayal, (b) identifies risk factors for its occurrence, (c) elucidates the mechanism(s) by which they occur, and (d) examines how such behaviors are or are not responded to effectively by institutions. To conduct such work, qualitative and quantitative instruments can be developed to both measure experiences of colleague betrayal and identify promising sites for intervention in therapist's professional training. Such measures could potentially be used alongside existing self-assessment measures (e.g., The Exploitation Index, Epstein & Simon, 1990; Epstein et al., 1992; The Boundary Violation Vulnerability Index, Celenza, 2011) designed to index early risk for boundary violations in psychotherapy. Such work may be used to inform the development of new training components and pedagogical innovations that are most effective at preventing colleague betrayal.

CONCLUSION

SBVs in therapy frequently represent a "dark little secret" within the helping profession. Identifying the multifaceted interpersonal, institutional, and cultural betrayals provides a nuanced understanding of the depth and breadth of their potential harm. As a type of institutional betrayal, colleague betrayal delineates the additional harm that SBVs have on colleagues, the organization in which it occurs, and the profession at large. Given the long-standing—albeit frowned-upon—history of SBVs in therapy, individual clinicians, institutions, and professional training programs are tasked with directly and consistently addressing all facets of SBVs—from the betrayals within the violations themselves, to those also done to the client, colleagues, trainees, the organization, and the profession. To reduce and ultimately eliminate betrayals related to SBVs, training in micro- and macrocosms in the field should be twofold: (a) empower professionals and trainees to identify colleagues' SBVs and follow ethical protocols for addressing them and (b) imbue all professionals and trainees with the skill and courage to respond appropriately when such violations are disclosed or witnessed. This two-pronged approach can increase the likelihood of meaningfully reducing or eliminating SBVs in therapy, while creating an ethical, supportive professional culture in which our field continues to self-correct. Because these violations can be so devastating and have such far-reaching deleterious consequences, specialized interventions and support for all involved parties should also be a professional priority.

REFERENCES

American Psychological Association. (2002). Ethical principles of psychologists and code of conduct. *American Psychologist, 57*(12), 1060–1073. https://doi.org/10.1037/0003-066X.57.12.1060

American Psychological Association. (2010). 2010 Amendments to the 2002 "Ethical principles of psychologists and code of conduct." *American Psychologist, 65*(5), 493. https://doi.org/10.1037/a0020168

American Psychological Association. (2017). *Ethical principles of psychologists and code of conduct* (2002, amended effective June 1, 2010, and January 1, 2017). https://www.apa.org/ethics/code/index.aspx

Brown, L. S. (2021). Institutional cowardice: A powerful, often invisible manifestation of institutional betrayal. *Journal of Trauma & Dissociation, 22*(3), 241–248. https://doi.org/10.1080/15299732.2020.1801307

Burstow, B. (2003). Toward a radical understanding of trauma and trauma work. *Violence Against Women, 9*(11), 1293–1317. https://doi.org/10.1177/1077801203255555

Burstow, B. (2005). A critique of posttraumatic stress disorder and the *DSM*. *Journal of Humanistic Psychology, 45*(4), 429–445. https://doi.org/10.1177/0022167805280265

Celenza, A. (1998). Precursors to therapist sexual misconduct: Preliminary findings. *Psychoanalytic Psychology, 15*(3), 378–395. https://doi.org/10.1037/0736-9735.15.3.378

Celenza, A. (2007). *Sexual boundary violations: Therapeutic, academic, and supervisory contexts*. Jason Aronson.

Celenza, A. (2011). *Sexual boundary violations: Therapeutic, supervisory, and academic contexts*. Jason Aronson.

Courtois, C. A. (2010). *Healing the incest wound: Adult survivors in therapy* (2nd ed.). W. W. Norton.

Courtois, C. A. (2017). Colleague betrayal: Countertrauma manifestation? In R. B. Gartner (Ed.), *Psychoanalysis in a new key book series. Trauma and countertrauma, resilience and counterresilience: Insights from psychoanalysts and trauma experts* (pp. 251–281). Routledge/Taylor & Francis Group.

Crenshaw, K. (1991). Mapping the margins: Intersectionality, identity politics, and violence against women of color. *Stanford Law Review, 43*(6), 1241–1299. https://doi.org/10.2307/1229039

Delker, B. C., Smith, C. P., Rosenthal, M. N., Bernstein, R. E., & Freyd, J. J. (2018). When home is where the harm is: Family betrayal and posttraumatic outcomes in young adulthood. *Journal of Aggression, Maltreatment & Trauma, 27*(7), 720–743. https://doi.org/10.1080/10926771.2017.1382639

Edwards, V. J., Freyd, J. J., Dube, S. R., Anda, R. F., & Felitti, V. J. (2012). Health outcomes by closeness of sexual abuse perpetrator: A test of betrayal trauma theory. *Journal of Aggression, Maltreatment & Trauma, 21*(2), 133–148. https://doi.org/10.1080/10926771.2012.648100

Epstein, R. S., & Simon, R. I. (1990). The Exploitation Index: An early warning indicator of boundary violations in psychotherapy. *Bulletin of the Menninger Clinic, 54*(4), 450–465.

Epstein, R. S., Simon, R. I., & Kay, G. G. (1992). Assessing boundary violations in psychotherapy: Survey results with the Exploitation Index. *Bulletin of the Menninger Clinic, 56*(2), 150–166.

Freyd, J. J. (1994). Betrayal trauma: Traumatic amnesia as an adaptive response to childhood abuse. *Ethics & Behavior, 4*(4), 307–329.

Freyd, J. J. (1996). *Betrayal trauma: The logic of forgetting childhood abuse.* Harvard University Press.

Freyd, J. J. (1997). Violations of power, adaptive blindness, and betrayal trauma theory. *Feminism & Psychology, 7*(1), 22–32. https://doi.org/10.1177/0959353597071004

Freyd, J. J., & Birrell, P. J. (2013). *Blind to betrayal.* John Wiley & Sons.

Freyd, J. J., DePrince, A. P., & Gleaves, D. H. (2007). The state of betrayal trauma theory: Reply to McNally—Conceptual issues and future directions. *Memory, 15*(3), 295–311. https://doi.org/10.1080/09658210701256514

Freyd, J. J., DePrince, A. P., & Zurbriggen, E. L. (2001). Self-reported memory for abuse depends upon victim–perpetrator relationship. *Journal of Trauma & Dissociation, 2*(3), 5–17. https://doi.org/10.1300/J229v02n03_02

Gabbard, G. O. (1994). Psychotherapists who transgress sexual boundaries with patients. *Bulletin of the Menninger Clinic, 58*(1), 124–135.

Gabbard, G. O. (1996). Lessons to be learned from the study of sexual boundary violations. *American Journal of Psychotherapy, 50*(3), 311–322. https://doi.org/10.1176/appi.psychotherapy.1996.50.3.311

Gabbard, G. O. (2017). Sexual boundary violations in psychoanalysis: A 30-year retrospective. *Psychoanalytic Psychology, 34*(2), 151–156. https://doi.org/10.1037/pap0000079

Gómez, J. M. (2019a). What's in a betrayal? Trauma, dissociation, and hallucinations among high-functioning ethnic minority emerging adults. *Journal of Aggression, Maltreatment & Trauma, 28*(10), 1181–1198. https://doi.org/10.1080/10926771.2018.1494653

Gómez, J. M. (2019b). What's the harm? Internalized prejudice and intra-racial trauma as cultural betrayal among ethnic minority college students. *American Journal of Orthopsychiatry, 89*, 237–247. https://doi.org/10.1037/ort0000367

Gómez, J. M., & Freyd, J. J. (2014, August 22). Institutional betrayal makes violence more toxic [OpEd]. *The Register-Guard,* p. A9.

Gómez, J. M., & Freyd, J. J. (2018). Psychological outcomes of within-group sexual violence: Evidence of cultural betrayal. *Journal of Immigrant and Minority Health, 20*, 1458–1467. https://doi.org/10.1007/s10903-017-0687-0

Gómez, J. M., & Gobin, R. L. (2019). Black women and girls and #MeToo: Rape, cultural betrayal, and healing. *Sex Roles, 82*, 1–12. https://doi.org/10.1007/s11199-019-01040-0

Gómez, J. M., Smith, C. P., & Freyd, J. J. (2014). Zwischenmenschlicher und institutioneller verrat [Interpersonal and institutional betrayal]. In R. Vogt (Ed.), *Verleumdung und Verrat: Dissoziative Störungen bei schwer traumatisierten Menschen als Folge von Vertrauensbrüchen* (pp. 82–90). Asanger Verlag.

Gómez, J. M., Smith, C. P., Gobin, R. L., Tang, S. S., & Freyd, J. J. (2016). Collusion, torture, and inequality: Understanding the actions of the American Psychological Association as institutional betrayal [Editorial]. *Journal of Trauma & Dissociation, 17*, 527–544. https://doi.org/10.1080/15299732.2016.1214436

Goren, E. R. (2017). A call for more talk and less abuse in the consulting room: One psychoanalyst–sex therapist's perspective. *Psychoanalytic Psychology, 34*(2), 215–220.

Hames-García, M. R. (2011). *Identity complex: Making the case for multiplicity.* University of Minnesota Press. https://doi.org/10.5749/minnesota/9780816649853.001.0001

Harsey, S. J., & Freyd, J. J. (2020). Deny, attack, and reverse victim and offender (DARVO): What is the influence on perceived perpetrator and victim credibility? *Journal of Aggression, Maltreatment & Trauma, 29*(8), 897–916.

Harsey, S. J., Zurbriggen, E. L., & Freyd, J. J. (2017). Perpetrator responses to victim confrontation: DARVO and victim self-blame. *Journal of Aggression, Maltreatment & Trauma, 26*(6), 644–663. https://doi.org/10.1080/10926771.2017.1320777

Hook, J., & Devereux, D. (2018a). Boundary violations in therapy: The patient's experience of harm. *British Journal of Psychiatry Advances, 24*(6), 366–373. https://doi.org/10.1192/bja.2018.26

Hook, J., & Devereux, D. (2018b). Sexual boundary violations: Victims, perpetrators and risk reduction. *British Journal of Psychiatry Advances, 24*(6), 374–383. https://doi.org/10.1192/bja.2018.27

Lamb, D. H., & Catanzaro, S. J. (1998). Sexual and nonsexual boundary violations involving psychologists, clients, supervisees, and students: Implications for professional practice. *Professional Psychology: Research and Practice, 29*(5), 498–503. https://doi.org/10.1037/0735-7028.29.5.498

Monteith, L. L., Bahraini, N. H., Matarazzo, B. B., Soberay, K. A., & Smith, C. P. (2016). Perceptions of institutional betrayal predict suicidal self-directed violence among veterans exposed to military sexual trauma. *Journal of Clinical Psychology, 72*, 743–755. https://doi.org/10.1002/jclp.22292

National Center for Victims of Crime. (2012). *Crime information and statistics.* http://victimsofcrime.org/library/crime-information-and-statistics

Norris, D. M., Gutheil, T. G., & Strasburger, L. H. (2003). This couldn't happen to me: Boundary problems and sexual misconduct in the psychotherapy relationship. *Psychiatric Services, 54*(4), 517–522. https://doi.org/10.1176/appi.ps.54.4.517

Peltz, M. L., & Gabbard, G. O. (2001). Speaking the unspeakable: Institutional reactions to boundary violations by training analysts. *Journal of the American Psychoanalytic Association, 49*(2), 659–673. https://doi.org/10.1177/00030651010490020601

Pope, K. S., Levenson, H., & Schover, L. R. (1979). Sexual intimacy in psychology training: Results and implications of a national survey. *American Psychologist, 34*(8), 682–689. https://doi.org/10.1037/0003-066X.34.8.682

Rousmaniere, T. (2019). *Mastering the inner skills of psychotherapy: A deliberate practice manual.* Gold Lantern Books.

Sarkar, S. P. (2004). Boundary violation and sexual exploitation in psychiatry and psychotherapy: A review. *Advances in Psychiatric Treatment, 10*(4), 312–320. https://doi.org/10.1192/apt.10.4.312

Simon, R. I. (1999). Therapist–patient sex. From boundary violations to sexual misconduct. *The Psychiatric Clinics of North America, 22*(1), 31–47. https://doi.org/10.1016/S0193-953X(05)70057-5

Slochower, J. (2015). Don't tell anyone. *Psychoanalytic Psychology, 34*, 170–192.

Smidt, A. M., & Freyd, J. J. (2018). Government-mandated institutional betrayal. *Journal of Trauma & Dissociation, 19*(5), 491–499. https://doi.org/10.1080/15299732.2018.1502029

Smith, C. P., Cunningham, S., & Freyd, J. J. (2016). Sexual violence, institutional betrayal, and psychological outcomes for LGB college students. *Translational Issues in Psychological Science, 2*(4), 351–360. https://doi.org/10.1037/tps0000094

Smith, C. P., & Freyd, J. J. (2013). Dangerous safe havens: Institutional betrayal exacerbates sexual trauma. *Journal of Traumatic Stress, 26*(1), 119–124. https://doi.org/10.1002/jts.21778

Smith, C. P., & Freyd, J. J. (2014). Institutional betrayal. *American Psychologist, 69*(6), 575–587. https://doi.org/10.1037/a0037564

Smith, C. P., & Freyd, J. J. (2017). Insult, then injury: Interpersonal and institutional betrayal linked to health and dissociation. *Journal of Aggression, Maltreatment & Trauma, 26*(10), 1117–1131. https://doi.org/10.1080/10926771.2017.1322654

Smith, C. P., Gómez, J. M., & Freyd, J. J. (2014). The psychology of judicial betrayal. *Roger Williams University Law Review, 19*(2), 451–475.

Strasburger, L. H., Jorgenson, L., & Sutherland, P. (1992). The prevention of psychotherapist sexual misconduct: Avoiding the slippery slope. *American Journal of Psychotherapy, 46*(4), 544–555. https://doi.org/10.1176/appi.psychotherapy.1992.46.4.544

Wright, N. M., Smith, C. P., & Freyd, J. J. (2017). Experience of a lifetime: Study abroad, trauma, and institutional betrayal. *Journal of Aggression, Maltreatment & Trauma, 26*(1), 50–68. https://doi.org/10.1080/10926771.2016.1170088

PART **V** RESPONDING TO SEXUAL BOUNDARY VIOLATIONS IN PSYCHOTHERAPY

18

TREATING CLIENTS WHO HAVE BEEN SEXUALLY ABUSED BY A THERAPIST

TYSON D. BAILEY AND LAURA S. BROWN

Therapy provides a powerful space in which to explore emotions, thoughts, identity, and experiences in the context a relationship in which trust and safety can be built and deepened over time. In fact, the connection between therapist and client has consistently been shown to be one of the most robust predictors of positive psychotherapy outcome (Norcross & Lambert, 2011, 2018). However, when therapy shifts from close, empathic connection to sexual communication and contact, the fundamental ethical principles creating the safe container of the therapeutic process have been broken (American Psychological Association, 2017; Pope, 1988, 1990, 1994, 2001; Schoener, Milgrom, Gonsiorek, et al., 1990; Summers, 2017). Myriad harms emerge from therapist sexual abuse (TSA), which are well documented in the literature (Gabbard, 2017; Pope, 1994, 2001; Schoener, Milgrom, Gonsiorek, et al., 1990; see also chapters in this text), and commonly result in clients' not ever returning to therapy, whether or not they recognize the harm or need treatment. When a client does choose to take that risk, the treating therapist must be ready to experience a level of anguish, ambivalence, and

https://doi.org/10.1037/0000247-018

Sexual Boundary Violations in Psychotherapy: Facing Therapist Indiscretions, Transgressions, and Misconduct, A. Steinberg, J. L. Alpert, and C. A. Courtois (Editors)

difficult relational dynamics that are not generally encountered outside of this treatment context.

Sexual behavior or contact in therapy creates a severe rupture in which the healing aspects of the relationship become compromised and tainted, creating a situation in which *any* therapist is now inherently suspect, and it is extremely difficult for trust to be (re-)established in a subsequent treatment relationship. Additionally, many of those sexually abused by a therapist do not attribute their ongoing and often deepening distress to the therapist's misconduct (which may not be recognized as such, may continue to be identified as love or part of the treatment, may be maintained on an ongoing or ambient basis, or may become an ongoing obsession); they may approach a new therapist with a narrative of self-blame, shame, connection to or protection of the prior provider, profound grief, and a longing to return to the relationship if it has ended (Luepker, 1990a, 1990b; Pope, 2001). It is for these reasons that we concur with the long-standing conceptualization of sexual boundary violations in therapy as abusive, akin to incest in its dynamics given the inherent power imbalance and the often parent–child nature of the transferential relationship We begin by briefly describing how the effects of collective shame may distort expectations of the frequency of TSA. We then focus on general guidelines for subsequent treatment, including management of transference and countertransference reactions, as well as the critical role of ongoing and consistent consultation for the therapist. Finally, we address the manner in which this information comes to our attention and discuss outcomes and actions the client may decide to take.

PUSHED INTO THE SHADOWS: TABOO CONVERSATIONS AND COLLECTIVE SHAME

Sexual feelings on either side of the therapeutic dyad are common, yet even acknowledging this fact may be sufficient to surface feelings of shame and a tendency to hide for both client and therapist (Pope et al., 1993). The shroud of shame increases exponentially when these experiences become overt sexual comments, advances, or behavior and shame then becomes one of the many major difficult emotions important to address in follow-up treatment (Slochower, 2017). Further, these reactions are likely to be intensified for individuals with a history of incest victimization (as well as other forms of child sexual abuse), which also appears to pose a unique risk for revictimization based on observational research and anecdotal information from those working with this population (Kluft, 1990) and the dynamics associated with incestuous abuse.

When it is discussed, literature pertaining to sex within the therapy dyad often uses terms such as *sexual boundary violations* or *therapist misconduct*. Although these phrases provide some sense of what happened, they fall short in accurately describing the gravity of the abuse. They also tend to minimize the level of damage caused by this particular betrayal trauma (Freyd, 1997), with effects similar to those of rape and incest (Luepker, 1990b; Pope, 1990; see also Chapter 13). The therapist who sexually abuses and exploits clients "obliterates the special space that defines [therapy]" (Summers, 2017, p. 178), using therapy in a way that is self-serving and harmful and that perpetrates a serious betrayal of trust that goes well beyond the individual victim (Demos, 2017). In some states, TSA is a form of criminal sexual assault that can result in jail time and requirement to register as a sex offender (for a listing of these states, see Chapter 3).

THERAPIST SEXUAL ASSAULT AND ABUSE: NOT A PROBLEM OF THE PAST

The "first wave" of information about sexual assault and abuse by therapists was in the 1980s and 1990s when studies, articles, chapters, and books on the topic were published and there was discourse in the public domain. When considering the dearth of more recent publications associated with this topic, one might hope that TSA has ceased and that therefore, it is unlikely for a victim to seek later therapy. The lack of research and published disciplinary data creates further difficulties in fully understanding the current scope of this problem. For example, the Association of State and Provincial Psychology Boards (2017) database has shown that psychologists continue to be reported for sexual-related offense; however, the 82 cases over the past 4 years solely include those who were disciplined by a state board. Unfortunately, the authors are not aware of any other organization that provides an overview of disciplinary actions for other mental health professionals, and there is no database of cases that were not reported to disciplinary boards, were settled out of court, or were never disclosed. However, an internet-based organization, Therapist Exploitation Link Line (TELL; see Chapter 15), has reported receiving increased reports of such abuses and assaults over the years of its existence and that reports have increased since the advent of the #MeToo movement (Wohlberg, 2019).

As with other forms of sexual abuse or assault, particularly by a known or trusted perpetrator, report rates are low. This is due to several factors, including the client's fear of being disbelieved or stigmatized and a paradoxical attachment to and protection of the abusive therapist, among others, as well as settlements with nondisclosure agreements. The latter have received increased attention in recent years as they have been a primary means of silencing victims and covering up all kinds of sexually abusive behavior. Of those clients who decide to seek follow-up treatment, only 12% decided to make a formal report to the authorities or a formal complaint to a licensing board or ethics office (Pope & Vetter, 1991); it is unclear whether this is still the case at this time. In any event, it is likely the available numbers drastically underrepresent the total number of clients who have experienced some form of TSA or exploitation (particularly since the Pope & Vetter, 1991, sample solely included information about clients who sought follow-up treatment with a psychologist).

TREATMENT AFTER ABUSE IN PREVIOUS PSYCHOTHERAPY

Therapy in the wake of any trauma is a complex, multifaceted process, particularly when the event(s) are interpersonal in nature and involve a fundamental betrayal (Freyd, 1997) by a powerful and beloved other with whom the victim has an ongoing relationship of some sort. This process becomes even more fraught when the harm was perpetuated by a therapist whose role is to heal and protect and not exploit. When sexual contact takes place, the entire relationship component of psychotherapy and the field as a whole are tainted (Demos, 2017; Pope, 2001; Schoener, Milgrom, & Gonsiorek, 1990). When the therapist is redefined as "the rapist," reentering treatment for any reason, much less to discuss what happened with a previous therapist, who may still be (paradoxically it seems) loved and grieved for, may seem impossible. For those clients who chose to work through the grief, anguish, ambivalence, shame, and consequences of these violations to their lives, it is critical that subsequent therapists not make assumptions about how these experiences have affected clients' lives nor presume to know a priori about the relationship and its significance (Luepker, 1990a). These clients, like incest survivors, may love and long for the therapist–perpetrator and so may see no harmful effects of TSA (Luepker, 1990a), what Freyd and colleagues described as *betrayal blindness*, a common response to betrayal trauma (Freyd, 1997). Given the transference and countertransference reactions that frequently emerge when treating a victim of TSA and the range of client responses to these experiences, it is necessary to allow clients' stories to unfold at their pace, with a general therapeutic focus in the interim on maintaining safety, regulating emotions and, in due time, providing psychoeducation (Schoener, Milgrom, & Gonsiorek, 1990). Because, as in incest and other forms of sexual abuse, the abusive therapist may have sworn the client to secrecy and placed the burden of blame and loyalty on the client they have betrayed, the story may emerge slowly; subsequent therapists must be patient.

Therapists treating TSA must remain mindful and accepting of the reality that most typical therapeutic interventions have been rendered suspect (Pope, 1994). For example, the routine gathering of information may feel like an enactment of therapist voyeurism. Empathy may be perceived and received as seduction. Paradoxically, for the client still in the stage of self-blame and idealization of the prior therapist, the new therapist's identifying the sexual boundary violation as such may counter what the client thinks to be the problem, not the prior therapist's exploitative behavior; this identification may itself feel like a betrayal of all the client holds dear. Clients may leave therapy with a subsequent therapist if their idealizing love of the abuser is not recognized and respected or if it is challenged too soon or directly. There is often a certain "Alice in Wonderland" quality to the initial stages of therapy with the survivors of such violations. Therefore, it is imperative that clinicians who treat survivors be grounded in the extant knowledge base regarding dynamics and challenges of such treatments, learn effective strategies for grounding themselves, think carefully, and regularly check in with the client to reduce the likelihood of yet another trauma reenactment (Luepker, 1990a; Pope, 1994).

ENTERING THE TREATMENT PROCESS LABYRINTH

It is a rare occurrence for a client to immediately report sexually exploitative behavior of a previous therapist when entering treatment. Whether this is due to a desire to hide the information due to shame, protect the previous therapist, or not conceptualize the behavior as a problem, it is more common for this information to be presented in an "oh, by the way" format after spending some time with the new therapist than to be a presenting issue a client discusses in the early parts of treatment (Luepker, 1990a; Pope, 1994). Once TSA becomes part of therapy, the authors (and other colleagues they have consulted with or provided consultation to) have found the recovery journey, already a winding and often daunting path for trauma survivors, becomes even more difficult to maintain. This may be especially true for individuals who have a history of other traumatic events, particularly incest survivors, who are likely to carry a vulnerability to being exploited by a beloved person in a powerful position (Courtois, 2010; Freyd, 1997; Kluft, 1990). Indeed, the Ninth Circuit Court of Appeals, in the case of

Simmons v. United States (1986), ruled that sexual boundary violations in therapy were precisely analogous to incest and that a therapist could thus not claim that such a relationship had been consensual, drawing on the second author's testimony in that matter on behalf of the plaintiff.

COMPOUNDED LOSS AND (RE)VICTIMIZATION

Survivors of sexually exploitative therapy frequently experience multilayered loss that may or may not be consciously recognized. Although some of the losses have been identified (e.g., sense of safety within therapy, loss of the relationship itself), many others can be experienced as a result of TSA. For instance, marriages or other romantic relationships may end when the abuse is disclosed or discovered and a spouse or partner experiences the sexual boundary violation within treatment as a major betrayal and an affair. Child custody issues can arise in those states where a parent's adulterous conduct may be considered. Friendships may be pushed away when friends or family of either the therapist or the victimized client name what is happening as having been a major breach of trust. Even when a survivor of an abusive therapist can identify what happened as a violation, many have experienced further betrayal when reports were made to institutions that failed in their protective functions or further perpetuated the trauma via victim-blaming, shaming, disbelief, or exonerating the abusive therapist.

DON'T JUST DO SOMETHING, SIT THERE: WADING THROUGH THE AMBIVALENCE

For clients who reenter therapy, distrust of both the helping professional and themselves are common themes, even when the previous relationship is viewed only as a love affair or even continues; in fact, when this is the case, the client may have been warned against a new therapist's judgment, just as incest victims are warned by perpetrators that should they tell, they will be blamed or disbelieved. This fear of judgment drastically increases the ambivalence about treatment and forming a new therapy relationship (Luepker, 1990a; Pope, 1994; Schoener, Milgrom, & Gonsiorek, 1990). In fact, Pope (2001) noted that "extreme ambivalence can be one of the most debilitating consequences of sexual involvement with a therapist" (p. 955). This is likely due to ambivalent attachment to the previous therapist who may be both loved and hated, depending on myriad factors. The second author has worked with several individuals who were suing sexually abusive therapists yet expressed guilt at "ruining" the therapist's life, grief for the loss of the special relationship, and confusion as to whether they had a right to lodge a complaint. Subsequent therapists are a trigger for these clients. A person who was mildly avoidant before the abusive therapy may come into the subsequent therapist's office prepared for the worst and behaving consistently with those fears in ways that may seem incomprehensible until the entire story unfolds.

Thus, there is a strong likelihood of encountering this group of clients in the precontemplation stage of change (Norcross et al., 2011) in regard to discussing the harm perpetrated by their previous therapist, particularly whether the "relationship" continues or there is ongoing contact. This may lead to a state that we have come to refer to as *anticontemplation*. Although we have conducted no research on this phenomenon and have only anecdotal reports and personal observations, this construct describes the palpable increased level of energy associated with pushing back against almost everything in therapy while client conducts tests of trustworthiness. Instead of the "problem, what problem?" narrative of precontemplation, the survivors of abusive therapy in anticontemplation know what the problem is: It's you, their next therapist, although you may not know that yet. They do not want to be in your office but are feeling desperate and overwhelmed enough that they have capitulated and reentered treatment. They do not want to connect—and in many cases actively disengage. They want you to keep your distance, emotionally and otherwise (with several of the second author's clients insisting that she move her chair to as far away in the room as possible). And yet they know that they need help and often feel shame and self-hatred for having been "weak" for having engaged with the previous therapist and needing to return to the "danger zone" of therapy. Thus, the therapist is put in a paradoxical situation in the same way the client is experiencing it.

It is critical for clinicians to hold space for this ambivalence and parallel process. This is a particularly important stance in general but particularly with regard to suggesting or initiating any nonmandated action against the prior therapist (Pope, 1994). The urge on the part of the subsequent therapist to "do something" and punish the previous therapist for their transgressions can be powerful—and understandable. Importantly, the client often does not necessarily share this urge. Following a client's lead on whether and what, if anything, to do about the abusive therapist can be a particularly difficult set of experiences for therapists to manage when considering the common reactions clinicians go through in response to learning about a colleague sexually exploiting one or many clients (Nicholson, 2010; Schoener, Milgrom, & Gonsiorek, 1990). Among other things, we feel anger, shame, and the desire to rescue or protect and for revenge; we lose track, temporarily, of our regard for client autonomy and adulthood (e.g., Pope, 1994). We may also experience our own grief if the perpetrator is a colleague we have admired—or even been trained or mentored by—or one we have supervised or have offered consultation.

Thankfully, the universal mandate to maintain confidentiality supersedes the obligation to report a colleague's unethical behavior in the authors' home state, which is true throughout most of the United States and Canada (for a listing of states where reporting is mandated, see Chapter 3). Preempting the client's right to decide whether or what to report is another form of disempowerment and invalidation that can perpetuate overall distress. Hence, the critical nature of consultation with someone knowledgeable about one's jurisdiction's reporting laws when working with individuals who have been sexually abused by a previous therapist (as we discuss later in the chapter). In the event that a report is mandated, this information should be imparted to the client by means of the treatment contract or informed consent document at the onset of treatment with all clients, as well as in verbal discussion at the point of intake and throughout the treatment. It should be recognized, however, that even in those states with mandatory reporting, subsequent therapists are unable to report if the client declines to share the prior therapist's name. One of us worked with such a client who was careful never to call the previous therapist by anything but her first name.

It should also be noted that reporting requirements can be different in different states and jurisdictions and that the therapist must follow the requirement of the state(s) where licensed. When mandated reporting is not required, clinicians often describe the distress associated with holding this information confidential as similar to having a client who is actively suicidal, which is often considered one of the most significant fear-related stressors associated with clinical practice (Brigham, 1989; Pope & Tabachnick, 1993).

An example of the difficulties inherent in dealing with this are illustrated by a case from the second author's consultation practice in which a client disclosed full information to her new psychotherapist, including the name and practice location, of a sexually abusive prior treatment provider. This occurred in a state requiring mandatory report of impaired or unethical behavior by another mental health professional. Although the therapist had the information about this sort of mandated reporting in their disclosure statement, believed the client was sufficiently informed as to the risks inherent in sharing the abusive therapist's name, and engaged in a collaborative manner with the client in making the mandated report after several weeks of consultation with experts, the effects of the reporting process were destructive to the therapy. The client dropped out shortly after the report was made and identified the reporting as more painful and harmful to them than anything the prior abusive therapist had done.

Thus, therapists must take all possible steps to mitigate the disempowering effects of such mandatory report laws while meeting legal requirements, a careful balancing act. Although their stated purpose is to protect the public, an unintended side effect can be to infantilize the survivors of abusive therapists and to disempower them by taking away the decision-making process, timing, and location of action (Schoener, Milgrom, & Gonsiorek, 1990). Involuntary and ill-timed disclosures and reports can be made by others in the client's life, such as a spouse or partner, as a means of punishment and retribution (toward the therapist, the client, or both), in some cases reporting and seeking legal redress for their own injuries and damages. This too can be extremely distressing and destabilizing for the client, especially when the motive is revenge and when the client is not involved in the decision to disclose or report. Any reporting to the media and media coverage would add yet another layer.

RISK MANAGEMENT: AN EVER-PRESENT CONCERN

Literature suggests that suicidal ideation, plan formation, and intent to engage in nonsuicidal and suicidal self-directed violence are common in the wake of TSA, although specific data are lacking (Luepker, 1990a; Pope, 1994). It is more critical to evaluate each client's level of risk and conduct a detailed suicide assessment in the treatment of this population than it might be in general practice. Although many clinicians are well versed in assessing suicide risk, it is a fundamentally different experience when the client has difficulty maintaining trust in the clinician or the process of psychotherapy and thus is more likely to withhold information about intentions and vulnerabilities. Risk is further exacerbated by the significant fluctuations in mood, high degree of ambivalence, and impaired ability to think or concentrate, all of which are common reactions to experiencing and acknowledging the betrayal associated with TSA (Pope, 1994), similar to what is seen in survivors of complex trauma (Courtois & Ford, 2013; see also Chapter 14 of this volume on the topics of attachment, grooming, and betrayal in incest and other forms of relationship-based abuse).

It is noteworthy that there are a number of cases reported in the literature and in forensic contexts of therapists whose rationalization for sexual involvement with a client was to prevent suicide. Their countertransference fear was so strong that they sought to manage the suicidal risk by attempting to rescue the patient through sexual interaction. In one forensic matter in which the second author served as an expert, the abusive therapist applied this rationale to six clients, all of whom confirmed that they had in fact told their therapist that they might kill themselves if the therapist did not have sex with them. This did not excuse the abusive therapist's behavior; in fact, each of his victims reported an increase in suicidality following on his initiation of sexual contact. A survivor of childhood sexual abuse may in fact experience feelings of rejection or abandonment when a therapist is clear about not being sexual, as not being venal or seducible, or as not expecting sex as the "price of the relationship." This distortion of relationship was stated emphatically by one of the second author's clients during an exchange about why no sex would happen in this new therapy: "If you won't have sex with me, it means that you hate me and think I'm disgusting."

Identifying the meaning that the client ascribed to the prior sexual contact is thus an important component of the subsequent therapy and in managing responses. For example, suicidality may increase in acuity as the client comes to reappraise the previous relationship as abuse, rather than as love or specialness (especially if the client learns that the therapist was sexual with other clients as well). It may also escalate as a consequence of the ending of the previous treatment or the personal and sexual relationship, often by the therapist and not uncommonly in an abrupt, unempathic, and hurtful manner that can leave the client devasted and result in traumatic bereavement. Unlike other more commonplace losses and due to its taboo nature, it can also fit the category of *ambiguous loss*, of the type that is often secret and that has no place to be aired or grieved and no one to understand (Boss, 2006). Furthermore, reactions can be aggravated by an unplanned discovery, disclosure, or reporting by third parties. It can be activated by a media or other reporting of the therapist having been sexually involved with other patients, serially or concurrently. At whatever point the "scales fall from the victim's eyes," enormous anguish, depression, grief, shame, self-blame and betrayal (among other reactions) can cause suicide to look like a good option.

TRANSFERENCE DYNAMICS WHEN THE PREVIOUS EXPLOITATIVE THERAPY ENTERS THE ROOM

Although clinicians are generally accustomed to intense transference dynamics associated with caregivers and parental figures, particularly in clients with histories of attachment trauma and incest (e.g., Courtois & Ford, 2013), it is often a subjectively different experience to work with a client whose abusive and confusing beloved and betraying figure was the last treatment provider (Luepker, 1990a; Pope, 1994). The harm becomes additive and has been done by *one of us*. For clients, this fundamental betrayal of the therapeutic process calls into question the safety and validity of all of the relational aspects of therapy, which constitute such a large percentage of what makes therapy work, especially with this population. Unless the subsequent therapist is prepared to openly discuss the matter of trust, and more specifically, that there is no reason why the client should have it or for the new therapist to expect it and why the new therapist is willing to patiently earn it, then the subsequent therapy is unlikely to go well, or last long (Luepker, 1990a; Pope, 1994; Schoener, Milgrom, & Gonsiorek, 1990; Summers, 2017).

Luepker (1990a) suggested discussing the adaptive nature of distrust after being harmed and how it makes sense that this experience would be present in follow-up treatment, which is consistent with how the issue of trust is addressed in trauma treatment more broadly, especially with survivors of complex trauma (e.g., Courtois & Ford, 2013). Empowering the survivor of therapist abuse by discussing ways in which they can assess and test the subsequent therapist, and then demonstrating not only the fortitude to embrace but also welcome such tests, makes for more effective and potentially healing treatment.

MY COLLEAGUE(S) WOULD NEVER! COUNTERTRANSFERENCE REACTIONS

One of the most commonly reported reactions to clients disclosing sexual abuse by a previous therapist is disbelief, followed closely by outrage, on the part of the next therapist (e.g., Pope, 1994). When left unchecked and unmetabolized, these reactions can lead to a variety of problematic behaviors on the part of the new therapist that are likely to cause further distress or harm to the client. For instance, the first author experienced his first disclosure about therapist sexual abuse as a trainee in graduate school. He experienced the air in the room suddenly disappear, followed closely by intense rage about the other clinician's behavior, even though the therapist was not a known colleague. He attended consultation with the second author, his supervisor at the time, pitchfork at the ready. Without the mindful guidance of numerous hours of consultation, there is a strong likelihood he would have followed these emotions and created another significant, irreparable rupture in the therapeutic process. The client in this matter, who has remained in treatment with the first author for close to a decade at the time of this writing, has repeatedly expressed how important the time immediately after disclosure was to their remaining engaged in treatment as they worked to help her decide whether to make a report and how to reconnect with therapy in a meaningful and healing way.

Luepker (1990a) noted that "professionals need to work out their frustration with unethical practitioners through professional consultation, not during a client session" (p. 111) and not with the client. Such consultation should not be a one-time occurrence. This is especially true for therapists new to working with this population and its idiosyncratic issues, dynamics, and reactions that resemble those of other incest and sexual abuse survivors but differ from them as well. After all, we rarely know the person who incestuously abused our clients; we often personally know or have a professional connection to the abusing therapist. The second author, after having served as the expert in a client's board proceedings, has run into the offender therapist—from whom she still receives hateful stares—in the grocery store on a regular basis for more than 20 years now. This, despite having confessed to everything the client had reported in the proceedings. Perhaps her reaction masks her shame or perhaps not.

On a personal level, therapists working with survivors of TSA are likely to have repeated encounters with the multiple ways in which our colleague groomed them, abused their trust, and exploited their vulnerability as they become more willing to share additional details of what happened. The emotions that arise while being a witness to these stories, including disgust and anger, may become particularly painful when aberrant forms of abuse are reported and we, our client, and the abusive therapist share membership in a target group (e.g., culture, religion, sexual orientation). In such cases, not only has the prior therapist betrayed our profession, they have also betrayed our group and perhaps made it more difficult for the client to find safe spaces, particularly if their former therapist has more standing or credibility.

Subsequent therapists must be exquisitely balanced in not scapegoating the abusive therapist while at the same time interrupting clients' narratives of self-blame and shame and in perhaps not even using the terms *abuse* or *unethical* until the client introduces or otherwise indicates a readiness for them. Therapists must separate the behavior of the perpetrator from the feelings the client may have about the behavior and the relationship, in recognition of that they are likely to be confounded and ambivalent. Exploring the client's feelings may help bring about some clarity about what happened and empower clients to decide how to label the prior therapist's behaviors. One of the second author's clients wisely stated that she needed her to be the anchor that is holding down the fact that her former therapist's involvement with her and the sexual contact was unethical and wrong. She further said she needed to be able to express her feelings and for the subsequent therapist to be able to accept all of them—and her for having them. She vacillated between extreme emotions of love and hate for some time and, over time, came to her own conclusions and resolution. She decided to report the abuse to the police and had quite of bit of evidence that supported her claim, including photographs, emails, texts, letters, and her driver's license which listed her therapist's home address as hers. She was deemed credible, the therapist was charged, and the case progressed almost to trial when the therapist entered a plea of "nolo contendere" to second-degree sex abuse. The therapist was required to undergo a sex offender evaluation, register as a sex offender, perform community service, and serve probation for a period of time. The court's finding and sentence proved to be a satisfying and validating outcome for the client, who had come to that course of action on her own accord.

The urge to "intrusively advocate" for action is a common pull when working with those who have been abused by a previous therapist and involves pressuring or pushing a client toward action or a solution (Sonne & Pope, 1991). Wanting the offender to be called to account and to be punished is not an abnormal response for the subsequent therapist. However, if it is the only response, it obviates the complexities of the client's relationship with the previous therapist, denying the client's love, grief, and confusion. As is often the case when sexual abuse or assault has occurred within the context of a family or intimate relationship, survivors have feelings of love, loyalty, and care for the person who has exploited and harmed them (e.g., Courtois & Ford, 2013; Freyd, 1997). They are likely to blame themselves for what happened and are often uncertain about wanting someone to be punished. Usually, what they want most is for the perpetrator to be stopped so they don't offend against someone else. As mentioned earlier, being knowledgeable about the options for actions against the prior therapist can be helpful. It is important for a subsequent therapist to know what, if any, statute of limitations is present when bringing a regulatory board complaint or a lawsuit. Many states now have "delayed discovery" rules, which toll the statute of limitations until such time as the client fully understands that what was done was a violation that harmed them. Thus, careful note-taking indicating how such awareness unfolds for the client may preserve their rights long past general statutes for tort claims in civil lawsuits. In most states, there appears to be no statute of limitations on regulatory board complaints (S. Frankel, personal communication, November 2012) or on criminal complaints.

How this information is shared, however, is crucial. Telling a client to "let me know if there's anything you want to know from me about the legalities of this" puts the timing of receipt of information into the client's hands. Taking initiative to "educate" the client too early can be an enactment of counter-transference under the guise of sharing information (Pope, 1994). The subsequent treating therapist's task is to follow the client's lead knowing that the opportunity to bring a complaint or lawsuit may pass and tolerating that knowledge; however, it can be important to convey information about a time limitation in the form of informed consent so the client knows of any decision-making limitations. The opportunity to empower this client will not pass and at times takes precedence over external and artificially imposed legal and regulatory timelines (Luepker, 1990a; Pope, 1994; Sonne & Pope, 1991). Subsequent therapists may soothe themselves with the knowledge that most jurisdictions do not have a statute of limitations for licensing board complaints and do have long ones for criminal complaints of sexual violations. In mid-2019, New York State took the lead to remove a statute of limitation from all sexual assault complaints.

SELF-DISCLOSURE: GENUINENESS, MISTAKE, OR SEDUCTION?

Therapist self-disclosure is a commonly used intervention in some schools of psychotherapy (Brown, 2018). Genuineness-based self-disclosure, which refers to in-the-moment disclosure of therapist feelings and thoughts about the client, is well supported by research on psychotherapy outcome and is considered an important tool of schools of psychotherapy ranging from feminist to existential to relational psychoanalysis (e.g., Henretty et al., 2014), although a recently published meta-analysis found that, at present, it is a promising intervention that has insufficient research (Norcross & Lambert, 2018). Despite this latter finding, in general, this type of disclosure may be even more helpful for those who have experienced trauma (e.g., Dalenberg, 2000), yet there is a need to consider this intervention more carefully, particularly when the abuse was perpetrated by a therapist. When working with individuals who have experienced therapist sexual abuse, it is critical to remember that "even the most simple, accepted, and well-meaning interventions can cause serious problems when important contextual factors are ignored" (Pope, 1994, p. 13). Therapist self-disclosure and boundaries are such issues.

TSA often begins under the guise of therapist self-disclosure (Luepker, 1990b; Pope, 1994; Schoener, Milgrom, & Gonsiorek, 1990). Therapists may begin to overdisclose information about their own life, including issues such as the state of their marriage or relationship, their loneliness, or their wish for a better sex life. They may also begin to make statements such as "I am attracted to you; of course we cannot/should not act on this," "You are special to me, so perhaps we will act on this," "If we end therapy, we can act on this" are all reportedly made by therapists who went forward to overt sexual contact with their clients (e.g., Pope, 1994). Clients report these utterances to be confusing, seductive, and powerful; "If he/she would risk his/her career for me, he/she must love me very much" is a common theme described by survivors. This misuse of self-disclosure taints what has the potential to be a powerful and healing intervention. Survivors of abusive therapy may have difficulty discerning whether the next therapist's self-disclosure is a helpful intervention or the warning sign that is a prelude to another dual relationship and boundary violation (Luepker, 1990b; Pope, 1994; Schoener, Milgrom, & Gonsiorek, 1990).

Even for therapists who regularly practice self-disclosure as part of their practice or due to their therapeutic orientation, it is critical to consider the specifics of the context when evaluating whether to self-disclose with someone who has been exploited by a previous provider (e.g., Bailey, 2018). This is likely to be particularly important if an urge to self-disclose arises when it is not a customary intervention for the therapist (G. Schoener, personal communication, July 16, 2017). In some cases, it might signify that the client is skilled in eliciting personal information as a means of taking care of the therapist and that this relational style needs to be identified and changed. Many formerly abused individuals have learned to caretake others as a survival or adaptation strategy and may be able to discern therapist needs before the therapist is even aware of them (Courtois, 2010; Courtois & Ford, 2013).

CONSULTATION: DO NOT ENGAGE IN TREATMENT WITHOUT IT

Whenever we run into an ethically difficult situation, we regularly practice the three Cs: consult, consult, and (just when you think you are done) consult again. Managing one's personal emotions can be extremely difficult in the face of learning that a colleague has sexually exploited a client, particularly when the person is known personally or is well respected in the community, or even someone who is part of one's own circle of therapists (for a detailed example, see Nicholson, 2010). Our own feelings about the event and its impact on the client's life may interfere with our ability to engage in mindful analysis of the most effective and therapeutic interventions or to evaluate whether our behavior is experienced by the client as helpful. We must simultaneously be mindful of our own responses and seek the support of consultation in developing strategies for managing them in the service of the therapy and our client (Pope, 1994; Pope & Keith-Spiegel, 2008). Further, accurate assessment of the client's treatment needs can be hampered if the therapist's reactions are "verbalized and/or acted out to the point where they interrupt a client's need to resolve her or his feelings, they may threaten to undo the therapeutic stance necessary to help the clients" (Luepker, 1990a, p. 161). Consultation provides a space for clinicians to discuss the full extent of their personal reactions and to discharge them while receiving personal support, reducing the chances of countertransference dynamics creating problems. They can also anticipate and explore options about how to respond outside of actual sessions.

I DID NOT SIGN UP FOR THIS

As noted earlier, it is rare, although not unheard of, for survivors of sexually abusive therapy to initiate a subsequent treatment by announcing that they had a sexual relationship with their previous therapist, even if they are aware of the damage that has been done. There are many reasons for this. At times, the client is still in the relationship and has been sworn to silence by the abusing therapist. At times, they have been threatened with being "outed" to a spouse or employer; in one case from the second author's forensic practice, a therapist did just that, and wrote a letter supporting sole custody for the other parent. Furthermore, the client may not think they were abused. Because of how confusing this kind of violation is likely to be, and because of the shame that the survivor often carries about what happened or their feelings of loyalty and protectiveness toward the previous therapist, the story of the abuse is often convoluted, even obscured, and frequently unfolds slowly over time (Pope, 1994; Schoener, Milgrom, & Gonsiorek, 1990). This is not to say that therapists need to be searching for these stories. Rather, it is important to understand that it is more common for the details to arise months or even years after the initiation of follow-up treatment. In one case known to the authors, a man confided to his therapist that he believed his wife had experienced TSA before their marriage and had developed posttraumatic symptoms as a result. He then communicated this perception to his wife. She did not believe it and entered her own treatment reporting that she was only there because of her husband and his therapist's beliefs. It subsequently took her years to identify the relationship as having been abusive and highly damaging, even though the behavior she described was particularly egregious and highly compulsive on the part of the therapist who had been very nurturing to her at the outset of her treatment. She continues to remain puzzled regarding her loyalty to this therapist.

In the interim and without the story, the subsequent therapist may be puzzled by what is happening (or not happening) in therapy. The client may be extremely reactive to apparently innocuous statements or actions by the therapist. In an experience from the second author's practice, she was in practice with her spouse, resulting in both names being on the voicemail message. The client was outraged "that you have your sexual partner's name on your voicemail." In a case from the second author's consultation practice, a therapist became pregnant and the client became furious that "you are exposing me to your sexuality." Although many clients are activated in some way by information that suggests their therapist has a life outside of the office (thus the custom in some schools of psychotherapy for the analyst to remove their wedding ring or other revealing objects), the degree and intensity of the activation, and the apparently unreasonable rage, might suggest that the client has a history of therapy abuse that has yet to be disclosed. Not considering this possibility may lead to misassessment of the client. Not knowing that this material is posttraumatic may confuse the therapist into characterizing the client as being paranoid or as having other personality pathology. Even when, and if, therapists in such situations come to know the nature and the details of the abuse by a prior therapist, they are likely to take projections personally and sometimes be surprised or hurt by them (Pope, 1994, 2001).

Therapists will also want to disbelieve what they are hearing, especially when the named abusive therapist is a friend, colleague, or respected member of the professional community (Nicholson, 2010; Pope, 1994). The second author worked clinically and forensically with more than 20 women who had been sexually abused over a multidecade period by a man who founded a doctoral program and was highly esteemed by hundreds of colleagues and trainees within a particular spiritual community of which all were members. This context made it nearly impossible for his victims to report until the first woman came forward publicly. All of these women had sought subsequent treatment within the same community of psychologists founded by their abuser. Tragically, all the women had been disbelieved and experienced shaming and suppressive responses from those previous therapists.

Even when the facts of the case are nonbizarre (i.e., when the only thing that has occurred is otherwise unremarkable sex with or without a romantic relationship of some sort between two adults), it can be difficult for a subsequent treatment provider to believe that it was harmful. Subsequent providers may rationalize and minimize; "this was sex between consenting adults" is the most frequent strategy for distancing from the reality that the power dynamics of therapy obviate the possibility of true consent, just as a child cannot consent to being sexual with an adult even if they said "yes" (McNulty et al., 2013; Pope, 1994). When cases involve bizarre or extreme behavior and sexual contact (i.e., a therapist calling out a sexualized ego state for sex with a client with dissociative identity disorder, having the client move into the therapist's home and care for their children, insisting a client cut off contact with friends and family, or having three-way sex with them and their spouse—all facts from cases on which the second author has been a forensic expert), therapists can have a hard time believing these accounts. As we have learned through sometimes painful experience, "every time you think you have seen or heard everything, think again and expect the unexpected." In this circumstance, therapists often question their own or their client's reality and their responses. It helps to know that circumstances such as these do occur and that careful listening that is neither suggestive nor suppressive (Courtois, 1999) is needed. As therapists with heightened awareness of matters of consent and power in all things sexual increasingly populate our professions, we hope that these new clinicians will bring this more thoughtful and sophisticated understanding of these issues to their responses to these clients. All of this is to underscore that disbelief and collusion with minimization will deepen the harm of the prior abuse (Kluft, 1990).

In addition to a carefully balanced and nonjudgmental stance, resilience and emotional hardiness may be even more essential in work with these clients. Although these are characteristics that inform good practice, it becomes particularly necessary to martial them in the face of the larger challenges that emerge when our role and we as individuals represent possible danger to a client. Working through our grief and rage at the damage done to the client by the previous therapist and the subsequent profound ambivalence that enters our office can make it possible to be present and hold the space for the survivor to work through the abuse and to make the space for *their* grief, rage, love, and confusion; in other words, to make the therapy about the client's needs, it must comprise the opposite of what was done to them by the previous therapist (Luepker, 1990a; Pope, 1994; Schoener, Milgrom, & Gonsiorek, 1990; Slochower, 2017).

In short, working with survivors of abusive therapists is a form of cultural competence that requires the same degree of humility, awareness of bias, and willingness to meet clients where they are. These are the same behaviors that we attempt to bring to all our work, but it will likely be more challenging with this subpopulation of trauma survivors.

FORENSIC ISSUES: KNOW YOUR ROLE

In some instances, clients decide they wish to make a criminal report or to take legal action, usually in the form of a civil suit. In these cases it is essential to clarify to all parties that the therapist cannot serve as both fact witness (i.e., treating therapist who will focus solely on statements associated with treatment) and expert evaluator (i.e., individual who can provide an objective opinion on damages based on subject expertise; Strasburger et al., 1997). The role of the therapist here is to give "just the facts" to any investigators— be they regulatory, criminal, or in the course of civil discovery. Therapists should do everything in their power to protect the therapy. Given the nature of these cases, it is important to be firm with attorneys that a forensic expert must be brought into play and resist the urge to serve in both capacities, despite the frequently persuasive arguments of counsel that this will save the client money or that they never hire experts. Therapists must hold firm to that boundary and not testify in a dual role as both therapist and expert.

If a therapist is called on to testify as a treatment provider, it is necessary to collaborate with the client to protect the treatment and to prepare for the potentially deleterious effects of having the therapy exposed in the legal setting (Pope, 1994). Details of this topic are beyond the purview of this chapter; however, if a therapist's countertransference includes a fear of being pulled into the legal system as a subsequent treater, they must guard against being overly discouraging of the client's decision to take legal action. Being a plaintiff in a lawsuit or a victim or witness in a criminal or regulatory proceeding is hard work and contains many opportunities for distress. If the subsequent therapist's stance in response to these challenges is to be other than fully empathic due to their own fear of litigation and attorneys, that countertransference acting out can be as harmful to the subsequent therapy as is any intrusive advocacy. Seeking consultation from a clinician who has experience in navigating the forensic realm is critically important in helping to reduce the likelihood of further harm.

CONCLUSION

Working with clients who have been sexually abused by a previous therapist creates a unique set of challenges to any subsequent therapeutic relationship. Therapists must contend with their own feelings and be especially mindful of their clients' ambivalent emotions toward the previous therapist and the relationship within which the sexual contact occurred, particularly when the perpetrator is personally known or well respected (Demos, 2017;

Nicholson, 2010; Slochower, 2017). Therapists must be open to hearing how the client understands the relationship, what prompted it, whether it is ongoing, or whether sexual or other types of contact occur episodically, and, if not, how it ended and what has transpired since them. Learning about why the client decided to reengage in psychotherapy is also important. A range of counter-transference reactions on the part of the subsequent therapist needs to be identified and monitored in an ongoing way because not doing so can lead them to engage in behavior that is not healing and that perpetuates, or might exacerbate, the distress and mistrust in the therapist and in the psycho-therapeutic endeavor (Luepker, 1990a; Pope, 1994; Schoener, Milgrom, & Gonsiorek, 1990). For example, subsequent therapists in a zeal to be unlike the previous therapist may be "too helpful" and violate the client's boundaries in other ways. A client of one of the authors recounted how her therapist, without first discussing it with her, insisted that their sessions be conducted outdoors rather than in the office because "that would be good for her" and she wouldn't feel entrapped. The client felt extremely vulnerable being out-side of what she perceived as the safety and privacy of the clinical setting and ended the treatment without discussing the reasons with the therapist. Obviously, communication and empowerment are critical.

We cannot overemphasize the importance of consultation when working with survivors of therapist sexual abuse. The multiple layers of transference and countertransference that are present, particularly when external sys-tems such as boards or courts come into play, are enough to challenge even the most experienced among us. No matter whether clients conceptualize the exploitative relationship as harmful, their symptoms often tell a differ-ent story. Betrayal trauma is trauma, even when it is not yet recognizable to its target. This is the reason that all mental health programs must teach that sexual contact within a therapy relationship is a violation of the code of conduct of all mental health professions (as well as criminally illegal in many states and provinces). Therefore, the authors concur with Pope's (1994) statement on this behavior: "It is the therapist who *always and with-out exception* bears the professional responsibility to refrain from engaging in sex with a patient" (p. 59, emphasis added), as well as with Courtois (2015): "First, do no *more* harm."

REFERENCES

American Psychological Association. (2017). *Ethical principles of psychologists and code of conduct* (2002, amended effective June 1, 2010, and January 1, 2017). https://www.apa.org/ethics/code/index.aspx

Association of State and Provincial Psychology Boards. (2017). *ASPPB disciplinary data system: Historical discipline report.* https://cdn.ymaws.com/www.asppb.net/resource/resmgr/dds/dds_historical_report_2017.pdf

Bailey, T. D. (2018). Therapist self-disclosure with chronically traumatized clients. In G. Danzer (Ed.), *Therapeutic self-disclosure: An evidenced-based guide for practitioners* (pp. 157–163). Brunner-Routledge. https://doi.org/10.4324/9780203730713-20

Boss, P. (2006). *Loss, trauma, and resilience: Therapeutic work with ambiguous loss.* W. W. Norton.

Brigham, R. E. (1989). *Psychotherapy stressors and sexual misconduct: A factor analytic study of the experience of non-offending and offending psychologists in Wisconsin.* Wisconsin School of Professional Psychology.

Brown, L. S. (2018). *Feminist therapy* (2nd ed.). American Psychological Association.

Courtois, C. A. (1999). *Recollections of sexual abuse: Treatment principles and guidelines.* W. W. Norton.

Courtois, C. A. (2010). *Healing the incest wound: Adult survivors in therapy* (2nd ed.). W. W. Norton.

Courtois, C. A. (2015). First, do no more harm: Ethics of attending to spiritual issues in trauma treatment. In D. F. Walker, C. A. Courtois, & J. D. Aten (Eds.), *Spiritually oriented psychotherapy for trauma* (pp. 55–76). American Psychological Association. https://doi.org/10.1037/14500-004

Courtois, C. A., & Ford, J. D. (2013). *Treatment of complex trauma: A sequenced, relationship-based approach.* Guilford Press.

Dalenberg, C. J. (2000). *Countertransference and the treatment of trauma.* American Psychological Association. https://doi.org/10.1037/10380-000

Demos, V. C. (2017). When the frame breaks: Ripple effects of sexual boundary violations. *Psychoanalytic Psychology, 34*(2), 201–207. https://doi.org/10.1037/pap0000119

Freyd, J. J. (1997). Violations of power, adaptive blindness, and betrayal trauma theory. *Feminism & Psychology, 7*(1), 22–32. https://doi.org/10.1177/0959353597071004

Gabbard, G. O. (2017). Sexual boundary violations in psychoanalysis: A 30-year retrospective. *Psychoanalytic Psychology, 34*(2), 151–156. https://doi.org/10.1037/pap0000079

Henretty, J. R., Currier, J. M., Berman, J. S., & Levitt, H. M. (2014). The impact of counselor self-disclosure on clients: A meta-analytic review of experimental and quasi-experimental research. *Journal of Counseling Psychology, 61*(2), 191–207. https://doi.org/10.1037/a0036189

Kluft, R. P. (1990). Incest and subsequent revictimization: The case of therapist–patient sexual exploitation, with a description of the sitting duck syndrome. In R. P. Kluft (Ed.), *Incest-related disorders of adult psychopathology* (pp. 263–289). American Psychiatric Publishing.

Luepker, E. T. (1990a). Clinical assessment of clients who have been sexually exploited by their therapist and development of differential treatment plans. In G. R. Schoener, J. H. Milgrom, J. C. Gonsiorek, E. T. Luepker, & R. M. Conroe (Eds.), *Psychotherapists' sexual involvement with clients: Intervention and prevention* (pp. 159–176). Walk-In Counseling Center.

Luepker, E. T. (1990b). Sexual exploitation of clients by therapists: Parallels with parent–child incest. In G. R. Schoener, J. H. Milgrom, J. C. Gonsiorek, E. T. Luepker, & R. M. Conroe (Eds.), *Psychotherapists' sexual involvement with clients: Intervention and prevention* (pp. 73–80). Walk-In Counseling Center.

McNulty, N., Ogden, J., & Warren, F. (2013). "Neutralizing the patient": Therapists' accounts of sexual boundary violations. *Clinical Psychology & Psychotherapy, 20*(3), 189–198. https://doi.org/10.1002/cpp.799

Nicholson, S. W. (2010). Too close to home: Countertransference dynamics in the wake of a colleague's sexual boundary violation. *Canadian Journal of Psychoanalysis, 18*(2), 225–247.

Norcross, J. C., Krebs, P. M., & Prochaska, J. O. (2011). Stages of change. *Journal of Clinical Psychology, 67*(2), 143–154. https://doi.org/10.1002/jclp.20758

Norcross, J. C., & Lambert, M. J. (2011). Psychotherapy relationships that work II. *Psychotherapy, 48*(1), 4–8. https://doi.org/10.1037/a0022180

Norcross, J. C., & Lambert, M. J. (2018). Psychotherapy relationships that work III. *Psychotherapy, 55*(4), 303–315. https://doi.org/10.1037/pst0000193

Pope, K. S. (1988). How clients are harmed by sexual contact with mental health professionals: The syndrome and its prevalence. *Journal of Counseling and Development, 67*(4), 222–226. https://doi.org/10.1002/j.1556-6676.1988.tb02587.x

Pope, K. S. (1990). Therapist–patient sex as sex abuse: Six scientific, professional, and practical dilemmas in addressing victimization and rehabilitation. *Professional Psychology: Research and Practice, 21*(4), 227–239. https://doi.org/10.1037/0735-7028.21.4.227

Pope, K. S. (1994). *Sexual involvement with therapists: Patient assessment, subsequent therapy, forensics.* American Psychological Association. https://doi.org/10.1037/10154-000

Pope, K. S. (2001). Sex between therapists and clients. In J. Worell (Ed.), *Encyclopedia of women and gender: Sex similarities and differences and the impact of society on gender* (Vol. 2, pp. 955–962). Academic Press.

Pope, K. S., & Keith-Spiegel, P. (2008). A practical approach to boundaries in psychotherapy: Making decisions, bypassing blunders, and mending fences. *Journal of Clinical Psychology, 64*(5), 638–652. https://doi.org/10.1002/jclp.20477

Pope, K. S., Sonne, J. L., & Holroyd, J. (1993). *Sexual feelings in psychotherapy: Exploration for therapists and therapists-in-training.* American Psychological Association. https://doi.org/10.1037/10124-000

Pope, K. S., & Tabachnick, B. G. (1993). Therapists' anger, hate, fear, and sexual feelings: National survey on therapists' responses, client characteristics, critical events, formal complaints, and training. *Professional Psychology: Research and Practice, 24*(2), 142–152. https://doi.org/10.1037/0735-7028.24.2.142

Pope, K. S., & Vetter, V. A. (1991). Prior therapist patient sexual involvement among patients seen by psychologists. *Psychotherapy: Theory, Research, & Practice, 28*(3), 429–438. https://doi.org/10.1037/0033-3204.28.3.429

Schoener, G. R., Milgrom, J. H., & Gonsiorek, J. C. (1990). Therapeutic responses to clients who have been sexually abused by psychotherapists. In G. R. Schoener, J. H. Milgrom, J. C. Gonsiorek, E. T. Luepker, & R. M. Conroe (Eds.), *Psychotherapists' sexual involvement with clients: Intervention and prevention* (pp. 95–112). Walk-In Counseling Center.

Schoener, G. R., Milgrom, J. H., Gonsiorek, J. C., Luepker, E. T., & Conroe, R. M. (Eds.). (1990). *Psychotherapists' sexual involvement with clients: Intervention and prevention.* Walk-In Counseling Center.

Simmons v. United States of America, 805 F.2d 1363 (9th Cir. 1986).

Slochower, J. (2017). Don't tell anyone. *Psychoanalytic Psychology, 34*(2), 195–200. https://doi.org/10.1037/pap0000082

Sonne, J. L., & Pope, K. S. (1991). Treating victims of therapist–client sexual involvement. *Psychotherapy, 28*(1), 174–187.

Strasburger, L. H., Gutheil, T. G., & Brodsky, A. (1997). On wearing two hats: Role conflict in serving as both psychotherapist and expert witness. *The American Journal of Psychiatry, 154*(4), 448–456. https://doi.org/10.1176/ajp.154.4.448

Summers, F. (2017). Sexual relationships between patient and therapist: Boundary violation or collapse of the therapeutic space? *Psychoanalytic Psychology, 34*(2), 175–181. https://doi.org/10.1037/pap0000115

Wohlberg, J. (2019). What you should know first: A history of TELL. In Therapy Exploitation Link Line (Ed.), *TELLing it like it is: When therapists abuse and exploit*. https://www.therapyabuse.org/ebook-TELLing-It-Like-It-Is.pdf

19

SUPERVISION AND CONSULTATION WITH THERAPISTS WHO HAVE ENGAGED IN SEXUAL MISCONDUCT

GARY R. SCHOENER

Assessment, counseling, and psychotherapy are all taught largely through an apprenticeship model. As such, supervision is key to earning a graduate degree, to being prepared for practice, and to being licensed. It is also one of the most commonly prescribed solutions by licensure boards, ethics committees, and employers to prevent reoccurrence of problems. This chapter focuses on supervision and consultation as they may influence the problem of sexual misconduct by therapists.

As central as it is to psychology and other psychotherapy and counseling fields, the art and practice of supervision has developed largely the past 3 decades. The literature on supervision has grown dramatically and can provide key preparation for those whose careers began before the topic was covered in training programs (e.g., Barnett et al., 2007; Campbell, 2000; Falender & Shafranske, 2004; Haynes et al., 2003; Powell, 1993). There is also an excellent text on the ethics of supervision and consultation that is well worth reviewing (Thomas, 2010).

The Association of State and Provincial Psychology Boards (ASPPB) published guidelines for supervision in the education and training leading to

https://doi.org/10.1037/0000247-019
Sexual Boundary Violations in Psychotherapy: Facing Therapist Indiscretions, Transgressions, and Misconduct, A. Steinberg, J. L. Alpert, and C. A. Courtois (Editors)

licensure as a health service provider in 2015 that were recently redrafted (ASPPB, 2018a) and for mandated supervision connected with board discipline (ASPPB, 2018b). Both are essential reading if one is to undertake either role. If one is undertaking the supervision of persons from professions other than psychology, it is critical to seek out similar guidelines from the relevant licensure board federations (e.g., Association of Social Work Boards) and professional associations (e.g., National Association of Social Workers; Council on Social Work Education) and to see literature in that field (e.g., O'Donoghue, 2004) as well as to be aware of contributions by professionals in related fields (e.g., Strean, 1993, is a social worker). Lastly, thinking and understanding about these activities and issues continue to evolve, making it important for supervisors to maintain an awareness of those conversations and literature (e.g., Kress et al., 2015).

Despite the importance of supervision and consultation in the training and oversight of the work of psychotherapists and the seriousness of sexual misconduct in the context of this work, there has been scant literature on the role of supervision in the prevention of sexual misconduct situations. This topic has only been examined in a few publications (Celenza, 2007; Conroe & Schank, 1989; Powell, 1993; Schoener, 1989b; Schoener & Conroe, 1989). It has been raised as an issue in assessment of impairment in psychologists (Brodsky, 1986; Lamb & Catanzaro, 1998; Schwebel et al., 1994), in graduate students and interns (Forrest et al., 1999; Schoener, 1999), as well as in the prevention of boundary violations in general (Epstein, 1994; Gutheil & Brodsky, 2008). However, specific research on predictors of sexual misconduct is lacking, and in at least one study, boundary crossings did not differentiate psychologists who had sex with clients from those who did not (Borys, 1988). Sexual misconduct can occur with students, novices, those in midcareer, or with very senior, experienced professionals.

During its more than 50 years of operation, the Walk-In Counseling Center (WICC) in Minneapolis has consulted in more than 2,000 cases of professional sexual misconduct. In terms of work with offending professionals, this has involved assessing offenders and designing rehabilitation or supervision plans. WICC staff members have advised both employers of therapists and licensure boards and have evaluated situations when there were problems in supervision. Beyond my work on this problem as a WICC staff member, I have served as an expert witness in civil suits and criminal, employment, and licensure cases involving sexual misconduct in which I have assessed and testified as to causal elements, including but not limited to the role of supervision.

On the basis of experience in our agency, supervision has seen widespread use as part of rehabilitation efforts directed at psychotherapists who have engaged in sexual misconduct. The vast majority of such situations involved disciplinary processes authorized by an ethics committee, licensure board, or an employer and as such represent a special supervisory challenge (Celenza, 2007; Celenza & Gabbard, 2003; Cobia & Pipes, 2002; Frick et al., 1995; Gartrell et al., 1989; Gutheil & Brodsky, 2008; Irons & Schneider, 1999; Strean, 1993; Thomas, 2005, 2011; Thomas & Hung, 2018).

Less commonly discussed but of critical importance is the supervision of trainees and students who are struggling with personal impairment or competence issues that can play a role in sexual misconduct (Behnke, 2014; Forrest et al., 1999; Schoener, 1999; Vacha-Haase et al., 2019). Sexual boundary crossings can be the result of general emotional breakdown or life struggles faced by trainees or by their lack of knowledge or experience conducting psychotherapy.

LEGAL RISKS

A supervisor has legal responsibility for the professional conduct of the supervisee under the legal theory of *respondeat superior*, also known as *vicarious liability* (ASPPB, 2018a; Bisbing et al., 1995; Caudill, 1997; Gutheil & Brodsky, 2008). Supervision of a professional who has a history of misconduct can carry an even greater risk. There have been efforts by state licensure boards to create immunity for supervisors who are providing mandatory supervision at the direction of a regulatory body, but these have not come to pass because such an arrangement would open the licensure board up to a civil suit if things do not go well. In fact, the examples of immunity provisions the ASPPB provides refer to immunity from civil action *by the supervisee—not by any client who claims harm by the supervisee* (ASPPB, 2018b, pp. 39–41).

Even if one follows all the best practices, there is still considerable risk. I am aware of many cases where a supervisor followed the best practices for a supervisory relationship and yet sexual misconduct occurred. One such case resulted in a substantial award against a psychologist-supervisor from whom the existence of the client was hidden and who had thus not supervised the case (Schoener & Conroe, 1989, p. 479). The term "supervisor" carries that responsibility, even if one is not directly supervising the case in question (Bisbing et al., 1995).

With regard to civil liability for the transgressions of a consultee (as opposed to a supervisee), the provision of consultation carries no such risk. However, if the consultation is an ongoing arrangement, one needs to be careful that this is not supervision under a different name. When one is in a consultative role, there is always the reality, as there is in a supervisory relationship, that the consultee is providing an account of the client relationship that is inaccurate in terms of specific events, the quality and intensity of feelings, the degree to which boundaries have been crossed, and other relevant information that might alter the consultant or supervisor's input and advice. Clinicians typically seek advice from practitioners with whom they have a friendly connection, and it is not uncommon for those acting as consultants to assume that no serious mistakes have been made. WICC has seen dozens of cases in which practitioners presented a case to their consultation group and colleagues, then later realized they had asked too few questions and failed to critically examine a case in which sexual misconduct eventually occurred.

In the literature on the supervision of professionals who have sexually offended against clients, several resources are worth consulting before undertaking such a task. Specific resources that examine the supervision of professionals who are under disciplinary order are helpful (e.g., ASPPB, 2018b; Cobia & Pipes, 2002; Thomas, 2005, 2010, 2014; Thomas & Hung, 2018). Also helpful are discussions specifically focused on supervision of professionals who have sexually offended (Celenza, 2007; Frick et al., 1995; Gonsiorek, 1995; Gonsiorek & Schoener, 1987; Plaut, 2001; Schoener, 1989a, 1989b, 1989c; Strean, 1993; Thomas, 2011).

Unfortunately, the literature contains examples of misconduct that followed inadequate and ineffective rehabilitation efforts (e.g., Bates & Brodsky, 1988), and there is no systematic analysis in the literature regarding what went wrong in these circumstances. In our consultative experience at WICC, the factors that continually emerge are a failure to have effectively assessed the degree of impairment or the severity of the practice issues. In many cases the problems presented by the supervisee are too great to be corrected sufficiently by supervision to allow for safe practice in a given setting. Public safety and the integrity of our work in the medical and mental health professions requires that we assess risks carefully as we construct supervision plans to enable someone to (return to) practice.

SUPERVISION AS PART OF A REHABILITATION PLAN

Even when a licensure board action orders supervision of a professional who has engaged in sexual misconduct, there may not have been a state-of-the-art assessment of the licensee. The same is true when an employer requires it. Supervision should be part of an overall rehabilitation plan, as illustrated in Figure 19.1. The supervision plan itself should be based on a careful and extensive assessment of the supervisee to be (Celenza, 2007;

FIGURE 19.1. Overview of Rehabilitation of the Impaired Professional

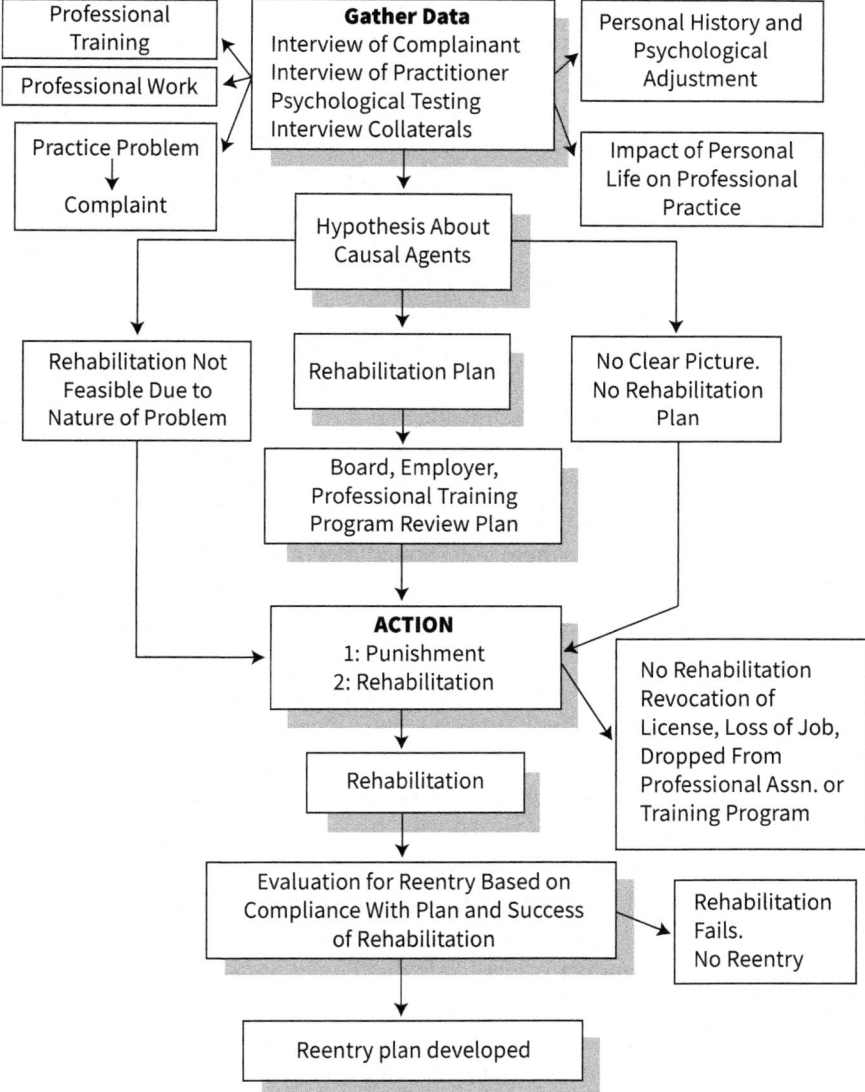

Note. From *Psychotherapists' Sexual Involvement With Clients: Intervention and Prevention* (p. 407), by G. R. Schoener, J. H. Milgrom, J. C. Gonsiorek, E. T. Luepker, and R. M. Conroe, 1989, Walk-In Counseling Center. Copyright 1989 by Walk-In Counseling Center. Adapted with permission.

Gartrell et al., 1989; Gonsiorek, 1995; Gonsiorek & Schoener, 1987; Schoener, 1995). It should be noted that an oft-cited claim from a major professional liability program that there is an "80% recidivism" rate in sexual misconduct cases, has been clarified to refer to situations in which rehabilitation is attempted absent an independent evaluation, clear treatment plan, and follow-up (Gonsiorek, 1995).

Moreover, it is critical that the supervisor have a clear picture as to the extent and severity of the sexual misconduct and how it occurred (including whether the relationship and sexual contact continue), what factors played a role in the case, whether it is the only case or the only one to come to light, and what role supervision is to play in the potential rehabilitation. Depending on whether the practitioner is also going to be in personal therapy or some sort of other treatment (e.g., for addiction) and what sort of cross-communication will be occurring between treatment providers is important. Releases of Information and clear lines of communication need to be established between those involved in the rehabilitation plan.

The organizational setting may have played a role in the original offense (White, 1995, 1997), and certainly there are organizational settings that can increase the risk of future misconduct (i.e., working in isolated settings with less supervision or where role boundaries are not well defined). In addition, it is critical to assess the relative risk of particular roles or the degree to which one can effectively supervise activities. Physical changes in the service setting, such as adding windows on doors or requiring video-taping, are of unknown effectiveness in preventing misconduct. Even the use of direct observation in monitoring plans does not provide the level of safeguard that one might assume, and misconduct can occur even with a monitor in the room (Schoener, 1989a). In instances where it is believed that the supervisee needs to be literally watched, it is critical to question whether that person should be allowed to practice.

There are several common myths in the assessment of relative safety in a given setting. First, use of an assignment to a correctional institution as a place where misconduct is less likely due to the numerous external constraints is misguided. WICC staff know of several such situations in which misconduct by a professional under supervision occurred in the correctional setting, partly a by-product of a challenging clientele who can be skillfully manipulative. Second, gender of clients is not always an effective safeguard in that some practitioners have misbehaved with clients of different genders, including same sex. Third, the age of the client who might be victimized can be varied, and limiting service to particular age groups is not a guarantee or deterrence. A practitioner who has sexually transgressed with an adolescent may still be a risk when assigned to a geriatric setting. The dynamics underlying the offending are clearly at issue with practitioners who are so impulse-driven and exploitive. Again, it is evident that individuals such as these should not be allowed to practice.

ASSESSMENT OF THE POTENTIAL SUPERVISEE

There are several models for assessment of professionals who have engaged in sexual misconduct, each of which may be especially helpful in a given case (Celenza, 2007; Gabbard, 1995a; Gonsiorek, 1995; Irons & Schneider, 1999; Schoener, 1995; Strean, 1993). Sexual misconduct situations are highly variable, and as such the composition of the evaluation and the instruments used may vary considerably.

All assessments begin with the collection of as much detail as possible on the professional relationship in which the sexual misconduct occurred. This usually involves examination of any treatment records and, in some situations, can involve input from the victim, from complaint letters to diaries to even one or more interviews of the victim. Multiple interviews with the professional being assessed are typical because sexual perpetrators, as a group, are prone to deny, rationalize, or minimize their behavior—or blame it on the victim. It is important to review any charging documents (in the case of legal action or a licensing board complaint) before meeting with the professional who is being evaluated.

The personal adjustment and emotional health of the professional are critical elements and may be assessed using a comprehensive psychosocial assessment as well as interviews with the practitioner's personal therapist (if there is one) or a past therapist. Over the years WICC staff have typically used psychological testing such as the Minnesota Multiphasic Personality Inventory–2 (MMPI-2; Butcher et al., 1989), and at times projective testing or other instruments as indicated. The testing should be done by an experienced examiner or a specialist in this population. For example, if there are indications of general sexual impulsivity or compulsivity issues, an evaluation by a specialist is needed. Although typically this involves one of several survey instruments, in some instances, psychophysiological tests such as the Abel Screen may be used (a test that measures autonomic responses to nude images of persons of different genders and ages). Likewise, if drug or alcohol abuse seems to play a role in the case, an addictive disorders assessment is indicated.

As family and relationship problems or other personal stressors may be involved, interviews with spouse/partners or family members (with attention to their distress as a result of the sexual transgression and any consequences—e.g., separation or divorce, effect on any children, pregnancy as a result of the family struggles, family illness, recent losses of any sort, legal charges, financial struggles) are very helpful in some cases. As noted earlier, interviews with past supervisors or professional colleagues can also be helpful.

Overall, the most critical issue in the assessment is the construction of a theory as to how and why the misconduct occurred. The focus needs to be on a coherent picture of the factors which played a role, and from that one can generate a plan for potential rehabilitation.

A wide range of factors have been found to have played a role in sexual misconduct by therapists. The failure to maintain professional boundaries or the violation of boundaries can take a great range of forms and occur for a wide variety of reasons. On the one hand, this can involve overinvolvement with clients including social contacts outside of the professional relationship, gifts, excessive therapist self-disclosure, for example. On the other, overly distant or abstinent therapists, those who do not maintain an awareness of countertransference responses including anger and resentment towards the client, might resort to sexual boundary violations due to these unacknowledged feelings. Dynamics that are anger-based may be an indication of underlying psychopathy and result in aggressive sexual interactions involving various forms of sadomasochism. Some factors that may have brought about a crossing of boundaries include inadequate training (in general or about professional boundaries), inadequate supervision or a failure to utilize it, lack of awareness of transference/countertransference, lack of insight into personal vulnerabilities, excessive need for client approval, emotional immaturity and lacunae in social judgment, compulsive exploitation of others due to narcissistic or sociopathic personality, impaired judgement due to organic brain injury or secondary to drug or alcohol abuse, or situational breakdown in the supervisee's personal life.

Divorce, relationship problems, death of a spouse or companion or parent, sibling or child all figure prominently in some cases, as does a decline due to illness or aging. Practitioners who have engaged in misconduct include those who are emotionally needy, with low self-esteem and high dependency needs, including high needs for client acceptance. Within this grouping is Gabbard's (1995b) "lovesickness"—the neurotic practitioner who can be highly dependent on the client. This type of situation is also described in the concept of the "wounded healer" (e.g., Irons & Schneider, 1999). It is important to note that some offenders in this category have a longer standing problem that Gabbard (1995b) described as "masochistic surrender" with a history of being dominated in relationships and feeling frustrated about it; these individuals allow a client to manipulate and dominate and then are consumed by resentment about it.

It should be obvious from the preceding lists of variables that supervision alone cannot necessarily significantly affect the underlying cause of the boundary violations. It is often the case that the offender needs in-depth personal psychotherapy that identifies and processes those issues and variables that led to the collapse of the treatment boundary. Ideally, an assessment will have been done to rule out conditions that cannot easily be changed, but this is not always the case. In failed supervisions, the most common factor seems to have been an inadequate initial assessment and plan in the first place and ongoing assessment and reporting over the course of the supervision to whoever mandated the supervision.

RECORD KEEPING

There are a great many models for record keeping in connection with supervision (ASPPB, 2018a, 2018b; Brantley, 2000; Falender & Shafranske, 2004; Luepker, 2012; Schoener, 1989c; Thomas, 2010). With regard to the supervision of therapists who have a history of sexual or other misconduct, the supervisor's records are important and thought needs to be given to record keeping. A licensing board or third party might specify how and what is to be documented in a supervisory note. The supervisee should be given informed consent about many issues but particularly that the content of sessions is not confidential and that reports will be made to whoever mandated supervision on their required timetable. A release of information form should be signed by the supervisee. Besides memorializing the supervision sessions, records should help keep the supervision on track and provide documentation of assignments, attendance, and general compliance by the supervisee. The supervisee's overall status and attitudes and motivation should be monitored and noted as well. Supervision sessions could be taped, but I am not clear what that would accomplish as a safeguard because it is contact outside of sessions that plays a role in setting up the sexual misconduct in the first place. Anything pertinent that is denied or kept hidden should be documented.

CONTRACTING FOR A SUPERVISORY RELATIONSHIP

In recent years, there has been a growing focus on the development of a supervisory contract. Thomas (2010) provided an analysis of informed consent as part of contracting for supervision. When one is in a supervisory relationship, a contract is essential to ensure that duties are defined for both parties. Proceeding informally without a contract carries with it the same liability and responsibility but provides the supervisor with far less protection.

Supervision, like other professional duties and tasks, requires an assessment and "game plan." One has the duty to gather background on the supervisee—from them, their training program, and former supervisors—to gain a preliminary assessment as to their strengths, weaknesses, and supervision needs. This goes beyond the hiring process and the activities of human resources. Job descriptions may play a role, but they rarely define the content of the supervisory interaction.

All supervisees should be directly asked the following:

1. What are their past supervision experiences—good and bad? If bad, did they involve any form of sexual boundary crossing or misconduct on the part of the supervisor?

2. What have they found helpful in terms of supervision methods?

3. Are there any past complaints or problems on their part in maintaining professional boundaries or in performing in the professional role?

4. Are there current problems or concerns that might limit their effectiveness or ability to perform? (Note that inquiry related to their problems or mental health history must be focused on implications for practice.)

5. Do they have any clients with whom they are unqualified to work or with whom they have significant problems?

6. What do they hope to get out of this supervisory experience, and what does their training program or employer expect?

If the supervisee is on probation or the supervision is a requirement of continued employment or licensure, then the supervisor must obtain all data about the background of the situation to know precisely what the original practice problems were and what the board, employer, or other party expects the supervision to accomplish. It is critical to determine (a) whether the plan makes sense and, as a practical matter, can be achieved; (b) whether your setting is an appropriate one for the practitioner to work in; and (c) whether you are qualified to provide such supervision to this person. A stipulation and order from a regulatory body or a contract with a human resources department of an employer often reveals only part of the story and can at times be misleading, so a careful and comprehensive assessment is in order before accepting the supervision. The potential supervisor should keep in mind that their license will be on the line if an infraction occurs.

In several cases for which WICC provided consultation, the evaluation of the practitioner determined that the sexual misconduct had occurred in the context of long-term therapy that was very much like a friendship. William Schofield's (1986) fine book, *Psychotherapy: The Purchase of Friendship*, first published in 1964, provided useful background for examining the situation. The therapist, a very senior practitioner who was well known, had a practice that evolved into long-term cordial relationships with clients that were social in content. The practitioner acknowledged that he enjoyed these relationships and that they "were not really psychotherapy," although they met in the office for an hour as one might do in traditional psychotherapy. The evaluator concluded that there was a question as to whether this therapist would be able to conduct standard psychotherapy and recommended to a licensure board that a supervised internship was required to determine this. Simply supervising his practice was not sufficient to ensure public safety. The evaluator took the position, and I agreed, that if an internship-type experience with that high level of oversight and training component could not be found, the practitioner should not return to practice.

It is important to note that those prominent in the field represent some special challenges in assessment and planning for supervision. There is some tendency to honor long service and professional contributions as well as personal and professional power and privilege, and it is no surprise that an evaluator often cannot be found in the practitioner's local area or even perhaps the same state. Furthermore, senior practitioners can often speak about psychological issues with a good deal of acumen, perhaps allowing them to obfuscate their behavior and its motivation and seriousness. It is easier for an evaluator to believe that a given case was a "perfect storm" or some sort of an anomaly in an otherwise sterling career. Unfortunately, many well-known and senior clinicians are among the offenders we have evaluated, and sometimes it turns out that they have successfully obscured other signs of trouble or questionable work from the past or there have been rumors or complaints about their behavior that were not responded to or taken seriously, given their status. In a situation like the case mentioned earlier, it is possible that the specific supervisory situation that assessment dictates can simply not be found for a senior figure in the field.

Under any type of supervision, the plan of supervision needs to include and elucidate the same elements: (a) types (group or individual), frequency, and length of meetings; (b) whether records are to be reviewed by you before, at, or after the meeting, as needed and which cases will be reviewed; (c) how cases will be discussed and selected; (d) whether you will expect a full accounting for the supervisee's caseload; (e) how and when the supervisee can contact you for an emergency and who your backups are; (f) any costs or fees; (g) any reporting duties to their training program, licensing board, or other parties; (h) disclosure of your own reporting duties and practices; (i) ground rules as to things that you consider essential to be informed of; (j) any expectations as to attendance at other meetings, review of manuals, continuing education, or anything else that is an expectation of supervision; and (k) your record-keeping requirements and expectations, including any requirements for taping (audio or video) and observation.

A great many methods can be used as tools in the supervisory relationship. An overview of them can be found in any of the major texts (e.g., Campbell, 2000, pp. 69–88; Haynes et al., 2003, pp. 81–107). The nature of the tasks being supervised, the experience of the supervisee, and many other factors dictate how one best undertakes the task. Unfortunately, selective reporting by the supervisee can lead to an inaccurate assessment of a given situation and is characteristic of both trainees (Ladany et al., 1996) and practicing professionals (Pope et al., 2006). Even the use of direct observation is not always a guarantee that the supervisor will be fully informed as to what is going on in a therapy session (Schoener, 1989a).

Signs of potential problems in the work of a supervisee are grounds for scrutiny of the work. Some of these danger signals cannot be observed by a supervisor unless they are on-site and able to observe or obtain feedback from support staff. Obviously, excessive arguing or difficulty getting along would be signs that the supervisory relationship is not working out. Other signs seen in cases we have examined include situations in which a supervisee takes on a case for which they do not have adequate training, fails to refer or strongly resists referring a client who needs a special service (e.g., alcoholism counseling), shows signs of a significant drinking or drug use problem or of anxiety or depression, is overly sensitive to criticism, angers easily, is preoccupied with sexual issues, has boundary problems with colleagues, begins withholding information or resists discussing a case, has contacts outside the professional setting with a client or spouse, begins to argue for extension of the length of treatment or frequency of contacts, or breaks rules for the client.

Sometimes inquiries by a client or by a relative or friend of a client signal that there may be poorly handled boundaries. Abnormal numbers of phone calls, messages, or letters can also signal excessive involvement. Other staff may note that the supervisee's interaction with a client seems unusual (e.g., excessive joking in the waiting room), or it becomes evident that there is far more self-disclosure than is typical. Supervisees may repeatedly emphasize how much they have in common with a given client, or they may appear to "dress up" for the appointment.

SUPERVISING A PRACTITIONER UNDER DISCIPLINARY ORDER

Mandated supervision as an intervention for disciplined professionals is finding its way into professional journals (e.g., Celenza, 2007; Cobia & Pipes, 2002; Thomas, 2005, 2014; Thomas & Hung, 2018). The following case example is a composite from a number of supervisory situations which is illustrative of some of the challenges in such a role with a disciplinary referral:

> Dr. X expressed positive feelings about beginning the supervision that was mandated by the licensing board but then was not cooperative in finding meeting times. At our first meeting, he interacted as though we were longtime colleagues and then asserted that he was pleased to be working with me. He indicated that he knew of my work and asked if he could borrow a copy of my book, and I responded that I was not comfortable with that. He exhibited resistance when I requested that he provide records of his therapy regarding the cases I would be supervising. I made it clear that was not negotiable.
>
> During the first meeting he diverted from the task at hand by trying to engage in conversation about various professional issues that were unrelated to the clarification of our relationship. I confronted this, but he would repeat it and then apologize for "bullshitting" about these issues.
>
> After the supervisory relationship was underway and a case came up where Dr. X was discussing his attraction to a client, he asserted that he knew this was common in the field and then made a pointed inquiry into my own experience with this. I refocused him back on his feelings and experiences and emphasized that the purpose of supervision was on assisting him in his own work including the processing of feelings.
>
> At another point, I came to realize that there was one client's case that we never seemed to get to since he was always focused on other cases, and I had to insist that this case be reviewed in some detail and actually scheduled an additional session the same week to make sure this was done. It turned out that this case was in fact one in which transference and countertransference had become problematic. In another instance Dr. X had failed to respond appropriately to some texts and emails from a client, and I had to insist that this issue be dealt with promptly and in fact required that he contact the client before his next scheduled session with her, which was to be several weeks in the future.

Transference and countertransference may occur in any supervisory relationship but are especially likely in situations where the practitioner is forced into some sort of remedial supervision (Celenza, 2007; Gabbard, 1995b; Thomas & Hung, 2018). Thomas (2011) provided an interesting example of some of the challenges in supervision of a therapist following sexual boundary violations. Transference and countertransference in the relationship with the supervisee can present a challenge in managing the supervisory relationship. To the degree that the supervisor is an extension of the licensure board or employer disciplinary actions, the supervisor can drift into the role of a disciplinarian and watchdog. The supervisor can also be seen as a rescuer and absolver given that many disciplined professionals come for supervision in a traumatized state. Supervision may be seen as a place for confession and absolution, and rescue fantasies can occur.

A supervisor can be seen as an authoritarian parent, especially if the supervisee is one who has resentment of authority and a rebellious streak. This can trigger an authoritarian response from the supervisor. Those with a history of self-destructive and masochistic relationships may pity themselves sufficiently to bring on frustration in the supervisor, eventually leading to some punitive interaction. In addition, practitioners who have trouble managing boundaries in general will challenge the supervisory boundaries. To the degree that they can undermine these boundaries, they may show that even the supervisor has problems with boundaries.

Given the legal risks and all of the pitfalls in terms of dynamics, it is important that the supervisor be able to remain emotionally regulated, compassionate, and observant despite these challenges. Most therapists who have been through disciplinary actions by a licensure board or employer are wounded by the experience. They may have lost contact with friends and colleagues and had a loss of their self-esteem, personal as well as professional. They may also have lost a relationship or marriage in addition to the relationship with the patient. They may be struggling with shame and also have financial difficulties. Not every supervisor, even the most skilled, is cut out for this sort of role and its associated responsibilities. Furthermore, some such assignments cannot be carried out, and supervisors need to remember that it is their responsibility to terminate the relationship if they do not believe it is working out.

ROLES AND COMMUNICATION

Supervisors who are providing required supervision for licensure or those supervising in connection with a disciplinary order are often external to the agency or organization for which the supervisee works. In addition, parallel to the supervision, there may be some sort of rehabilitation or therapy going on. Finally, with those under disciplinary order there is always the potential of discovering a risk to public safety. As such, although the supervisor–supervisee relationship is a confidential one as an extension of the confidentiality of the relationship with the Supervisee's clients, there need to be some communication pathways defined and agreed to prior to the beginning of supervision.

However, as in all supervision, there is a challenge in having a trusting relationship with the supervisee when the reality is that the supervisor is also performing an oversight function. Supervisors can have an impact on one's salary, one's professional career and future, one's career and licensure status, and so on. At the same time, the most effective supervision involves the supervisee sharing things they are struggling with or that may constitute limitations (personal or professional) and mistakes they have made.

There needs to be clarity about communication with whoever has authorized or requested the supervision—licensure board, employer, or training program. There needs to be a clear understanding that supervisors have the right and responsibility to communicate if they believe that there may be a risk to client safety or the ability of the supervisee to adequately and safely perform job duties. This is beyond the usual requirement that there be quarterly reports about the supervision to a board, employer, or training program.

Depending on how a rehabilitation plan is structured, some periodic communication may be arranged between the therapist treating the practitioner and the supervisor. This is not always the case and not always needed, but in some instances may be helpful. This is most important when the supervisee's emotional stability is at issue or where psychopathy is suspected.

There needs to be an understanding, when supervision begins, as to what sort of report or set of recommendations will be required at the end of the formal supervision period. Beyond evaluating how well the supervision went based on the supervisor's view, it is important to communicate any recommendations moving forward. A key issue is whether supervision should continue, and if so in what fashion or manner?

PATHWAYS AND OUTCOMES

We have seen a wide range of cases and situations and an equally wide range of outcomes to supervisory relationships following sexual misconduct by therapists. Some illustrations may be helpful:

- Some therapists go through the contracting process and then decide to resign their position or surrender their license and leave the field.

- Some begin the process of supervision and other aspects of a rehabilitation program and stop midway through.

- Some disciplined professionals complete their rehabilitation but decide to change either the main thrust of their work or to take up research or evaluation work rather than therapy. This still gives them access to evaluees.

- Some begin to get into the same problems but avoid actual misconduct. However, they may be terminated from their job or choose to move on.

- Some do not get along with the supervisor or do not keep up with the accountability and change supervisors or drop out.

- Some develop considerable insight and clearly improve their skills— a number have commented that "getting into trouble" was a fortunate thing because it caused them to deal with personal issues (e.g., a failed marriage) or to face some personal challenges in therapy.

With regard to practice reentry, I have observed four types of case situations:

- The practitioner continues in the same position they had when the offense occurred. The issue in those cases is whether someone can eventually "graduate" from supervision. Sometimes the result is that the supervision continues for a long time.

- The practitioner continues in the same place of employment but with a limitation as to type of duties. These practitioners may be limited to evaluation, case coordination, or only allowed to see certain types of clients. It should be noted that in some instances, it is difficult to sort clients at intake so that one cannot reliably avoid certain types.

- The practitioner has a license suspended or revoked for months or years and then comes back into the field. Such persons have a serious challenge in terms of attaining employment. They often have an outside supervisor for licensure board requirements and also an internal supervisor. In such situations, there needs to be a clear understanding as to how the supervisors can collaborate. The supervision must take into account the supervisee's need to be updated. The supervisor may require that that therapist attend some continuing education to get up-to-date.

- Sometimes the practitioner is reentering the field but undertaking a different type of position. WICC staff members have worked with several who moved to the addictions field and required considerable updating and assistance in the transition. In some instances, this has involved assisting the person with regard to very different workplace dynamics.

SOME SPECIAL ISSUES

Practitioners facing disciplinary actions may have many challenges relating to the procedures of a board or employer, and supervisors may find themselves in unfamiliar territory that requires them to seek consultation themselves. Civil suits move far more slowly than criminal or administrative law procedures, so the challenges and stresses of civil litigation may also come into play. It is quite possible that access to the records of the supervision may be subpoenaed and a supervisor could also be asked to give a deposition in such a case.

The criminalization of therapist sexual contact with clients also brings with it a large number of challenges. The practitioner could be facing a sentence or practice limitations ordered by a criminal court. If the offense involves a minor, these consequences exist in all states and Canadian provinces. If the victim was an adult client, the sexual contact can be a criminal offense in about half of the states but only under very limited circumstances in Canadian provinces (Bisbing et al., 1995). With the advent of sex offender registries, offending therapists in a number of states may be publicly listed as sex offenders, something which can have a dramatic effect on them and their families.

The internet and social media provide avenues for public criticism and even stalking of a therapist. Some may be pursued for years and have current and future employers contacted by former clients, their relatives or spouses, or self-appointed advocates. This has made it difficult to use offenders as speakers in professional training programs. The Psychiatry Residency Program at Jefferson Medical College in Philadelphia developed a program that used offending therapists as speakers and reported that residents found this one of the most helpful parts of their training (Gorton et al., 1996).

Supervisors and even evaluators may find themselves being asked to assist a practitioner in thinking through such situations and weighing alternatives.

FINAL THOUGHTS

Over the past 50 years, WICC staff members have consulted in more than 2,000 cases of counselor or therapist sexual misconduct. We have followed the English-language literature on this topic and some of the non-English-language literature via translations. It has been our privilege to converse and consult about these issues in many settings around the world and to have had the benefit from collegial input, as well as experience with regulatory boards, professionals, professional associations, and victims of professional misconduct.

WICC staff members have seen graduate students and trainees have "near misses" and effectively use supervision to grow personally and professionally and become fine practitioners who go on to help many and, in some cases, to make major contributions. We have also seen careers end before they got going due in part to failed supervisory training relationships. Some were surprises, and some were not promising from the beginning.

In terms of sexual misconduct, WICC staff members have seen incidents end careers and result in harm to many besides the therapist and the client. In other cases, some practitioners "skate by" and do not receive any effective discipline, monitoring, or supervision and end up violating additional client victims. However, in some cases, offending professionals have been successfully rehabilitated and gone on to have long and productive careers.

Although sexual predators of all types make their way into the helping professions and are responsible for serious offenses, many sexual misconduct cases do not have generic sexual obsession and impulse control at their core. Problems in personal adjustment or handling the stresses of work in the field combine to provide a part of the causation in many cases, and the earliest warning signs are not about sex but rather about adjustment and impairment.

Transference and countertransference, which at times get scant attention in today's training and service provision, emerge as continuing challenges. In both cases, the challenge for the clinician is to recognize them and then to obtain appropriate consultation from colleagues, consultants, and supervisors to help sort through courses of action. In some instances, these issues have been shared with a personal therapist but not with those in a direct position to assist with practice through consultation or supervision.

With regard to the design of remedial supervision the most common error WICC staff members have seen is the failure to do a state-of-the-art comprehensive evaluation before designing a rehabilitation plan, and any plan for supervised experience or return to work.

With regard to the carrying out of either treatment or supervision of practitioners who have offended, the most common error is allowing for these remedies to end before the work is complete. When asked to review or give a second opinion, the number of supervisors or personal therapists who had supported a premature ending to the rehabilitation and who expressed relief when our staff concluded more was needed is huge. Many times, they would say "he's worked hard and come a long way and is 95% there" and acknowledge that more was needed for them to feel that the work was "100% done."

But they felt compelled to go along with the request to return to work or have the supervision requirement lifted.

The reality of this era is that there are many professionals facing serious financial challenges from huge college loan debts, many workplace pressures around productivity and payment uncertainties, and high visibility of board disciplinary actions published on the web. It is natural to want to support professionals struggling with these challenges. However, the price for a slip-up once one has already been disciplined is a high one, and it benefits nobody when corners are cut.

To the degree that we step up and try through research and reexamination of our work to improve our ability to form good consultative and supervisory relationships in which trust is high enough to have colleagues come for help and prevent problems, we can continue to grow in our understanding of sexual misconduct and other problems in helping relationships. We can also help struggling colleagues do better and avoid harm to clients as well as more clearly discern who should not hold a license and be providing psychological services.

REFERENCES

Association of State and Provincial Psychology Boards. (2018a). *Supervision guidelines for education & training leading to licensure as a health service provider.* https://www.asppb.net/page/guidelines

Association of State and Provincial Psychology Boards. (2018b). *Supervision guidelines—Mandated supervision—February 2018.* https://cdn.ymaws.com/www.asppb.net/resource/resmgr/guidelines/supervision_guidelines_manda.pdf

Barnett, J. E., Cornish, J. A., Goodyear, R. K., & Lichtenberg, J. W. (2007). Commentaries on the ethical and effective practice of clinical supervision. *Professional Psychology: Research and Practice, 38*(3), 268–275. https://doi.org/10.1037/0735-7028.38.3.268

Bates, C., & Brodsky, A. (1988). *Sex in the therapy hour.* Guilford Press.

Behnke, S. H. (2014). Remedial and disciplinary interventions in graduate psychology training programs: 25 essential questions for faculty and supervisors. In W. B. Johnson & N. J. Kaslow (Eds.), *The Oxford handbook of education and training in professional psychology* (pp. 356–376). Oxford University Press.

Bisbing, S. B., Jorgenson, L. M., & Sutherland, P. K. (1995). *Sexual abuse by professionals: A legal guide.* The Michie Company.

Borys, D. S. (1988). *Dual relationships between therapist and client: A national survey of clinicians attitudes and practices* [Unpublished doctoral dissertation]. University of California at Los Angeles.

Brantley, A. P. (2000). A clinical supervision documentation form. In L. VandeCreek & T. L. Jackson (Eds.), *Innovations in clinical practice: A sourcebook* (Vol. 18, pp. 301–307). Professional Resource Press.

Brodsky, A. M. (1986). The distressed psychologist: Sexual intimacy and exploitation. In R. R. Kilburg, P. E. Nathan, & R. W. Thoreson (Eds.), *Professionals in distress:*

Issues, syndromes, and solutions in psychology (pp. 153–171). American Psychological Association. https://doi.org/10.1037/10056-008

Butcher, J. N., Dahlstrom, W. G., Graham, J. R., Tellegen, A. M., & Kreammer, B. (1989). *The Minnesota Multiphasic Personality Inventory–2 (MMPI-2) manual for administration and scoring.* University of Minneapolis Press.

Campbell, J. M. (2000). *Becoming an effective supervisor: A workbook for counselors and psychotherapists.* Accelerated Development.

Caudill, O. B. (1997). Can therapists be vicariously liable for sexual misconduct? In L. E. Hedges, R. Hilton, V. W. Hilton, & O. B. Caudill (Eds.), *Therapists at risk: Perils of the intimacy of the therapeutic relationship* (pp. 269–273). Jason Aronson.

Celenza, A. (2007). *Sexual boundary violations: Therapeutic, supervisory, and academic contexts.* Jason Aronson.

Celenza, A., & Gabbard, G. O. (2003). Analysts who commit sexual boundary violations: A lost cause? *Journal of the American Psychoanalytic Association, 51*(2), 617–636. https://doi.org/10.1177/00030651030510020201

Cobia, D. C., & Pipes, R. B. (2002). Mandated supervision: An intervention for disciplined professionals. *Journal of Counseling and Development, 80*(2), 140–144. https://doi.org/10.1002/j.1556-6678.2002.tb00176.x

Conroe, R. M., & Schank, J. A. (1989). Sexual intimacy in clinical supervision: Unmasking the silence. In G. R. Schoener, J. H. Milgrom, J. C. Gonsiorek, E. T. Luepker, & R. M. Conroe (Eds.), *Psychotherapists' sexual involvement with clients: Intervention and prevention* (pp. 245–262). Walk-In Counseling Center.

Epstein, R. S. (1994). *Keeping boundaries: Maintaining safety and integrity in the psychotherapeutic process.* American Psychiatric Press.

Falender, C. A., & Shafranske, E. P. (2004). *Clinical supervision: A competency-based approach.* American Psychological Association. https://doi.org/10.1037/10806-000

Forrest, L., Elman, N., Gizara, S., & Vacha-Hasse, T. (1999). Trainee impairment: A review of identification, remediation, dismissal, and legal issues. *The Counseling Psychologist, 27*(5), 627–686. https://doi.org/10.1177/0011000099275001

Frick, D. E., McCartney, C. F., & Lazarus, J. A. (1995). Supervision of sexually exploitive psychiatrists: American Psychiatric Association district branch experience. *Psychiatric Annals, 25*(2), 113–117. https://doi.org/10.3928/0048-5713-19950201-11

Gabbard, G. (1995a). Psychotherapists who transgress sexual boundaries with patients. In J. C. Gonsiorek (Ed.), *Breach of trust* (pp. 133–144). Sage Publications.

Gabbard, G. O. (1995b). Transference and countertransference in the psychotherapy of therapists charged with sexual misconduct. *Psychiatric Annals, 25*(2), 100–105. https://doi.org/10.3928/0048-5713-19950201-09

Gartrell, N., Herman, J., Olarte, S., Feldstein, M., Localio, R., & Schoener, G. (1989). Sexual abuse of patients by therapists: Strategies for offender management and rehabilitation. In R. D. Miller (Ed.), *Legal implications of hospital policies and practices* (pp. 55–66). Jossey-Bass. https://doi.org/10.1002/yd.23319894106

Gonsiorek, J. C. (1995). Assessment for rehabilitation of exploitive health care professionals and clergy. In J. C. Gonsiorek (Ed.), *Breach of trust* (pp. 145–162). Sage Publications.

Gonsiorek, J. C., & Schoener, G. (1987). Assessment and evaluation of therapists who sexually exploit clients. *Professional Practice of Psychology, 8*, 79–93.

Gorton, G. E., Samuel, S. E., & Zebrowski, S. M. (1996). A pilot course for residents on sexual feelings and boundary maintenance in treatment. *Academic Psychiatry, 20,* 43–55. https://doi.org/10.1007/BF03341960

Gutheil, T. G., & Brodsky, A. (2008). *Preventing boundary violations in clinical practice.* Guilford Press.

Haynes, R., Corey, G., & Moulton, P. (2003). *Clinical supervision in the helping professions: A practical guide.* Brooks/Cole.

Irons, R., & Schneider, J. (1999). *The wounded healer: An addiction sensitive approach to the sexually exploitive professional.* Jason Aronson.

Kress, V. E., O'Neill, R. M., Protivnak, J. J., & Stargell, N. A. (2015). Supervisor's suggestions for enhancing counseling regulatory boards' sanctioned supervision practice. *Journal of Mental Health Counseling, 37*(2), 109–123. https://doi.org/10.17744/mehc.37.2.p658p5k07m830351

Ladany, N., Hill, C. E., Corbett, M. M., & Nutt, E. A. (1996). Nature, extent, and importance of what psychotherapy trainees do not disclose to their supervisors. *Journal of Counseling Psychology, 43*(1), 10–24. https://doi.org/10.1037/0022-0167.43.1.10

Lamb, D., & Catanzaro, S. (1998). Sexual and nonsexual boundary violations involving psychologists, clients, supervisees, and students: Implications for professional practice. *Professional Psychology: Research and Practice, 29*(5), 498–503. https://doi.org/10.1037/0735-7028.29.5.498

Luepker, E. T. (2012). *Record keeping in psychotherapy and counseling* (2nd ed.). Routledge. https://doi.org/10.4324/9780203128527

O'Donoghue, K. (2004). Social workers and cross-disciplinary supervision. *Social Work Research, XVI,* 2–7.

Plaut, S. M. (2001). Sexual misconduct by health professionals: Rehabilitation of offenders. *Sexual and Relational Therapy, 16*(1), 7–13. https://doi.org/10.1080/14681990125420

Pope, K. S., Sonne, J. L., & Greene, B. (2006). *What therapists don't talk about and why.* American Psychological Association.

Powell, D. J. (1993). *Clinical supervision in alcohol and drug abuse counseling.* Jossey Bass.

Schoener, G. R. (1989a). Problems in the use of direct observation in probation plans for professionals who have sexually exploited clients. In G. R. Schoener, J. H. Milgrom, J. C. Gonsiorek, E. T. Luepker, & R. M. Conroe (Eds.), *Psychotherapists' sexual involvement with clients: Intervention and prevention* (pp. 447–449). Walk-In Counseling Center.

Schoener, G. R. (1989b). The role of supervision and case consultation: Some notes on sexual feelings in therapy. In G. R. Schoener, J. H. Milgrom, J. C. Gonsiorek, E. T. Luepker, & R. M. Conroe (Eds.), *Psychotherapists' sexual involvement with clients: Intervention and prevention* (pp. 495–502). Walk-In Counseling Center.

Schoener, G. R. (1989c). Supervision of therapists who have sexually exploited clients. In G. R. Schoener, J. H. Milgrom, J. C. Gonsiorek, E. T. Luepker, & R. M. Conroe (Eds.), *Psychotherapists' sexual involvement with clients: Intervention and prevention* (pp. 435–446). Walk-In Counseling Center.

Schoener, G. R. (1995). Assessment of professionals who have engaged in boundary violations. *Psychiatric Annals, 25*(2), 95–99. https://doi.org/10.3928/0048-5713-19950201-08

Schoener, G. R. (1999). Practicing what we preach. The Counseling Psychologist, 27(5), 693–701. https://doi.org/10.1177/0011000099275003

Schoener, G. R., & Conroe, R. M. (1989). The role of supervision and case consultation in primary prevention. In G. R. Schoener, J. H. Milgrom, J. C. Gonsiorek, E. T. Luepker, & R. M. Conroe (Eds.), Psychotherapists' sexual involvement with clients: Intervention and prevention (pp. 477–493). Walk-In Counseling Center.

Schoener, G. R., Milgrom, J. H., Gonsiorek, J. C., Luepker, E. T., & Conroe, R. M. (Eds.). (1989). Psychotherapists' sexual involvement with clients: Intervention and prevention. Walk-In Counseling Center.

Schofield, W. (1986). Psychotherapy: The purchase of friendship [Ebook]. Transaction Publications. https://doi.org/10.4324/9781351307642

Schwebel, M., Skorina, J. K., & Schoener, G. (1994). Assisting impaired psychologists (rev. ed.). APA Board of Professional Affairs, American Psychological Association.

Strean, H. S. (1993). Therapists who have sex with their patients. Bruner-Mazel.

Thomas, J. T. (2005). Licensing board complaints: Minimizing the impact on the psychologist's defense and clinical practice. Professional Psychology: Research and Practice, 36(4), 426–433. https://doi.org/10.1037/0735-7028.36.4.426

Thomas, J. T. (2010). The ethics of supervision and consultation. American Psychological Association.

Thomas, J. T. (2011). Knocked off kilter: Supervising in the wake of sexual boundary violations. In W. B. Johnson & J. P. Koocher (Eds.), Ethical conundrums, quandaries, and predicaments in mental health practice (pp. 297–305). Oxford University Press.

Thomas, J. T. (2014). Disciplinary supervision following ethics complaints: Goals, tasks, and ethical dimensions. Journal of Clinical Psychology, 70, 1104–1114. https://doi.org/10.1002/jclp.22131

Thomas, J. T., & Hung, J. H. (2018). Disciplinary supervision: Ethical challenges for supervisors. In R. M. Leach & E. R. Welfel (Eds.), The Cambridge handbook of applied psychological ethics (pp. 531–551). Cambridge University Press. https://doi.org/10.1017/9781316417287.027

Vacha-Haase, T., Elman, N. S., Forrest, L., Kallaugher, J., Lease, S. H., Veilleux, J. C., & Kaslow, N. J. (2019). Remediation plans for trainees with problems of professional competence. Training and Education in Professional Psychology, 13(4), 239–246.

White, W. L. (1995). A systems perspective on sexual exploitation of clients by professional helpers. In J. C. Gonsiorek (Ed.), Breach of trust (pp. 176–192). Sage Publications.

White, W. L. (1997). The incestuous workplace: Stress and distress in the organizational family. Hazelden.

20 THE TREATMENT OF THERAPISTS WHO SEXUALLY OFFEND

PHILIP HEMPHILL, CHRISTINE A. COURTOIS,
MARK S. GOLD, ALEXIS POLLES, AND DREW EDWARDS

Sexual misconduct among health care professionals is a serious ethical, moral, and usually illegal event, with impacts that are devastating to all parties. In this chapter, we discuss risk factors and the assessment and treatment process for behavioral health professionals who have engaged in sexual misconduct. This issue is critically important on several levels, but none more so than the emotional injury inflicted on vulnerable individuals seeking professional help. The recent and unprecedented barrage of individuals coming forward with evidence of past sexual coercion, misconduct, and criminal abuse (e.g., the #MeToo movement) has shown a spotlight on the underreporting of sexual misconduct in many professional relationships and settings and the plight of victims and third parties (Langone, 2018). Yet there continues to be inadequate empirical investigation and evidence on the prevalence of sexual assault and misconduct in the health care professions, especially among psychotherapists. This, along with a lack of consensus on the basic question of what constitutes sexual misconduct among disciplines and in various jurisdictions, leaves information gaps that can be filled only with more rigorous study, prevention efforts, reduction of reporting barriers,

https://doi.org/10.1037/0000247-020
Sexual Boundary Violations in Psychotherapy: Facing Therapist Indiscretions, Transgressions, and Misconduct, A. Steinberg, J. L. Alpert, and C. A. Courtois (Editors)
Copyright © 2021 by the American Psychological Association. All rights reserved.

implementation and development of treatment strategies for both parties, and rehabilitation or punishment of offending therapists.

The authors collectively have more than 100 years' experience in a variety of academic and organizational leadership, state licensing and regulatory agencies, and the direct assessment, treatment, and monitoring of professionals with addiction, personality disorders, sexual offending, and professional boundary issues as well as their client-victims; this informs the clinical approaches presented here. Although no formal training or certification exists for this work, working with both victims and offenders has provided insight into the grooming tactics, cognitive distortions, primary defense mechanisms, relationship deficits, and the ability to bend one's professional ethics that allow perpetration to be justified by the offender. A background of addiction medicine, sexual addiction concepts, and sexual offending profiles provides a foundation for this approach while integrating a forensic lens. Although each professional struggling with these issues and disorders warrants a unique, personalized response, we present an overview of fundamental strategies drawn from our myriad backgrounds, experience, and publications in the field.

TYPES OF VIOLATIONS AND RANGE OF SEVERITY

Licensed therapists, regardless of specialty, are instructed and tested on professional ethics during their primary clinical education, and supervised clinical training is part of their pre- and postdegree training, commensurate with increased professional autonomy and responsibility. This training is designed to ensure clinical and ethical-moral competence within the scope of licensing regulations and the relevant profession's code of ethics. Boundaries are defined as the separation between appropriate versus inappropriate professional behavior between a clinician and a client, particularly regarding dual relationships of any type. These boundaries serve to define and frame normative therapeutic, social, and emotional margins between the parties. Current standards of professionalism are derived from long-standing ethical treatise, societal morality, fiduciary responsibility, and jurisprudence. At this time, however, the etiological factors, nuances, or patterns of behavior associated with sexual misconduct are not well elucidated in professional literature, nor have they been sufficiently analyzed to provide objective stratification of risk factors associated with causality, determinants of committing a sexual boundary offense, or the efficacy of identification, evaluation, and treatment strategies for an offending professional (Alpert & Steinberg, 2017).

A therapeutic relationship is established solely for the purpose of help-ing the patient move toward or attain mutually agreed-upon therapeutic objectives and outcomes. If the contract deviates from these objectives, it creates a nontherapeutic relationship and constitutes a violation of the clinician's' fiduciary responsibility. Two distinct types of boundary issues are discussed repeatedly in the clinical literature. A *boundary crossing*, a usually benign deviation from normal therapeutic activity that is nonexploitative (and, in some cases, is supportive of the therapeutic process) may set the stage for boundary violations and thus warrant interruption before it pro-gresses. Further along the continuum, a *boundary violation* is an activity or pattern of behavior that, at a minimum, compromises the therapeutic objectives, process, and outcome while placing the client at risk for harm. A boundary violation is when a therapist knowingly (often deliberately and with premeditation) or unwittingly trespasses on the client's emotional, social, occupational, physical, spiritual, or sexual space, whether malice was consciously intended or not. *Boundary violations always constitute unethical exploitation of the client in some way and are cause for investigation, inter-vention, and discipline of the professional.*

RISKS FOR BOUNDARY CROSSINGS AND VIOLATIONS

Indicators for engaging in boundary violations have been categorized in many studies; however, using these because absolute predictors or predic-tive profiles is problematic because the studies are not controlled, and many of the behaviors are common in general practice. Doing so indiscriminately increases the likelihood that the application of profile characteristics to situations will result in a high rate of false prediction that potential sexual boundary violations (SBVs) are likely to occur or have occurred. Consensus exists that the likelihood of a violation occurring may increase when limits or boundaries are disregarded, softened, tolerated, or become unclear (Gold, 2013). For example, sexual innuendo and remarks or jokes in the office set a permissive, unprofessional, and potentially hostile tone, a situation that may be minimized or ignored or allowed to pass without further scrutiny, even though it may cause discomfort and distress to all parties. These may lead to more serious behaviors and violations.

Studies of the myriad factors associated with SBVs can be grouped as follows: individual characteristics in the therapist and associated life and professional factors; the nature of the therapist's practice; and characteris-tics of the client and client expectations. We focus here on those involving the offending therapist because our emphasis is on their assessment and treatment. Among others, *primary individual characteristics* of therapists who commit SBVs are male gender (although a relatively recent study found female therapists accounting for 28.8% of client sexual abuse, likely due to more females practicing psychotherapy than ever before; Eichenberg et al., 2010) and older age, a lack of emotionally intimate relationships outside of work, a personal history of abuse, a history of neglect by a parental figure, and grandiosity regarding their role as authority figures responsible for others. Additional *personal findings* include having questions about or problems about sexual identity or orientation, sexual dissatisfaction, anxiety and guilt, and having career stresses and uncertainties (Halter et al., 2007). Other *primary personal and situational factors* related to boundary slippage and violations involve personal life crises, financial setbacks and difficulties, and professional and practice challenges. Some therapists struggle with isolation and loneliness and find a client who can be their confidante or comforter.

Although most therapists respond well to their training expectations as helping professionals, unfortunately some are not equipped with the internal resources that allow them to define their professional role identity or formation and may struggle with accountability to others, have unrealistic expectations, and poor self-appraisal skills. Moreover, they may have difficulties righting themselves in times of error or mistakes, avoid further professional development, have poor insight into therapeutic limitations, have struggles in transitions during their career, or be unable to restrain themselves.

Many professionals acknowledge that they have had sexual thoughts about or have felt attraction to clients, and in fact, these are quite normal, given the intimacy that can emerge in the therapeutic relationship (Pope et al., 1987). The boundary, of course, is not acting on the attraction and instead using these feelings and any complementary client feelings to better understand their issues and dynamics. It is unknown at present how many therapists act on their attraction; however, when they become aware of such feelings and any urge or temptation to act on them, discussing these with trusted mentors, colleagues, or in their personal therapy is important. Therapists who do not do so due to shame, viewing themselves as the expert or too experienced to need it (hubris), or, more seriously, due to immorality or criminal and predatory intent, increased their risk (Halter et al., 2007). Additionally, absent or poor training regarding sexual boundary issues and lack of awareness of guidelines and policies of the work setting, holding a professional license, and regulatory board responsibilities and functions are also frequent.

The therapist's belief that a "special" relationship exists with the client—a belief that usually develops gradually, supported by self-talk and rationalizations such as "I wish she were a friend and not a client," "I'm probably the only one who can help," "I knew from the start that there was something special between us and that our paths crossed to be together," "What could be wrong with having one drink together?" or "Having sex could be healing for him" creates risk. Conflicted roles have been described as "dual relationships," which may be inevitable in certain settings and communities and do not always lead to boundary crossings or boundary violations, nor are they always unethical. A pattern of rationalizing dual relationships may be easier for therapists working in addiction services, residential programs, rural or smaller practice environments, or other closed communities (e.g., religious cultural, ethnic, or sexual minority groups). It is the therapist's responsibility to provide guidance for how they and clients interact when they come into contact in outside settings.

Therapist Psychopathology

Additional variables and attitudes to consider include sexual entitlement, intimacy deficits, sexual preoccupation, hostility toward women or other groups, general lifestyle instability, general antisocial, predatory, or criminal attitudes, an inability to deconstruct problems and recognize the consequences of one's actions, and level of callousness and proneness to manipulative behavior. Cognitive impairments associated with a reduced ability to process complex and conflicting information, an overreliance on immediate salient social cues, and difficulty stopping a line of action once it is initiated may further increase risk.

MacDonald et al. (2015) developed a hypothetical risk model of both distal and proximal risk. *Distal experiences* include such as childhood adversities and resultant insecure attachment and early maladaptive schemas. These can then lead to proximal factors such as (a) a lack of emotional awareness and mindfulness, (b) impaired emotional regulation and impulse control, (c) lowered empathic capacity, and (d) social and professional isolation. Others *structural factors* include the demands of one's profession and role, core and ongoing training experiences, and organizational culture (whether in a group or solo practice setting), and geographic environment. *Proximal factors* including professional burnout create vulnerability. Vicarious traumatization and secondary traumatic stress are risks for those who treat trauma and, along with empathic strain, may lead to overidentification with clients on one hand and detachment from or aggression toward them on the other, both of which can create risk. These *intrapersonal and interpersonal factors* exist on a continuum and covary with the needs and characteristics of the heterogeneous group of therapists who commit SBVs. Significantly, MacDonald et al.'s study revealed an elevated sense of entitlement for those who violated boundaries, reflecting a perpetration dynamic found in grooming behavior (see Chapters 14 and 15, this volume) that includes intentional and purposeful erosion of professional boundaries.

Compulsive Sexual Behavior and Sex Addiction

The emotional health of the therapist and situational factors can all create risk, but these factors are not causal. Therapists who engage in abusive and predatory behaviors may or may not suffer from compulsive sexual behavior, recently described in the 11th revision of the *International Classification of Diseases* (World Health Organization, 2018) as characterized by a persistent pattern of failure to control intense, repetitive sexual impulses or urges, resulting in repetitive sexual behavior over an extended period of time (e.g., 6 months or more) that causes marked distress or impairment in personal, family, social, educational, occupational, or other important areas of functioning. Typically, a sexual response cycle includes (a) a triggering event or situation that can be any stressor the therapist is having difficulty coping with or managing; (b) an emotional state that is distinct and exacerbates a risk state; (c) preoccupation and fantasizing that excites the neurobiology of sexual reward; (d) a planning state that includes anticipatory reward, narrowing of focus, sexual craving, and activation of reward-seeking sexual behavior; and (e) the suspension and shutdown of the original trigger and emotional state when replaced by a few moments of calm and relaxation and the numbing of anxiety or fear following sexual gratification. The last step in the cycle is short-lived, and the cycle can be retriggered soon thereafter, resulting in reinforcement of these aberrant sexual behaviors whether by inappropriate fantasy, planning, or behavior. Therapists struggling with this condition are at increased risk for SBVs.

Patrick Carnes (2001), a pioneer researcher of sex addiction, developed a stratified listing of severity of sex addiction that included SBVs at work and professional SBVs as part of their compulsive and disordered sexual behavior. It is noteworthy that such offenses are at the more serious level of Carnes's system and may be occurring simultaneously with other offenses.

Sexual Offending and Sexual Deviance

When considering therapist boundary violations, familiarity with litera-ture on sexual offending and treatment (Schwartz & Cellini, 1995; Ward et al., 2006) that integrates numerous paradigms and theories can prove to be informative. Most of this literature suggests the possibility that some type of genetic, hormonal, chromosomal, or neurobiological process (along with the therapist's temperament, personality, and developmental history) and situational factors as contributory to sexually aberrant behavior (Blum et al., 2015). The risk–needs–responsivity model (Andrews et al., 2011) has been widely accepted as a standard for guiding treatment matching to not over- or undertreat the offensive behavior. It uses an actuarial assessment and a theoretical model based on protective factors within the context of a strengths-based, positive, and restorative approach. Factors associated with treatment, such as case management, drug screens, polygraph testing, workplace monitors, safe alterations of practice parameters, and anonymous client satisfaction surveys all contribute to enhanced outcomes. Given the variance in risks of offensive behaviors by therapists, a one-size-fits-all approach to treatment and recidivism is not suggested. More studies are needed within this domain to justify therapeutic matching, identifying traits of those who do not respond or who best respond increases opportunities for prevention.

REPORTING AND EARLY ASSESSMENT OF ETHICAL VIOLATIONS

At present, different states have individual laws about what constitutes a sexual violation, who constitutes a vulnerable and protected population, and whether mandatory reporting is required when a violation becomes known to another licensed professional. There are procedural differences between states once a report is made. Typically, a report to a licensing board by a client or a third party is followed soon after by an investigation con-ducted by a specially trained evaluator or the board's impaired professional group, or both, who contact the involved parties for more details. Action taken is dependent on the objective seriousness of the situation and some-times, unfortunately, based on the therapist's status and reputation. Some therapists are allowed to continue to practice during the investigation phase; however, they may be directed to no longer treat or have contact with the alleged client-victim(s) or any other complainants and to establish ongoing consultation and supervision with someone the board recommends. Where a situation of high risk is determined (e.g., incapacitating addiction or substance abuse, untreated major depression, bipolar disorder involving mania or major mood changes, or psychosis; extent and severity of the sexual violations; general life chaos, acute medical condition or advancing dementia [of self or close family members] and resultant inability to function; obsessive or compulsive contact with or stalking of the victim in texts and emails or in-person; and threats of violence or harm to or from self or others on the part of the therapist), it may result in immediate removal from practice and admission to an inpatient facility or a specialized program for impaired professionals for both emergency assessment and treatment.

Understandably, disclosure and reporting of sexual misconduct can be highly traumatic and shameful for the therapist and can literally be deadly. A review by Montgomery et al. (2015) of 876 physicians who were criminally charged with inappropriate sexual behavior revealed that 24 committed suicide, 83% of whom did so shortly after discovery or reporting. This fact argues for recognition of the vulnerability that accompanies disclosure and reporting, particularly when media or other public disclosure is involved. Early intervention should therefore routinely include immediate attention to issues of risk and violence to self and others and a comprehensive suicide assessment. When high risk is determined, immediate hospitalization might be indicated. Risk and safety assessments should be repeated and reviewed on a routine or as-needed basis, particularly during times of increased stress, adversity, or loss (i.e., being found guilty or jailed; losing family or other relationships and professional status) over the course of evaluation and treatment.[1]

Formal and Detailed Assessments

Formal assessments, especially for therapists who admit their transgressions and who hope to retain their license and return to practice, are usually conducted in a treatment facility or on an outpatient basis by mental health clinicians, psychiatrists, psychologists, addictionologists, and forensic and neuropsychologists who are independent of the board or the organization and who have had no previous experience with or relation to the offending

---

[1]Although our focus here is on the offending professional, it should be noted that client-victims also warrant assessment and other assistance at the time of reporting because they too may be extremely vulnerable and in need of immediate intervention. This is beyond the scope of this chapter but is an important consideration after a report is made and intervention begins.

therapist. Assessments are used to determine the circumstances of the violation(s) including severity and duration and degree to which it involved predatory behavior; the type and degree of psychopathology in the therapist; whether offending has occurred previously, serially, or concurrently; whether previous reports are on record; and recommendations regarding level of intervention and care needs. A brief screening instrument, PATHOS (Carnes et al., 2012), developed to classify which individuals are deemed appropriate for a formal psychosexual evaluation and therapeutic intervention, focuses on Preoccupation, feeling Ashamed, seeking Treatment, Hurting others, being Out of control, and Sad after acting out.

The evaluation of sex offenders in general and of professionals who engage in SBVs with clients requires specialized training and expertise. Opinions are based on principles of risk assessment, including the aforementioned specifics of the professional and the violation, knowledge of the limitations of assessment tools, history of and potential for recidivism, and potential benefits and limitations of treatment, supervision, and monitoring (Gold & Frierson, 2018). Because there is a lack of available published empirical data on benchmarks or indicators of treatment effectiveness of this population, assessment of potential recidivism must be made on a case-by-case basis; this occurs even in specialized evaluation centers that have significant experience in this treatment niche. The findings and recommendations are made to the licensing body or organization, which then considers the case and determines next steps and practice parameters. This can include immediate revocation of license; suspension from practice; requirements for treatment, education, and supervision for rehabilitation; other short- or long-term practice restrictions; or the filing of criminal charges, if not made previously.

Past Reports and Documentation

A starting point is gathering information is the sexual offender registry in all states where the practitioner trained and has practiced to determine whether any past offenses have been reported, investigated, prosecuted and resulted in a conviction. Additionally, the National Practitioner Data Bank (NPDB), a government repository that collects, stores, and discloses reported information concerning therapists, including criminal charges or ethical violations against a professional's license to practice, should be accessed to determine whether a previous report has been made (AbuDagga et al., 2016). Due to the nature of the NPDB reporting process and requirements, however, underreporting is the norm. Specifically, the reporting of medical and behavioral health professionals (such as nurses, massage therapists, psychiatrists, and counselors) in some states is optional and at the discretion of the relevant state's licensing board (AbuDagga et al., 2019), creating a loophole that allows offending (and disciplined) professionals to move to other states to practice when there is no record of their transgression in the national repository. Another loophole exists when professionals voluntarily surrender their licenses and are not then subject to official investigation or reporting to the NPDB. Thus, any offending party may be able to negotiate a voluntary disciplinary action in exchange for no official investigation or the posting of a violation on their public record. Moreover, only 25% of clinicians reported to the NPDB for a boundary violation had their license to practice revoked, while others were given lesser penalties, such as education, supervision, other remediation, treatment and monitoring—data that we consider shocking.

Fitness for Duty Evaluation

Such evaluations are required to assess whether a practitioner has a potentially unstable psychological, medical, psychosocial, or characterological status that could interfere with performing their job or role in a professional and bounded way. This type of evaluation differs significantly in process and scope from a routine psychiatric or psychological evaluation because it typically involves a more detailed sexual history regarding attitudes and experiences, whether the personality has been shaped by sexual or traumatic experiences, whether sex is used to meet nonsexual needs and is overvalued, whether sexual signals are misinterpreted and social skills are lacking, and development of a sexual genogram (Belous et al., 2012). Substance abuse and other addictions, particularly sexual addiction, are also evaluated in detail. Collateral information is especially important to obtain from the client-victim, a spouse or significant others, and current and previous employers, colleagues, and office staff because minimization, rationalization, and dissimulation (e.g., concealment of symptoms of mental illness, substance use disorder, addiction, or aberrant behavior) is common in those who offend and in addicts. A series of uniform questions such as type of relationship, relationship history, general temperament of the therapist, history of physical confrontations or verbal or physical aggression, level of responsibility for actions, providing insufficient or inadequate explanations for behaviors, client satisfaction ratings, flow of practice, and open-ended questions are used to assess these additional concerns. Finally, the use of polygraphs, notwithstanding questions about their reliability and validity, can be invaluable for initial evaluation and for ongoing monitoring (Association for the Treatment of Sexual Abusers, 2014; Finlayson et al., 2015). Simon and Gold (2010) further identified the importance of intelligence assessment within the forensic framework because it can provide the current status of functioning or may lead to further exploration of the explanatory pathology.

PSYCHOLOGICAL AND PSYCHIATRIC ASSESSMENT

The standard psychosocial assessment includes attention to developmental history in the following domains: identity, sexual and relational functioning, medical, psychiatric, vocational, and spiritual. A psychiatric evaluation reviews and utilizes these six dimensions for diagnostic clarification and mental status. The comprehensive psychological assessment should include the use of standardized personality instruments (i.e., Minnesota Multiphasic Personality Inventory-2, Personality Assessment Inventory); mood disorder screens (Beck Depression Inventory, State-Trait Anxiety Inventory); measures of cognitive, neurological, or executive functioning (Adjorlolo & Egbenya, 2016); trauma and posttraumatic stress; attention-deficit/hyperactivity; substance use; behavioral observations; and careful review of collateral documents and interviews. The Boundary Violation Index (Swiggart et al., 2008), an instrument measuring risk factors related to sexual boundary violations, was designed to assess for the thoughts, feelings, and behaviors associated with increased risk of physician sexual misconduct and is a valuable specialized assessment measure A Boundary Violation Index score of 6 or greater is suggested as the threshold at which individuals with a high probability of committing sexual boundary violation could be differentiated from those with a low probability of doing so.

Evaluation should also include attention to various defensive or oppositional characteristics that may constitute contributory risk factors or blind spots. These include such varied elements as avoiding consultation or supervision and resisting feedback due to being accustomed to being in control; resisting or withdrawing from feedback by means of rage, contempt, and aggression; maintaining secrecy due to fear of self-disclosure or exposure and stigma, punishment, or disapproval; manipulating rules to cover malfeasance or for other reasons; exhibiting self-aggrandizement, grandiosity, and lack of concern for others; exhibiting superficial compliance especially toward those authority; utilizing intellectualization and superiority as primary defenses; discounting their own feelings and needs; and overprotecting or overresponding to patients without setting limits due to fears of patient retaliation or suicide.

When an evaluation indicates significant psychopathology, including little or no recognition that the sexual contact involved a violation and a misuse of professional power and authority, little or no remorse or empathy for the client-victim or loved one(s), entitlement and grandiosity, serial offending, and aberrant sex and other behavior, the therapist's license may be permanently revoked. Depending on the state, criminal charges may be brought and, in some cases, the therapist jailed and made to register as a sex offender if found guilty. When the evaluation results in a finding of a treatable condition and a lack of serious psychopathology, then the individual can be referred to the appropriate level of treatment (i.e., residential, intensive outpatient, partial hospitalization, or outpatient program; individual and group treatment; supervision and monitoring).

TREATMENT

The first stage of treatment is to use the assessment to clarify treatment needs, strategies for care, setting the necessary boundaries (e.g., limiting access to specific individuals, including the client-victim or other clients or family members; technology, including sexual outlets; use of substances; payment, scheduling, and attendance requirements; clear demarcation of the role and limitations of the therapist or treatment team) while in treatment, giving informed consent and release of information (i.e., treatment notes and other material is not confidential and is available to the licensing board for which an open release of information is required), determining the level and source of the therapist's motivation (i.e., internal vs. external and the related stage of change), the differentiation of treatment from clinical supervision (an important distinction that some clients try to circumvent due to finances, time, or other contingencies; this is a warning sign because blending the two would create a dual relationship), and the expected length treatment. (For discussion of these issues as related to supervision of the offending therapist, see Chapter 19.) This process further serves to introduce the professionals who will provide treatment, either individually or as part of a team, and to communicate the philosophy, expectations, and contract for care. Relevant documents from the assessment process such as psychiatric evaluation, addiction assessment, psychological evaluation, neuropsychological evaluation, relationship and spiritual history, history and physical, (any) nursing assessment, victim statement, family history, sexual history, penile plethysmograph results, and polygraph testing should be discussed with the patient.

From the point of its initiation, therapy should include careful identification of the chain of events and antecedents leading to the violating behavior(s), including cognitive distortions and beliefs, distorted interests and ideas, and emotional and psychological conflicts. Assessment of the offending therapist's understanding of harm done and capacity for empathy for the victim(s); ongoing motivation for treatment; and any attempts to short-circuit, undermine, or manipulate it are also needed (Bloom et al., 1999). Treatment includes directed attention to co-occurring issues such as mood, anxiety, trauma-related disorders, addiction(s) and compulsions, developmental disorders, and personality characteristics or disorders. These co-occurring disorders have bidirectional impact and yet are primary disorders, with one not the result of the other. The best available evidence informs that viewing and treating addiction and all comorbidities as "co-occurring" illnesses each requiring their own concurrent or sequential treatment produces the best outcomes.

Treatment Interventions

No one treatment method or intervention is used. Schwartz and Masters (1994) were among the first to describe treatment of sexually violating and offending behavior with a "theory-knitting" construct and developed a forerunner integrated paradigm for treatment, with which we agree. They stated the following:

> The association with intense pleasure and other functional aspects of the symptoms result in addictive cycles which maintain and perpetuate deviant sexual behavior. Therefore, cognitive-behavioral, systemic, and 12-step approaches to treatment are required to control the symptomatology. Trauma-based approaches to treatment and cognitive restructuring are then useful in resolving the original issues for which the compulsivity symptoms had served as a functional distorted survival strategy. By blending therapeutic approaches, treatment efficacy improves dramatically. (pp. 23–24)

Given the long-term needs of offending therapists, use of a 360-degree feedback model in the assessment, treatment, and monitoring following a boundary violation has proven to be one of most effective deterrents to future offending (Martin & Hemphill, 2013; Swiggart, 2014). This model of a multirater system allows objective others, in addition to the offending therapist's self-report, to provide relevant information about and facilitate ongoing behavioral monitoring. Culling information from multiple sources gives a lenticular view of a violation, thus allowing a comprehensive intervention with four objectives: (a) to elucidate risk factors and stratify their predictive value to enhance intervention efforts and validate prevention strategies; (b) to enhance successful personal restoration of the offending professional and reintegration into practice if appropriate; (c) to use these data to better estimate outcome probability; and (d) to reduce recidivism. Assessing how the offending therapist responds to ongoing monitoring and feedback is also a determinant of whether they can safely return to practice (see Chapter 19 on supervision for discussion of the latter).

In the event that the relationship with the client-victim is ongoing, the offending therapist should be supported in ending it, an ending that may encompass loss and grief when strong emotional, romantic, and sexual ties were involved. When the client was the one who reported the malpractice to outside authorities or is the plaintiff in a lawsuit, the therapist is likely to feel betrayed and angry (and possibly blindsided) and may resort to blaming the client for causing their sexual involvement in the first place or for breaking their pledge of secrecy and nondisclosure. These feelings need to be expressed and issues of responsibility and any offloading of blame and shame onto the client confronted. Issues of future contact and communication between both parties should also be discussed and boundaries established.

In a similar vein but from the perspective of the spouse/partner or other family members, adjunctive family or couples counseling may help to address the extreme betrayal typically experienced by the practitioner's loved one after disclosure and associated actions. Couple counseling should involve a formal disclosure of the scope and severity of the violation and the extent of the infidelity to the victim-partner to help them be fully informed as they weigh their choices. The exposure of possible causes such as sexual addiction or an intimacy disorder can help both partners understand risk factors and how the behavior has hurt their relationship and help them to reconnect or, if necessary, part ways. Some spouses/partners choose to end the relationship due to the infidelity and the associated disregard of family obligations and well-being, and some as a result of other issues, such as shame. Thus, offending therapists may suffer more than one major loss consequent to the reporting of their behavior and benefit from additional support and possibly concurrent bereavement therapy.

Systems must be reviewed and evaluated to measure the risk of future behavior to support the victim, public confidence, and the offender. The competing needs that most professionals experience in their lives require a full reassessment. How does the therapist balance family and work roles? How do they define and regulate their sense of "self"? What is their ability to maintain their duties and obligation to their clients while being governed by their "code of conduct" and other life and relationship responsibilities? They must develop the skill of intentionality. If these factors are compromised, then decision-making and capacity for maintaining healthy boundaries are as well, and a return to practice (especially solo) is contraindicated. Instead, it might be recommended that they work in a group practice or within an organizational setting with ongoing monitoring or that they shift their career focus to an activity that does not involve direct client contact.

The use of peer support and therapy groups (in addition to individual therapy) has shown indications of effectiveness. Groups provide a unique forum for feedback to and from the self and others and for self-understanding from interacting with peers who "are in the same boat," who "have been there," and who can therefore provide unique perspective and support while simultaneously identifying and challenging cognitive distortions or other issues. It is important for such groups to be led (or optimally co-led) by therapists experienced with this population because these clients tend to be controlling and challenging (some are arrogant with regard to their professional or personal status and authority and might demonstrate contempt for or other disrespect of the therapists). Open releases of information between the group leader(s) and the individual's outside therapist and clinical supervisor (or any other adjunctive treatment provider such as a psychopharmacologist) are needed to support collaborative treatment and work against typical forms of client resistance, particularly splitting.

A relatively new treatment model, the good lives model (Ward & Brown, 2004), is a positive psychology approach that offers dynamic variables to consider when formulating recommendations, interventions, and monitoring after SBVs. Therapists can benefit from being goal-directed while (re)constructing their sense of purpose and meaning as they reconcile their behavior. The core idea of this model is the achievement of both primary and secondary "human goods," which enhances inclusion, mastery, and community that are valuable when assessing risk and preventing boundary violations. *Primary goods* are states of affairs, states of mind, personal characteristics, activities, or experiences that are sought for their own sake and are likely to increase psychological well-being if achieved. *Secondary goods* are the cognitive and behavioral means of fulfilling the primary goods, such as forming and maintaining relational bonds, caring for one's body and physical health, pursuing educational goals, practicing one's spirituality, or expressing one's creativity (Harris et al., 2019; Ward & Stewart, 2003).

Kendall et al. (2011) and Fronek and Kendall (2017) developed the Boundaries in Practice (BIP) Scale, a useful instrument to prepare a therapist for return to practice that both identifies the underlying skill set required to maintain professional boundaries and provides examples of practical decision-making processes. This model separates the therapist's *knowledge, comfort, experience, and ethical decision-making* into a segmented process to further understand areas of need and risk. Boundary vignettes are used to represent a variety of situations that might emerge in practice and walk an offending therapist through real professional issues and exchanges.

On the basis of all of the accumulated information, a comprehensive relapse prevention plan is developed that identifies triggers, high-risk situations, distorted schema, boundary crossings that on the surface are apparently irrelevant, and other lapses. Such a plan also includes courses of corrective action if the therapists begins to slip or relapse.

Outcomes: Monitored Rehabilitation, Reintegration, and Recidivism

The popular press has rightfully brought the issue of sexual abuse in professional settings into wider public awareness with a focus on licensing boards that do not respond to complaints in an adequate or timely manner, do not extend appropriate attention to victims or reporters, and, in the interim, allow boundary-violating professionals to continue to practice, putting the public at continued risk (Teegardin & Datar, 2016). The ultimate decision of whether an offending licensee continues in their field is the purview of the state licensing board, usually after receiving reports from the rehabilitative treaters. The subject of rehabilitation is controversial, with some advocating for a permanent loss of license in most cases and others arguing for rehabilitation. Many professional boards attempt to strike a balance in cases of boundary crossings and less serious sexual or other violations and give the offending therapist a chance at treatment or with ongoing supervision and monitoring. It appears that ongoing monitoring is effective in reducing future boundary violations, although some slippage, lapse, relapse, or even recidivism is to be expected. These must be reported to the licensee's board, which then determines whether more treatment, supervision, and education or professional restrictions, license revocation, or criminal charges are warranted.

An argument can be made that with proper and intense interventions and adequate follow-up, some therapists can work safely with clients (see Chapter 19) or in other areas of health care that do not involve direct patient care. This is not an attempt to condone the behavior, nor should it be an alternative to discipline by licensing boards or criminal prosecution when laws have been broken. That treatment, rehabilitation, and monitoring can be effective is supported by the results of one 40-year follow-up study of a physician's health program, which found that up to 90% of physicians reported (by self-report and external observers and victims) no further violations during the monitoring period (averaging 950 days; Brooks et al., 2012). The exception is the most egregious (and serial) offenders who have been identified as traumatic narcissists or psychopaths, have preyed upon clients, and exhibit little or no recognition of the harm caused, no empathy, or no remorse.

Calls for Prevention

There is definitely a mandate for regulatory bodies, professional organizations, supervisors, educators, colleagues, and other professionals to proactively engage in preventing or stopping these problems in the first place. Professional and personal modeling is powerful in influencing the behavior of trainees and early-career professionals, and so it must demonstrate boundary maintenance and personal limits and demonstrate how to manage conflict, emotions, professional–client and professional–professional interactions, and work–life balance. Educators, trainers, department chairs, supervisors, employers, and board members who serve as role models will be better prepared and able to fulfill this mandate if they themselves have obtained initial and ongoing continuing education training in this area. At present, several organizations offer such courses or credits online.

CONCLUSION

Although the focus of this chapter has been on treatment and intervention for the offending professional, the consequences for the victimized client and their needs must be continuously kept in mind, along with the protection of members of the public who are seeking psychotherapy. The wish of most victims is for the offender to be stopped and for them to get help. Yet in some cases, victims also seek justice, including punishment; appropriate administrative action including suspension, restriction, rehabilitation, monitoring, or loss of license; and compensation for their suffering. Too often, victims have complained of not being responded to with respect or understanding, being blamed or additionally shamed, or not being kept apprised of the status or outcome of their complaints. At the very least, professional licensing boards and health programs must ensure that reports and complaints are handled professionally and do not constitute a second injury for the victim, while providing due process for all.

A great deal remains to be done in professional training, practice settings, and at the level of licensing boards, other regulatory bodies, and state legislatures to prevent and then appropriately respond to reports of sexual improprieties and violations in psychotherapy. Those who evaluate and treat offending therapists, whether in formal impaired professional programs or independently as assigned by a licensing board, and those with expertise in understanding and treating sexually offensive behaviors have accumulated a body of information that can be used to assist the development of policy, procedures, and laws. To supplement this mostly clinically derived information, treatment approaches and their outcomes require additional research investigation and substantiation.

REFERENCES

AbuDagga, A., Carome, M., & Wolfe, S. M. (2019). Time to end physician sexual abuse of patients: Calling the U.S. medical community to action. *Journal of General Internal Medicine, 34*(7), 1330–1333. https://doi.org/10.1007/s11606-019-05014-6

AbuDagga, A., Wolfe, S. M., Carome, M., & Oshel, R. E. (2016). Cross-sectional analysis of the 1039 US physicians reported to the National Practitioner Data Bank for sexual misconduct, 2003–2013. *PLoS ONE, 11*(2), e0147800. https://doi.org/10.1371/journal.pone.0147800

Adjorlolo, S., & Egbenya, D. L. (2016). Executive functioning profiles of adult and juvenile male sexual offenders: A systematic review. *Journal of Forensic Psychiatry & Psychology, 27*(3), 349–375. https://doi.org/10.1080/14789949.2016.1141431

Alpert, J. L., & Steinberg, A. (Lu). (2017). Sexual boundary violations: A century of violations and a time to analyze. *Psychoanalytic Psychology, 34*(2), 144–150. https://doi.org.libproxy.tulane.edu/10.1037/pap0000094

Andrews, D. A., Bonta, J., & Wormith, J. S. (2011). The risk–need–responsivity (RNR) model: Does adding the good lives model contribute to effective crime prevention? *Criminal Justice and Behavior, 38*(7), 735–755. https://doi.org/10.1177/0093854811406356

Association for the Treatment of Sexual Abusers. (2014). *ATSA practice guidelines for the assessment, treatment, and management of male adult sexual abusers.*

Belous, C. K., Timm, T. M., Chee, G., & Whitehead, M. R. (2012). Revisiting the sexual genogram. *The American Journal of Family Therapy, 40*(4), 281–296. https://doi.org/10.1080/01926187.2011.627317

Bloom, J. D., Nadelson, C. C., & Notman, M. T. (Eds.). (1999). *Physician sexual misconduct.* American Psychiatric Association Publishing.

Blum, K., Badgaiyan, R. D., & Gold, M. S. (2015). Correction: Hypersexuality, addiction and withdrawal: Phenomenology, neurogenetics and epigenetics. *Cureus, 7*(9), c1.

Brooks, E., Gendel, M. H., Early, S. R., Gunderson, D. C., & Shore, J. H. (2012). Physician boundary violations in a physician's health program: A 19-year review. *Journal of the American Academy of Psychiatry and the Law Online, 40*(1), 59–66.

Carnes, P. (2001). *Out of the shadows: Understanding sexual addiction.* Hazelden Publishing.

Carnes, P. J., Green, B. A., Merlo, L. J., Polles, A., Carnes, S., & Gold, M. S. (2012). PATHOS: A brief screening application for assessing sexual addiction. *Journal of Addiction Medicine, 6*(1), 29–34. https://doi.org/10.1097/ADM.0b013e3182251a28

Eichenberg, C., Becker-Fischer, M., & Fischer, G. (2010). Sexual assaults in therapeutic relationships: Prevalence, risk factors and consequences. *Health, 2*(9), 1018–1026. https://doi.org/10.4236/health.2010.29150

Finlayson, A. R., Brown, K. P., Iannelli, R. J., Neufeld, R., Shull, K., Marganoff, D. P., & Martin, P. R. (2015). Professional sexual misconduct: The role of the polygraph in independent comprehensive evaluation. *Journal of Medical Regulation, 101*(2), 23–34. https://doi.org/10.30770/2572-1852-101.2.23

Fronek, P., & Kendall, M. B. (2017). The impact of Professional Boundaries for Health Professionals (PBHP) training on knowledge, comfort, experience, and ethical decision-making: A longitudinal randomized controlled trial. *Disability and Rehabilitation, 39*(24), 2522–2529. https://doi.org/10.1080/09638288.2016.1236152

Gold, J. A. (2013). Alligator hands. *Annals of Internal Medicine, 159*(7), 498–499. https://doi.org/10.7326/0003-4819-159-7-201310010-00013

Gold, L. H., & Frierson, R. L. (2018). *The American Psychiatric Association Publishing textbook of forensic psychiatry.* American Psychiatric Association Publishing.

Halter, M., Brown, H., & Stone, J. (2007). *Sexual boundary violations by health professionals—An overview of the published empirical literature.* Council for Healthcare Regulatory Excellence.

Harris, D. A., Pedneault, A., & Willis, G. (2019). The pursuit of primary human goods in men desisting from sexual offending. *Sexual Abuse, 31*(2), 197–219. https://doi.org/10.1177/1079063217729155

Kendall, M., Fronek, P., Ungerer, G., Malt, J., Eugarde, E., & Geraghty, T. (2011). Assessing professional boundaries in clinical settings: The development of the Boundaries in Practice Scale. *Ethics & Behavior, 21*(6), 509–524. https://doi.org/10.1080/10508422.2011.622186

Langone, A. (2018, March 8). #MeToo and Time's Up founders explain the difference between the 2 movements—And how they're alike [updated March 22]. *Time Magazine.*

MacDonald, K., Sciolla, A. F., Folsom, D., Bazzo, D., Searles, C., Moutier, C., Thomas, M. L., Borton, K., & Norcross, B. (2015). Individual risk factors for physician boundary violations: The role of attachment style, childhood trauma and maladaptive beliefs. *General Hospital Psychiatry, 37*(5), 489–496. https://doi.org/10.1016/j.genhosppsych.2015.06.002

Martin, M., & Hemphill, P. (2013). *Taming disruptive behavior.* American College of Physician Executives Press.

Montgomery, J., Hemphill, P., & Stone, A. C. (2015, April). *Suicide in physicians charged with criminal sexual behavior: An opportunity to intervene?* Annual Conference of the Federation of State Physician Health Programs, Fort Worth, TX.

Pope, K. S., Tabachnick, B. G., & Keith-Spiegel, P. (1987). Ethics of practice: The beliefs and behaviors of psychologists as therapists. *American Psychologist, 42*(11), 993–1006. https://doi.org/10.1037/0003-066X.42.11.993

Schwartz, B. K., & Cellini, H. R. (Eds.). (1995). *The sex offender: Corrections, treatment, and legal practice* (Vol. 1). Civic Research Institute.

Schwartz, M. F., & Masters, W. H. (1994). Integration of trauma-based, cognitive, behavioral, systemic and addiction approaches for treatment of hypersexual pair-bonding disorder. *Sexual Addiction & Compulsivity, 1*(1), 57–76.

Simon, R., & Gold, L. H. (2010). *The American Psychiatric textbook of forensic psychiatry*. American Psychiatric Association Publishing.

Swiggart, W. H. (2014). Assessment of a physician's workplace behavior. *Physician Leadership Journal, 1*(2), 28–33.

Swiggart, W. H., Feurer, I. D., Samenow, C., Delmonico, D. L., & Spickard, W. A., Jr. (2008). Sexual boundary violation index: A validation study. *Sexual Addiction & Compulsivity, 15*(2), 176–190.

Teegardin, C., & Datar, S. (2016). How well does your state protect patients? Doctors and Sex Abuse series. *The Atlanta Journal-Constitution.* http://doctors.ajc.com/states/

Ward, T., & Brown, M. (2004). The good lives model and conceptual issues in offender rehabilitation. *Psychology, Crime & Law, 10*(3), 243–257.

Ward, T., Polaschek, D., & Beech, A. (2006). *Theories of sexual offending*. John Wiley & Sons.

Ward, T., & Stewart, C. A. (2003). The treatment of sex offenders: Risk management and good lives. *Professional Psychology: Research and Practice, 34*(4), 353–360.

World Health Organization. (2018). *International classification of diseases* (11th rev.). https://icd.who.int/en

EPILOGUE

Prevention and Intervention

JUDITH L. ALPERT, ARLENE (LU) STEINBERG, AND CHRISTINE A. COURTOIS

In this volume, we have considered, among other issues, why sexual transgressions occur and why they occur with such frequency, why our mental health colleagues who obviously disapprove of these violations and know the damage that they cause are relatively tolerant and even dismissive of them, and what we can do to avoid or prevent such transgressions or to interrupt them if warning signs are present. We have also considered the harmful impact of such violations on the survivor, the therapist, associated others, and institutions and the profession at large.

Experts believe that even with adequate education and training, it is likely impossible to completely eliminate sexual boundary violations (SBVs) in treatment (Gabbard, 2017); however, there are other ways that we, as individuals, groups, and communities within the helping professions, can attempt to lessen its occurrence. We discuss various methods and issues in this epilogue and are hopeful that, along with the other material included in this book, they constitute a call to action for all.

https://doi.org/10.1037/0000247-021
Sexual Boundary Violations in Psychotherapy: Facing Therapist Indiscretions, Transgressions, and Misconduct, A. Steinberg, J. L. Alpert, and C. A. Courtois (Editors)

As indicated in the first chapter, although this text focuses primarily on SBVs in psychotherapy, boundary violations occur in related contexts, such as training, supervision, and service and employment settings, and many of the issues and dynamics are similar across settings. Also, such violations occur in other service contexts with other practitioners, such as massage therapists and clergy, in addition to mental health professionals. At the outset, it should be stated that while men and women (and non-binary gender therapists) may be violators in the therapy room and may also be victims, for purposes of this epilogue, we mostly refer to violators as men and victims as women because this remains the most common configuration.

Although we have covered many relevant issues in this text, there are others that require additional attention. One is the need to understand offending therapists in more depth in terms of their motivations and any personal characteristics or impairment that makes them vulnerable to erotic transference or as otherwise dangerous to clients. It is sometimes the case that indications of such problems emerge during training, yet many programs lack clear policies and procedures by which to address them or even to remove an unsuitable trainee. This may be due to fear of lawsuits filed by the trainee on the part of training programs and faculty members. A program may also be wary of being perceived as having train-ees with problems or as being overly rigid or punitive in how they deal with them. A second issue that demands more attention concerns licens-ing board members, legislators, and criminal justice personnel. They are all in need of specialized information and training regarding SBVs, and the system would benefit by the development of consistent standards of practice. Once a violation comes to light—whether through direct obser-vation, report, or complaint—means of investigation and intervention that are professional, equitable, and timely and intended to promote the rights and well-being of all parties with the least amount of administra-tive or procedural damage need to be developed and utilized. An exam-ple is the Association of State and Provincial Psychology Boards (2018) guidelines for board-mandated supervision of an offending therapist (see also Chapter 19, this volume, on supervision for discussion). More over-arching efforts by professional organizations like this one that are tasked with standards of practice, licensing, competence, reporting, and record keeping are needed.

We now move to discussion of efforts that are underway and that must be expanded in our attempts to curb sexual misconduct within psychotherapy.

EDUCATION AROUND TRANSFERENCE AND COUNTERTRANSFERENCE: THE CHALLENGE OF SEXUALITY IN THE TREATMENT ROOM

As has been emphasized throughout this book, well-intentioned therapists, regardless of theoretical orientation, are vulnerable to committing SBVs in psychotherapy. We may think that we have high moral standards, are cognizant of ethics, and would not commit this kind of violation. Nevertheless, we still err—it is not just bad or immoral professionals who lose their bearings. It happens to ordinary and generally ethical therapists, usually when a confluence of issues and vulnerabilities come together. Most violators are not criminal psychopaths or predatory and corrupt individuals who use the therapeutic relationship as an opportunity to seduce and exploit. In fact, Gabbard (1996) and Celenza (Chapter 4, this volume), both of whom have extensively studied these issues for decades, report that the majority of those who transgress are more similar to than different from the rest of us. However, there is little hard data on this issue, and research is indicated.

SBVs by psychotherapists can be thought of as a form of professional incest, highly taboo and damaging, high in betrayal, imbued in secrecy and silence, and indicative of serious role reversal and misuse of the patient. Training focused on boundaries, power differential, ethics, self-care, erotic transference and countertransference, and traumatic transference and enactment is indicated for mental health professionals in training and in practice. Understanding of these issues has become more sophisticated due to the development of knowledge about interpersonal violence and victimization and the overarching field of traumatic stress studies. This development is likely to continue. We have recently seen this positive development at work in the Harvey Weinstein trial when an understanding of victimization within asymmetric relationships of power and ambivalent attachments between victim and perpetrator was helpful in validating victim's reports.

In addition to more general education, there needs to be discussion about sexual feelings and desires arising within the treatment context and how therapists can identify and manage them without acting on them and damaging the client. It is important to consider erotic transference and countertransference and traumatic transference because their mishandling is often what precedes SBVs (Bolognini, 1994; Gabbard, 1996). There needs to be discussion about how to address erotic transference and countertransference. Some sexualized enactments, rather than being sexual desires, may actually be indicators of traumatic transferences and unresolved posttraumatic issues. Space is needed to process such experiences for those mental health professionals struggling to understand their client's traumatically based sexual enactments.

Two relevant examples follow. The first involves an enacted transference in the form of a client's kiss and inadequate discussion and response on the part of her supervisor. The second involves more assistance and discussion given to the therapist–trainee.

Example 1

Early in her training and at the end of the second therapy session, one of the authors of this chapter was kissed by her patient. It was clearly a kiss with sexual intent. The therapist immediately told her supervisor. His response was to tell her not to worry and that he would transfer this patient to a male intern. The new therapist-in-training felt shame. She thought that it was her fault and that she must have done something to provoke the patient's kiss. These issues were never discussed or resolved for her within that supervision. Although we hope it is less common to receive this type of "nonsupervision" today, in general, there continues to be inadequate training around erotic transference and countertransference as well as sexuality in treatment.

Example 2

This example also involves an author of this chapter. A male patient expressed his love for her (his therapist) early in his treatment. She was attracted to him as well. She told her supervisor, who was 87 years old and walked with a noticeable limp. The supervisor said to the therapist, "Don't take it so personally. You should see the gorgeous 20-somethings who have the hots for me." The supervisor also said that it is *the patient's right to try to seduce his therapist and that it is the analyst's obligation to analyze the behavior.* The supervisor made it clear that the patient's feelings of love and attraction for his therapist may well have come up with any other therapist. Transference was at work.

Given that there are many forms of both erotic transference and countertransference (i.e., erotic maternal, dependent or ambivalent, indulgent and caregiving, vengeful and hostile, aggressive or assaultive) and that sexuality can also be used as a defense against expression of other hidden feelings, as resistance to or distraction from deeper work, or as a means of communication as occurs in traumatic reenactments and enactments, what, at first glance, may be seen as erotic transference or desire may be much more complicated. In fact, these dynamics may have little to do with sexual feelings and a lot more to do with other issues, even though they are expressed in sexual terms or through sexual behavior. Most likely there is a lot more going on than sexual desire.

Erotic transference and countertransference and traumatic transference are relevant for *all* mental health professionals regardless of the therapist's theoretical orientation. Transference and countertransference are present in all treatments. Although attraction between therapist and patient is prevalent, there remain gaps in training about patient–therapist sexual attraction and erotic transference–countertransference, in the literature about the benefits of working ethically with such clinical issues, and in both training and literature as to how to work with issues of sexuality in the consulting room in general.

Since the beginning of the field of psychotherapy, psychoanalysts, more than any other group of therapists, have studied and written about issues concerning the holding environment, the maintenance of boundaries and the treatment frame, transference and countertransference, erotic transference and countertransference, traumatic reenacts, and SBVs. Freud (1915/1975) warned about SBVs in his article on transference. He noted that the analytic situation induces the patient to fall in love with her therapist, and he counseled analysts to keep countertransference in check. Despite this admonition, there were many violations. Carl Jung, Sandor Ferenczi, Erich Fromm, Freida Fromm-Reichman, Wilhelm Reich, Harry Stack Sullivan, and Karen Horney are just a few well-known "professional analytic grandparents" who were transgressors. Although psychoanalysts and psychodynamically oriented therapists have written and continue to write about SBVs, violations have not been found to be more prevalent among them (Alpert & Steinberg, 2017). Examples among other therapeutic orientations abound (see Chapters 5–9). In fact, psychoanalytic and psychodynamic therapists have lower prevalence rates of misconduct than therapists of other orientations (Celenza, 2007). This may be the case because psychoanalytic and psychodynamic therapists, in general, attend to transference and countertransference more than other therapists.

Research supports that sexualized or erotic excitement is a common occurrence in treatment (Pope et al., 1993). The patient may have sexual feelings for the therapist and vice versa. The sexual feelings may be mutual, and when this is the case, the situation is particularly challenging to manage therapeutically. Contemporary psychoanalytic thinking acknowledges that ongoing mutual enactments between the therapist and the patient can shape the erotic transference. Thus, countertransference is believed to be a joint creation, involving mutual influence and contributions from both patient and therapist (Aron, 1996).

Transference and countertransference have relevance for every type of treatment as they are always present in therapy, whether the therapist knows about it or practices from a psychoanalytic orientation. Why? Because the therapy process is relationship-based and its very nature promotes the emergence of unresolved transference-based issues often related to the reasons the client sought treatment in the first place. These are basic to psychotherapy, should be subject to discussion, and used to increase understanding and resolution.

Thus, sexuality can be present in the treatment, regardless of the type of psychotherapy offered. There are different ways patients might express their erotic feelings or desires. Some extreme examples include patients not wearing underwear and exposing themselves or "flashing" the therapist; masturbating in session; dressing or behaving in a highly sexualized manner; and even disrobing in session and offering themselves to the therapist. More commonly, however, patients express their longings and desires verbally or in writing and through other behaviors. In this digital age, some have even sent the therapist seductive texts and emails describing their love and desire or posting sexualized or pornographic videos or selfies. Other patients have researched the therapist's life, invading their privacy through trailing or stalking the therapist or family members or through other intrusive behavior. If they feel their attempts are rebuffed or rejected by the therapist, they may retaliate in some way (e.g., by trolling the therapist online, writing negative reviews, or making false allegations about sexual misconduct). Anything is possible, and in cases where therapists is threatened in some way, they may need to act to protect themselves, their careers, their livelihood, and their loved ones.

Although sexuality is often present in the treatment room in some way, there are not many case examples in the literature that illustrate ways to productively work with and process sexual attraction in treatment. "Publication anxiety" is the term Britton (1977) used to explain why there is a lack of writing in this area. This term refers to fear of recrimination and, possibly, exile by colleagues for daring to discuss such taboo issues in an open forum. Borys and Pope (1989) considered research findings and other writings on the topic having been suppressed or censored for many years due mainly to denial, distaste, disavowal, and coverup or protection of the perpetrator. Since Pope's observation, a good number of comprehensive and authoritative texts dealing with many facets of the issue have been published, although many of these do not contain detailed case examples. Yet some courageous mental health professionals have presented cases dealing with sexuality and the relational and ethical challenges they present (see, e.g., Celenza, 2014; Davies, 1994; Dimen, 2011; Gabbard, 1994; Jørstad, 2002; Pizer, 2017; Renn, 2012, 2013).

CASE EXAMPLES

This section presents two abbreviated cases and the response to each by the treating therapist. In both, the patient expresses love and desire for the therapist. The two therapists, who differ in the way they respond to their patient's pronouncement, explain why they reacted as they did. Brief discussion of these two cases follows the abbreviated case presentations. Our intent here is to promote discussion in education and training settings in graduate school, at the internship level, and in postdoctoral training. Dealing with erotic transference and erotic countertransference can be an important part of the work. The issues it raises are complicated, challenging, and confusing. They demand multilayered thought.

These two cases fall at different ends of the continuum with respect to how two therapists respond to their patient's erotic transference. At one end of the continuum is *therapeutic restraint*, or the therapist not disclosing his feelings despite the patient's request for him to do so. Gabbard (1996) chose to exercise restraint, believing that explicit self-disclosure of his sexual feelings would do more harm than good. His withholding of information allowed the release and exploration of the patient's representational world and maintained her sense of safety. On the other end of the continuum is a *less restrictive response* involving the disclosure of some information while, at the same time, maintaining boundaries. The self-disclosure of some degree of countertransference, is exemplified by Renn (2012, 2013), who discussed how he did so to mitigate against a patient feeling rejected and invalidated. He acknowledges that the approach he took, based on his knowledge of his patient and the relationship between them, was playful and flirtatious and, as such, had some risk associated with it. Gone wrong, it could have been devastating to the client; however, it worked out well, proved to be therapeutic, and helped uncover nuances of the patient's transference.

These cases are not offered as a recommendation as to how to respond to the challenges of sexual issues as they emerge in treatment because issues such as these are much too complicated for that. Rather, these cases ideally will be read and considered by therapists of all theoretical orientations, with the goal of supporting more sophisticated, knowledgeable, and informed interventions. What the cases clearly illustrate is that there are many ways to respond to erotic and traumatic transference–countertransference in therapy. The path chosen should be based, above all, on a consideration of ethics, the maintenance of professional boundaries, and the injunction to do no harm by misuse or exploitation.

Case 1

In his writings, Gabbard generally takes the position that explicit self-disclosure of the therapist's sexual feelings and the desire for a sexual liaison with the patient usually does more harm than good. The patient's response to the therapist's countertransferential love is complex and may lead to many different feelings, including stirring the patient's love or, alternatively, frightening the patient and leading to the shutting-down of erotic and other feelings.

Gabbard (1996) presented a case of a 30-year-old, never-married professional woman who developed an intense erotic transference to him during the first 2 years of her treatment. The case illustrates how disclosure can be countertherapeutic as well as counteranalytic. His patient expressed both erotic transference and anger. She was angry at his unavailability as a lover. Then something happened. The never-late-for-a-session therapist was late for a session with her. This resulted in her seeing the preceding patient. The patient was angry and then accused Gabbard of trying to make her jealous. Where was this intense jealousy from?

Her feelings related back to her sister, who charmed her father. Here she was once again, "the other female." This case illustrates how a patient's feelings of hostility, low self-worth, jealousy of a sibling rival, and lack of validation by her father made themselves known through erotic transference.

Gabbard acknowledged his contribution of lateness, which led to her seeing his earlier patient. He then helped her to see how the re-creation of her childhood rivalry with her sister for their father's love was the trigger. Also, he considered his own feelings and behavior. Why was he late? What was going on in *his* unconscious? Gabbard became aware of a feeling that his patient was dangerous and that he needed to protect himself and wanted retaliation.

A dream the patient had around this time was helpful to the work. In the dream, the patient was standing in a shower washing male genitals unattached to a body. Associations to the dream included her reading in the newspaper that prostitutes were being arrested and included the names of the men who visited them. She had another association: a fantasy of taking her therapist to the cleaners. All of this (and more) led to a powerful interpretation and to the recognition of the yearning as well as the enmity in her fantasy. He said: "I wonder if there is a wish in the dream, namely, that if you have the man's genitals, it assures you that he will come back for them" (Gabbard, 1996, p. 262). She could then discuss how her father said that no man would put up with her. She also discussed why she desired to seduce Gabbard (to bring him down). With this, the therapist understood why he sensed danger and felt the need to protect himself. He also became aware of his own unconscious hostility, leading to his lateness. The therapist was enacting a countertransference scenario. He became the patient's father, perhaps contributing unconsciously to the meeting of his two patients.

In summary, although the patient acknowledged that she could not have the therapist, she expressed her wish for him to acknowledge that he found her sexually attractive and would be interested in her if he were not her analyst. To this, Gabbard remained silent. The patient then continued and indicated that seduction, for her, wasn't really sexual. Rather what she wanted was some form of validation, which she never got from her father. The patient agreed with Gabbard's interpretation that she would have felt worse had she been able to seduce him. Gabbard also reflected on his own countertransference—namely, his rivalry with his brother for his mother's affections. This also contributed to his reactions to the patient.

Gabbard points to the climate of safety necessary to do this work and holds that self-disclosure of countertransference feelings of love or affection (or even other emotions such as anger and hostility) can be problematic. If self-disclosures, he holds that the therapist must be clear about his agenda. In this case, Gabbard chose to limit what he disclosed. At the same time, he was able to use his feelings in understanding both his patients' transference enactments and his own countertransference, including feelings of hostility and the need to protect himself. These feelings only became known to him when the patient requested that he self-disclose.

Gabbard (1996) illustrated how the analyst's countertransference influenced the patient's transference desires. He stated clearly that the therapist's participation may shape, suppress, or encourage the patient's erotic transference and identified such factors as the therapist's expectations, needs, theory, personal characteristic, anxiety, and countertransference as playing a role. Specifically, he made the point that the therapist plays a role in whether transference love is or is not reciprocated, as well as the degree to which it may be reciprocated. He also pointed out that the patient might also have a seductive influence on the therapist.

Case 2

In Renn's (2012, 2013) case, attachment issues were important to his 38-year-old patient, who, expecting abandonment and loss, experienced attachment as dangerous. Although the patient's history is relevant with respect to how the therapist chose to deal with her erotic transference, suffice it to say that she had an insecure attachment to her parents, a cumulative developmental trauma history, and an intergenerational transmission of fear. At the same time, the patient paradoxically wanted a more personal and a sexual relationship with the therapist. In addition, she indicated that she was afraid that she was too much for him. Undoubtedly, all of this played a role in how Renn chose to respond to her erotic transference, which became apparent a few years into the treatment.

The patient wondered aloud what it would be like to have sex with him. While Renn did not tell her whether he was attracted to her sexually, in the end he said, "Although I'm old enough to be your father, the thought of spending a romantic weekend with you in York sounds very appealing. It's such a damned shame I'm your therapist, isn't it?" (Renn, 2013, p. 143). Whether he was physically attracted to her remained a mystery to her—and to us, for that matter—as he intentionally did not disclose that information. As he pointed out, such disclosure could have moved them from the playful "as if" quality of the interaction and into a sexual enactment.

Renn noted that when this issue had come up previously, he had responded to his patient with restraint and a more emotionally distant response indicating that having a personal relationship would destroy the therapeutic one. This time, he felt the need to do something different for the work to progress, believing that it was safe and timely and that the patient could hear what he said, as it was meant, and that it would be therapeutically useful. He was trying to find a balance between emotional detachment on one hand and, on the other, an emotionally contained personal disclosure— all the while recognizing and respecting treatment boundaries. Renn chose the riskier side of self-disclosure but did not transgress boundaries in doing so. He was trying to avoid hurting or humiliating his patient, and he felt he understood the dynamics well enough, knew where he would and would not go, and understood that his patient needed emotional honesty at that moment. Also, he knew his response had to be heartfelt rather than defensive or judgmental and that the way he said what he said, including tone of voice and facial expression, were crucial.

Renn was cognizant that his comment might be viewed as wrong by many therapists when taken out of context. We add that some might find it unsuitable even in context and that readers might want to debate this.

Some might be concerned that it was a countertransference enactment or that what he said constituted acting out or being inappropriately seductive. Yet, while stating his understanding that relational psychoanalysis forbids any form of sexual relations with patients, Renn made it clear he was trying to avoid a frozen emotional detachment. He did not want to replicate the constricted pattern of communication that the patient had grown up with. He was confident that the patient knew they were relating in the pretend mode where it was safe to play with highly charged material. Having seen her two times a week for 5 years, he felt that he knew his patient and, at the same time, knew the consequences were significant had he misjudged.

What was the impact of this intervention between Renn and his patient, which was tailored for this particular patient at this particular time given her issues and therapeutic history?

An important focus of a relationally oriented analyst is mutuality and the humanness of the connection. What Renn did was unique to this therapeutic situation and resulted in what he called a "now moment." Emotional honesty, a new connection, and a demarcated experience were provided. Following his playful limit-setting comment in which he made clear that sex would not follow ("Damned shame I'm your therapist, isn't it?"), something important happened between them. There was a meeting of minds, of sorts. Humor and verbal expression of his thoughts and fantasies deepened their work and their therapeutic relationship and resulted in an increased sense of trust and feeling of safety. He had responded authentically while, at the same time, enabling her to feel safe, recognized, and appreciated. Rather than loss, abandonment, and rejection, there was honesty, playfulness, recognition, and boundary maintenance.

Renn is an experienced therapist who is knowledgeable around the issues relevant to erotic transference and countertransference. His intervention likely would have been much more dangerous with a less sophisticated or unethical therapist who was intent on sexually engaging with the patient and was testing her with his admission. Renn made a crucial recommendation, stressing the importance of regular, ongoing supervision and consultation, which he seemed to utilize, and the avoidance of isolation in clinical work, especially when engaging in a more direct and relational ways regarding sexuality. However, as discussed and as illustrated throughout this volume, being a well-trained and senior therapist does not necessarily prevent SBVs. In fact, such training or seniority can stir a sense of grandiosity and entitlement and lead to an encroachment of standards and boundaries. In this case, it did not, and the therapy instead was maintained and deepened.

BOTTOM LINE: DISCUSSION OF THE TWO CASES

Gabbard (1996) wrote that while limited therapist self-disclosure can be useful in some treatments, he does not support the disclosure of sexual feelings. Therapists sometimes reveal sexual feelings to a patient in what is usually a misguided effort to make them feel more secure. Gabbard identified problems that can result from doing so, including a shutting down of discussion in the representational realm and a disruption of the patient's sense of safety. Moreover, learning of the therapist's sexual feelings has the possibility of overwhelming a patient and can lead to a bad outcome.

In contrast to Gabbard's position, Renn (2013) presented a case in which *guarded* self-disclosure based on knowledge of the client and their relationship moved the treatment forward. As stated at the beginning, whether to disclose or not to disclose deserves consideration and is case dependent.

There are challenges in dealing with sexuality in treatment, especially when the sexual attraction is mutual. Supervision or consultation is often needed at these times to understand what is happening, retain the role and function, access the language to talk about it with the patient, contain anxiety, and maintain boundaries.

Nonsexual boundaries may also be crossed or violated in treatment. These are more common and may lead to SBVs. Boundary crossings that begin as nontoxic or inconsequential can increase and intensify and lead to unethical and destructive behavior. The literature is replete with examples.

Therapists need to learn how to use supervision and supervisors need to learn how to offer supervision that includes permission to discuss sexual feelings and desire in a setting of acceptance and confidentiality. The very information that a supervisee may feel he cannot share with his supervisor is the very information that should he shared. Supervisors need to encourage the therapists to share concerns of this type and to listen for this material. It needs to be discussed. In addition, one could even make a case for the therapist informing the patient about the third party (supervisor, colleagues) hearing about their sessions. In that way, both patient and therapist know that they are not alone together and that others are "watching."

In summary, we suggest ongoing training that focuses on boundaries, power differential, ethics, self-care, erotic transference and countertransference, and traumatic transference and enactment. Explicit and ongoing permission to discuss sexual feelings as they emerge within a treatment and how to therapeutically and safely deal with erotic transference and countertransference are needed in training, supervision, and consultation. An example of a means to consider these issues is provided by Steinberg and

Alpert (2017). They present vignettes, and the reader is encouraged to consider each of the four issues presented (hugging a patient posttermination, sex with a patient 2 years posttermination, and terminating a patient when the therapist feels overwhelmed or at risk). The vignettes are followed by a discussion among some senior therapists. We offer these as examples for how therapists and trainers can deliberately include such issues in their education, training, supervision, and consultation efforts.

Although not specifically the focus of the present chapter, other issues demanding education and training include vulnerabilities inherent in the process of psychotherapy; ethics, ethical challenges, and ethical dilemmas; ethical decision-making; dynamics of victimization such as grooming, betrayal trauma, and trauma bonding; the therapist's vulnerabilities related to life quality, personal and career satisfaction, characterological and other personal issues, and self-care; the consequences of transgressions for all involved parties; innovative individual and communal prevention and intervention efforts, including standards for response; and legal and criminal justice issues.

We recognize that although education around erotic transference–countertransference and enactments is important, it is not enough. Therapists and other involved professionals such as lawyers, judges, administrators, licensing boards, and policymakers need specialized information and training regarding the damaging impact of the abuse on the patient and all associated third parties, as Strasburger et al. (1990) suggested. They must be involved in developing policies and procedures that are equitable to all parties and that emphasize their ongoing well-being. These can then be conveyed in a variety of ways including required continuing education, regular educational programs, ethical standards and standing committees with clearly written guidelines, standards, record-keeping, and procedures. Clearly, not every patient develops erotic or romantic transference, even as they may come to love the therapist. Given that there is an interplay between the reality of everyday life and transferential reality, there are many possibilities as to how transference presents.

ADDITIONAL WAYS TO THINK ABOUT PREVENTION AND INTERVENTION

Bystanders and Communal Responsibility and Response

The primary betrayal involved in SBVs is that perpetrated by the violator. Secondary betrayals (the "second injury" as discussed in texts on victimology) are often described by victim–survivors as worse that the original violation. The harmful role of bystanders has been considered by several authors (e.g., Demos, 2017; Dimen, 2016; Slochower, 2017) who have grappled with the recurrent and significant issue of the collective bystander silence or inaction. Case studies and reports describe the impact of both the sexual misconduct and a community's silence, avoidance, and failure to act (Honig & Barron, 2013). This phenomenon occurs commonly whether SBVs are suspected, observed, or reported. Clearly, a case can be made that those who are not directly involved but know should take some form of action, possibly determined after consultation with others. Psychoanalysts and other therapists are often connected to an institute where they trained and may supervise, teach, attend talks and otherwise engage with each other. When boundary violations become known, the community may hear rumors but may be unclear about what actually happened. Legal and other constraints might limit open discussion and the naming of the alleged violator. The issue may result in a great deal of conflict among members. For those who disclose or report abuse, there is concern about the ramifications, including retaliation or shunning for being a whistleblower. Other members may seek to protect the alleged violator for any number of reasons, among them that they are in denial or that they lack information about SBVs and their dynamics. Also the violator may be powerful, and there may be fear of retaliation. They may be unsure about what happened or they may want to protect his other patients or supervisees from learning the "dark side" of someone they respect, need, lean on, and often idealize. They may also want to protect the reputation of their beloved (if he is, and he often is) violator-therapist as well as the reputation of their institute and their profession. There may be concern that there will be a lawsuit with repercussions to the profession or to the institute's finances or reputation. Many bystanders do not intervene because they lack certainty, self-assurance, or knowledge. Perhaps the alleged transgressor is protected by other members he had been previously sexually involved with or abused, or perhaps other members know that they, too, could possibly fall down the slippery slope and be a violator. Other possible reasons for nonintervention include previous violations and the previous victim's concern that these violations may become known. Thus, some members become gossipmongers, sitting in judgment or anger (Slochower, 2017). Honig and Barron (2013) elaborated on many of these points.

The idea of bystander response and intervention was founded on the assumption that bystanders, although often silent, passive, unknowing, and uninvolved, can be of assistance when educated and called to action. This communal perspective emphasizes collective behavior and responsibility.

So, contrary to the typical response, when a bystander such as a coworker sees something or has something reported to them, they respond to interrupt and intervene and to prevent further transgressions. In this way, the potential or actual victim is assisted by someone who not only notices or has information but acts based on that noticing. For example, they might ask the involved therapist about something they have observed or heard that seems "off" to them, such as furtive behavior, boundary changes, and excitement about and overinvolvement with a particular client. They might need to go further and challenge suspected therapist's denials and rationalizations (that are sometimes offered with great defensiveness and even hostility and threats toward the questioner) and to give assistance and consultation. They might also question and offer support to the affected client and not be thrown off course by a client's denial or protection of the therapist. In accordance with their organization's policies and procedures and the reporting laws of their state or jurisdiction, they must also weigh whether they need to make a report within or outside of the organization.

Such a change of response by community members comes with increased understanding of the dynamics of SBVs and a resultant shift in social norms, including more understanding of victimology and a lessening of victim-blaming. Accordingly, accountability and responsibility for intervention, prevention, and even rehabilitation belong to all; however, it is understood that some members of the community hold positions of greater power, accountability, and responsibility. Those in leadership and supervisory positions and those more established in the profession need to be mindful of the possibility of transgression and be willing to investigate and take other action when it is indicated. They bear the responsibility to take reports seriously and to take other necessary actions such as suspending an accused therapist pending an investigation, removing the therapist if allegations are credible or founded, attending to the needs of the client-victim and to other members of the organization, and indicating an understanding that the repercussions can have an impact on everyone in the community. Indeed, they can be and often are widespread.

Institutional Betrayal

Discussion of institutional and other forms of betrayal were included elsewhere in this book (see Chapters 14 and 17). *Institutional betrayal*, a concept identified and labeled by Smith and Freyd (2014), occurs when harm is caused by the actions of agents of an institution or a group to an individual who is a member of or dependent on that institution or group. Over time, both trauma victims and transgressors have reported being betrayed by institutions invested in protecting their reputations. Denial, silencing, and coverups as exemplified by scandals in the Catholic Church and other religious organizations, colleges and universities, and the military. Families as a group may also betray victims by not believing them or not intervening to effectively protect them.

How institutions deal with transgressions needs to be reconceptualized. More sophistication regarding dynamics and nuances of the typical abuse scenario is indicated. For example, colleagues often deny that a valued colleague or mentor could possibly be a violator. But, as Gentile (2018) pointed out, a more nuanced understanding based on evidence is that someone's reputation, credibility, and professional output as an influential theorist or a very competent therapist does not mean they cannot be a transgressor. These are not mutually exclusive but *are* hard to reconcile. Consent is another issue that has been reconceptualized. Although it was formerly the case that organizations based their determinations of sexual misconduct on the issue of consent (freely given, adult to adult), such a view did not take into account issues of unequal power and whether the ability to give consent from a position of lesser power is even possible. At present, it is accepted that power within the context of psychotherapy is not equal, and consent to sexual contact on the part of the client is therefore not possible. Moreover, the typical grooming dynamics that render the victim overly dependent on the therapist, as well as confused and uncertain about their personal agency, can result in ambivalent attachment and trauma bonding. These have the effect of further confounding the issue of responsibility, with client-victims often holding themselves out as the responsible party while exonerating the therapist.

In sum, it is necessary for organizations to continue to find ways to responsibly respond to and protect all parties when abuse is alleged. When they do not do so, they add the proverbial insult to injury, increasing the damage. Rather than continuing to protect the institution and its reputation or personnel, it is the true victims who need sensitive response and protection.

Ethics Codes

Although we could address numerous issues with respect to ethics codes, we focus on the one we, as clinicians, consider to be primary: the issues associated with erotic transference and countertransference and SBVs. Since the power differential between therapist and patient exists beyond termination (Gabbard, 1994; Gabbard et al., 2001), a case can be made that ethics codes of some professions do not adequately take this into account. Nor do they attend to the dynamics of transference and countertransference. For example, Principle (b) of 10.08 of the American Psychological Association (APA's; 2017) *Ethical Principles of Psychologists and Code of Conduct* states the following:

> Psychologists do not engage in sexual intimacies with former clients/patients even after a two-year interval except in the most unusual circumstances. Psychologists who engage in such activity, following cessation or termination of therapy and of having no sexual contact with the former patient, bear the burden of demonstrating that there is not potential for harm or exploitation.

It is unclear how the 2-year point was determined. Is research available that supports this interval? We have been unable to locate any.

Licensing Boards, Laws, and Social Policy

We believe most professional licensing boards in the United States need additional training and resources to work more productively and therapeutically with the complex issues they confront when SBVs are reported. Board members need to know more about how abusers manipulate and exploit vulnerabilities, especially in cases where the patients were previously abused and traumatized. They also need to know more about how to effectively assess and intervene in such cases. Over the years, many complainants have reported being treated poorly and unfairly in what can be described as another form of institutional betrayal by boards to whom they looked to for protection and intercession. There has been victim blaming. Labels such as "borderline personality disorder" or hysterical, seductive, or vengeful woman, and archaic thinking such as "those with mental illness lie or don't know what is real or are mistaken" or "it really was an affair" are some of the responses that have been reported. Not believing and blaming women for abuse has a long history (Alpert, 1995; Herman, 1992). Herman (1992) pointed out that throughout the history of the field, survivors of child sexual abuse as well as other victims of interpersonal trauma have been misunderstood, doubted, and provided inadequate care. To all of the identified victim groups (wife battering, incest, child sexual abuse, rape, and others), we include victims of therapist SBVs. Perhaps now, in the midst of the changes wrought by the #MeToo movement and in the aftermath of the guilty verdicts in the Bill Cosby and Harvey Weinstein trials, the dynamics of abuse by those more powerful toward those in less powerful and dependent conditions, including those with fiduciary duties to their clients, will be better understood and lead to ongoing changes. Women will certainly be the prime beneficiaries of these changes in understanding, as will all victims regardless of gender or gender identity.

Although agencies are charged with protecting the public and providing oversight and adjudication of cases of sexual exploitation and sexual misconduct by professionals, it often seems to be the case that the organizational and cultural structure of professional occupational licensing and regulatory agencies do not have policies and procedures based on (a) foundational knowledge about trauma and victims and (b) an understanding of the dynamics of how SBVs occur, especially within the context of erotic transference and countertransference and traumatic transference and enactment. At present, there are few, if any, differentiated processes, policies, or victim advocacy programs for consumer-victims of sexually abusive therapists. Complaint processing and adjudication often place already vulnerable and traumatized victims in situations that demand that they steer what is often an extended bureaucratic political nightmare that takes place behind closed doors in isolation and usually without adequate support. It is not surprising that some, if not most, consumer victims of SBVs report being retraumatized by the complaint and investigative process itself. Many are subjected to disbelief or held to be coresponsible for their own abuse. The investigations may lag for years without periodic updates from the regulatory organization, leaving them in a sort of limbo since their lives may have been totally upended and interrupted. It is now recognized that support services and victim advocates are needed for those who report misconduct. All parties—victims as well as the accused—should have the right to be present and to be heard at all critical stages of judicial proceedings. Clearly, change is needed in laws, regulations, and processes in order to adjudicate cases and assist both victims and violators.

There are various groups that lobby state legislatures, licensure boards, and professional organizations and work to make the public more aware of the problem of SBVs by therapists, to develop ways to prevent future exploitation, and to compensate victims for damages. Some (e.g., Haspel et al., 1997) hold that the civil, criminal, reporting, and injunctive relief statutes now in effect are an important step in decreasing SBVs in treatment. It is too early, however, to know their impact because there is little research on this to date. Changes are needed in law and policy that are consistent with advancing administrative commitment to trauma-informed policies, agencies, screenings, training and education of employees, and the conducting of organizational evaluation, as suggested by Harris and Fallot (2001) and other trauma survivor advocates.

BOOK AND CHAPTER THEMES

Numerous themes emerge and reemerge in the chapters of this book. Here, as we wrap up this chapter and the text, we list and restate some of them:

- Psychotherapy is a relationship with an asymmetry in power between therapist and client. Therapists are enjoined to understand this. Therapists should not abuse their position of greater power against the patient in any way.

- Transference and countertransference exist regardless of a therapist's theoretical orientation. SBVs occur within all theoretical orientations as well. The mishandling of erotic and trauma-based transferences can be fueled by, for example, therapist personal or characterological issues; lack of training, inexperience, and naivete; attempts to be needed or in control; and other work and situational issues.

- Significant damage to the patient, the therapist, family members, organizations, colleagues, and the profession takes place when sexual and other boundaries are violated especially when the transgressions are reported or otherwise become known.

- Being a mental health professional or trainee does not protect against becoming a victim of SBVs.

- Both the therapist and the client involved in a sexual relationship require support in the aftermath of disclosure or reporting or in any administrative, legal, or criminal proceeding.

- Individual supervision, peer group supervision, consultation, excellent training and institutional structure do not prevent SBVs but, ideally, lessen their occurrence or the damage caused.

- Being a well-trained and senior therapist does not prevent SBVs. In fact, such training or seniority can lead to a sense of grandiosity and greater entitlement in some, and age- and stage-related anxieties may be contributory to transgressions.

- Institutes and colleagues often deny, minimize, or rationalize sexual transgressions in a form of collective shrouding. It is difficult to accept that a valued and esteemed colleague has erred and easier not to. This is an additional injury to abused patients whose reports are dismissed or downplayed or who are disbelieved or blamed.

- Therapists do not consistently enforce their own ethics and principles and seem to be uncomfortable assuming the role of whistleblower or intervener. The focus seems to be more on protecting and excusing violating colleagues due to discomfort, disbelief and "benefit of the doubt," and denial. Training and role-play would be useful to assist colleagues in discussing these difficult issues with one another and with a transgressor-colleague. Therapists must be ready to report allegations or observations of a colleague's misconduct and must be aware of their state's mandatory reporting requirements. They also need to know how to work with these issues when clients disclose as well as how to work competently and compassionately with clients when they disclose.

- Members of professional licensing boards require specialized training in investigating and responding to reports of sexual misconduct. Standard interjurisdictional procedures and a standard national reporting mechanism would be of great benefit. Some professional groups have begun to address the need for more standardization (i.e., the Association of State and Provincial Psychology Boards, 2018, document on mandated supervision described in Chapter 19, this volume, on supervision).

- When reports are made to a professional licensing board, they must be investigated with great attention to timeliness and intervention appropriate to the gravity of the allegation. Investigations should not drag on for years as many do, in the process creating more hardship for both accused therapist and client-victim. Ongoing and timely communication with all parties regarding the status of the investigation should also be standard practice. Finally, there need to be clear standards about whether and when a reported therapist can continue to practice and under what conditions.

- There is consistency across the ethics codes of various professional organizations with regard to current treatment: They prohibit sexual relations between mental health professionals and clients. However, some of the codes across professional organizations differ with respect to post-termination sexual relations. Some, such as the American Psychoanalytic Association and the American Association of Sex Educators Counselors and Therapists, extend this prohibition into perpetuity, whereas others, such as APA and the National Association of Social Workers (NASW), offer latitude, with APA indicating a 2-year posttermination phase. In the event that former therapist and client become romantically or sexually involved, both APA and NASW place the burden on the therapist to demonstrate lack of exploitation, coercion, or manipulation.

CONCLUSION

Although it is difficult for us to ignore, we have been trying to not know what we know, which is that SBVs occur in some treatments. Historically we have ignored or denied abuse by therapists. We continue to do so. Although it may be impossible to totally eliminate sexual misconduct in treatment, we can work to minimize its occurrence and make ongoing attempts to eradicate it. One way, as indicated in this chapter, is by means of increased therapist and therapist-in-training education around issues of transference and countertransference. There needs to be supervision and consultation around these issues as well. Some other ways discussed in this chapter include focusing on bystander intervention, ethics codes, standards and training of licensing boards, and social policies and laws.

As mental health professionals dedicated to healing, we must monitor ourselves and our own. We can no longer afford to not know what we indeed do know. These are our #WeToo moments in support of and in response to the #MeToo movement.

REFERENCES

Alpert, J. L. (Ed.). (1995). *Sexual abuse recalled: Treating trauma in the era of the recovered memory debate*. Jason Aronson.

Alpert, J. L., & Steinberg, A. (2017). Sexual boundary violations: A century of violations and a time to analyze. *Psychoanalytic Psychology, 34*(2), 144–150. https://doi.org/10.1037/pap0000094

American Psychological Association. (2017). *Ethical principles of psychologists and code of conduct* (2002, amended effective June 1, 2010, and January 1, 2017). https://www.apa.org/ethics/code/index.aspx

Association of State and Provincial Psychology Boards. (2018). *Supervision guidelines—Mandated supervision—February 2018*. https://cdn.ymaws.com/www.asppb.net/resource/resmgr/guidelines/supervision_guidelines_manda.pdf

Aron, L. (1996). *A meeting of minds*. The Analytic Press.

Bolognini, S. (1994). Transference: Erotised, erotic, loving, affectionate. *The International Journal of Psycho-Analysis, 75*(1), 73–86.

Borys, D. S., & Pope, K. S. (1989). Dual relationships between therapist and client: A national study of psychologists, psychiatrists, and social workers. *Professional Psychology: Research and Practice, 20*(5), 283–293. https://doi.org/10.1037/0735-7028.20.5.283

Britton, R. (1977). Making the private public. In I. Ward (Ed.), *The presentation of case material in clinical discourse* (pp. 11–28). Karnac.

Celenza, A. (2007). Academic and supervisory contexts. In *Sexual boundary violations: Therapeutic, supervisory, and academic context* (pp. 65–76). Jason Aronson.

Celenza, A. (2014). *Erotic revelations: Clinical applications and perverse scenarios*. Routledge. https://doi.org/10.4324/9781315773056

Davies, J. (1994). Love in the afternoon: A relational reconsideration of desire and dread in the countertransference. *Psychoanalytic Dialogues, 4*(2), 153–170.

Demos, V. C. (2017). When the frame breaks: Ripple effects of sexual boundary violations. *Psychoanalytic Psychology, 34*(2), 201–207. https://doi.org/10.1037/pap0000119

Dimen, M. (2011). Lapsus linguae, or a slip of the tongue? A sexual violation in an analytic treatment and its personal and theoretical aftermath. *Contemporary Psychoanalysis, 47*(1), 356–79. https://doi.org/10.1080/00107530.2011.10746441

Dimen, M. (2016). Rotten apples and ambivalence: Sexual boundary violations through a psychocultural lens. *Journal of the American Psychoanalytic Association, 64*(2), 361–373. https://doi.org/10.1177/0003065116640816

Freud, S. (1975). Observations on transference love. In J. Strachey (Ed. & Trans.), *The standard edition of the complete psychological works of Sigmund Freud* (Vol. 12, pp. 157–173). The Hogarth Press. (Original work published 1915)

Gabbard, G. O. (1994). On love and lust in erotic transference. *Journal of the American Psychoanalytic Association, 42*(2), 385–403. https://doi.org/10.1177/000306519404200203

Gabbard, G. O. (1996). The analyst's contribution to the erotic transference. *Contemporary Psychoanalysis, 32*(2), 249–273. https://doi.org/10.1080/00107530.1996.10746952

Gabbard, G. O. (2017). Sexual boundary violations in psychoanalysis: A 30-year retrospective. *Psychoanalytic Psychology, 34*(2), 151–156.

Gabbard, G. O., Peltz, M. L., & COPE Study Group on Boundary Violations. (2001). Speaking the unspeakable: Institutional reactions to boundary violations by training analysts. *Journal of the American Psychoanalytic Association, 49*(2), 650–673.

Gentile, K. (2018). Assembling justice: Reviving nonhuman subjectivities to examine institutional betrayal around sexual misconduct. *Journal of the American Psychoanalytic Association, 66*(4), 647–678. https://doi.org/10.1177/0003065118797138

Harris, M., & Fallot, R. D. (Eds.). (2001). *New directions for mental health services: Using trauma theory to design service systems.* Jossey-Bass/Wiley.

Haspel, K. C., Jorgeson, L. M., Winncze, J. P., & Parsons, J. P. (1997). Legislative intervention regarding therapist sexual misconduct: An overview. *Professional Psychology: Research and Practice, 28*(1), 63–72. https://doi.org/10.1037/0735-7028.28.1.63

Herman, J. (1992). *Trauma and recovery.* Basic Books.

Honig, R. G., & Barron, J. W. (2013). Restoring institutional integrity in the wake of sexual boundary violations: A case study. *Journal of the American Psychoanalytic Association, 61*(5), 897–924. https://doi.org/10.1177/0003065113501868

Jørstad, J. (2002). Erotic countertransference: Hazards, challenges and therapeutic potentials. *Scandinavian Psychoanalytic Review, 25*(2), 117–134. https://doi.org/10.1080/01062301.2002.10592737

Pizer, B. (2017). "Why can't we be lovers?" When the price of love is loss of love: Boundary Violations in a clinical context. *Psychoanalytic Psychology, 34*(2), 163–169.

Pope, K. S., Sonne, J. L., & Hollyroyd, J. (1993). *Sexual feelings in psychotherapy: Explorations for therapists and therapists-in-training.* American Psychological Association. https://doi.org/10.1037/10124-000

Renn, P. (2012). *The silent past and the invisible present: Memory, trauma, and representation in psychotherapy.* Routledge. https://doi.org/10.4324/9780203126868

Renn, P. (2013). Moments of meeting: The relational challenges of sexuality in the consulting room. *British Journal of Psychotherapy*, *29*(2), 135–153. https://doi.org/10.1111/bjp.12017

Slochower, J. (2017). Don't tell anyone. *Psychoanalytic Psychology, 34*(2), 195–200. https://doi.org/10.1037/pap0000082

Smith, C. P., & Freyd, J. J. (2014). Institutional betrayal. *American Psychologist*, *69*(6), 575–587. https://doi.org/10.1037/a0037564

Steinberg, A., & Alpert, J. (2017). Sexual boundary violations: An agenda deserving more consideration. *Psychoanalytic Psychology*, *34*(2), 221–226.

Strasburger, L. H., Jorgenson, L., & Randles, R. (1990). Mandatory reporting of sexually exploitative psychotherapists. *Bulletin of the American Academy of Psychiatry and the Law*, *18*(4), 379–384.

Index

Brooks, E., 381
Brown, L. S., 142, 151, 224, 225, 306
Brownfain, J. J., xv
BTT. *See* Betrayal trauma theory
Burke, Tarana, 10
Business relationships, with therapists,
    58–59
Bystanders
    of clergy sexual abuse, 163, 165, 172,
        173
    in personal narratives of survivors,
        292–293
    SBV response and intervention by,
        397–399

C

California, 38, 164–165
Cambridge Hospital, 73
*The Capacity for Empathy, Regression and
    Ego Boundaries* (Celenza), 70
Caretaking, 144, 247, 269–273, 333
Carnes, Patrick, 370
Caruth, C., 250
Case examples
    abuse of power in feminist therapy,
        149–150
    abusive relationship dynamics,
        265–272
    betrayal trauma, 298–300, 304–305
    erotic idealization, 97–102
    erotic transference response, 391–395
    ethical judgments about digital
        technology use, 187–188
    ethical misconduct, 189–191
    ethical mistakes involving technology,
        188–189
    grooming process, 249–250
    involving noncishet dyads, 231–233
    mandated supervision, 355
    sociocultural context for sexual
        boundary violation, 208–211
CBT. *See* Cognitive behavioral therapy
Celenza, Andrea, 69–89, 387
    clinical work and writing of, 71–72
    on countertransference management,
        87
    on criminal charges for offenders, 77
    on disciplines/theoretical orientations
        of offenders, 83–85
    on erotic transference and counter-
        transference, 78–81

on gender/sex differences for offenders,
    81–82
on #MeToo Movement and abuse
    reporting, 88–89
on motivation of offenders, 74–75
on offenders/victims from marginalized
    communities, 82–83
on patients impacted by SBVs, 72–73
on prevention of SBVs, 85–86
on prognosis for mental health field,
    86–87
prominence of, in psychoanalysis, 70
on rehabilitation of offenders, 75–77
on support and consultation for treating
    therapists, 87–88
on treating offenders, 77–78
work in area of sexual boundary
    violations by, 69–71
Celibacy, vows of, 162
Charismatic leaders, sexual misconduct by
    in clergy, 163–164, 171
    in feminist therapy, 145–148
    in gestalt therapy, 118–120
Charles, M., 92
Child abuse, 8, 158, 280–281. *See also*
    Child sexual abuse
Children
    conception of, by clergy, 164–165
    prohibited relationships for therapists
        with child clients, 30–31
    sexual violations involving, 7–9
The Child Safeguarding Policy Book
    (Tchividjian & Berkovits), 178, 180
Child sexual abuse, 9
    betrayal trauma in, 251
    boundary maintenance after, 328
    by clergy, 176, 178
    feminist research on, 144
    grooming in, 244
    personal narrative of, 280–281
    shame about sexual feelings after, 320
    victim-patient survivors of, 253–254,
        320, 328
Christianity, 165
Chung, R. C.-Y., 227
Cisgender–heterosexual dyads (cishet dyads)
    defined, 221
    therapy outside of. *See* Noncishet dyads
Citizens Commission on Human Rights
    International, 38–39
Civil liability, in consultation, 345–346
Civil negligence suits, 195

Devereux, D., 305
Diagnoses
    discrediting victim-patients with, 275
    for professional boundary violators,
        62–63
*Diagnostic and Statistical Manual of Mental
    Disorders* (American Psychiatric
    Association), 222
Dialectical behavior therapy (DBT), 110
Differently special clients, 266–267
Digital technology, 185–200
    ethical standards on, 193–195
    expressing sexual feelings using, 390
    risk management for, 195–199
    themes of boundary challenges
        involving, 191–193
    types of boundary violations involving,
        189–191
Dignity, 210
Dimen, M., 215, 244
Direct observation, 348, 354
Disbelief, 166, 172, 329, 335–336
Disch, Estelle, 294, 295
Disciplinarian role, for supervisor, 356
Disciplinary action
    resources on supervision under, 346
    special issues for supervisees facing,
        359
    supervision of therapist under, 344,
        346, 355–356
    trends in, APA Ethics Committee, 39–40
Disciplines, of offending therapists, 83–84
Disclosure
    effects of, for offender, 372
    sociocultural context for, 213
    in subsequent treatment, 323–324,
        326–327, 329–330, 334–335
Discomfort, in grooming process, 245
Discontinuity models, 308
Discrimination, 213
Disempowerment, 325–327
Disenchantment, 258
Disenfranchised grief, 258–259
Disengagement, in anticontemplation
    stage, 325
Dissociation, 254, 281, 291
Dissociative identity disorder, 254
Distal factors, in hypothetical risk model,
    369
Distancing, after sex talk, 136
Distress signal, erotic idealization as,
    92–93

DNS hijacking, 193
Documentation, 53, 373–374
Dorahy, Martin, 151
Drescher, J., 226
Drum, K. B., 186
Dual relationships
    altruistic motives in, 192
    for behavioral health professionals, 185
    boundaries to prevent, 366
    for clergy, 160, 165
    in closed communities, 369
    disciplinary actions involving, 39
    ethics codes on, 23–25, 29
    in gestalt therapy, 119, 122
    and grooming, 247
    for incest/CSA survivors, 253
    intimacy in, 191
    in LGBQ and gender-expansive
        communities, 229–230
    nonsexual, 39
    personal gain from, 192
    in professional relationships, 58–59,
        63–64
    rationalization of, 369
    in supervision, 240
    unanticipated circumstances leading
        to, 193
Duthie, R. F., 197–198
Duty to help, 47
Dyad-specific vulnerabilities, 6
D'Zurilla, T. J., 112

E

Early assessment, of ethical violations,
    371–375
Early behavior stage of grooming,
    245–246
Eber, M., 250
Education
    for SBV prevention, 5–6, 86, 387–391
    sexual misconduct in field, 48
Educational tools, in ethics codes, 21
Egalitarian relationship
    as defense for SBVs, 145–147
    in feminist therapy, 142, 143, 150
    FTI Ethics Code on, 148
Ego-syntonic SBVs, 228
Electronic communications
    boundary confusion related to, 200
    confidentiality of, 199
    in grooming process, 189–191, 196–197

About the Editors

Arlene (Lu) Steinberg, PsyD, is an adjunct associate professor at Ferkauf Graduate School of Psychology, where she supervises clinical psychology graduate students and teaches psychological counseling to rabbinic students. She is also a practicing psychoanalyst in New York City and a psychotherapy education consultant at the Icahn School of Medicine at Mount Sinai, New York. She is the author of several articles and chapters on trauma and coedited the 2017 special issue of *Psychoanalytic Psychology* on sexual boundary violations with Dr. Judith L. Alpert. Dr. Steinberg is past treasurer of Division 39 (Society for Psychoanalysis and Psychoanalytic Psychology) of the American Psychological Association, is currently serving her second 3-year term as Division 39 representative on the APA Council of Representatives, and is chair of Divisions for Social Justice.

Judith L. Alpert, PhD, is a professor of applied psychology at New York University and faculty and clinical consultant at the NYU Postdoctoral Program in Psychotherapy and Psychoanalysis. She has edited six books and numerous journal articles in the area of trauma and women's issues and has a focus on sexual abuse trauma. She coedited the 2017 special issue of *Psychoanalytic Psychology* on sexual boundary violations with Dr. Arlene (Lu) Steinberg. She practices psychoanalysis and psychoanalytically oriented psychotherapy in New York City. She was the first president and a founding member of Division 56 (Trauma Psychology) of the American Psychological Association (APA). Dr. Alpert is the recipient of the Award for Scholarship from Division 39 (Society for Psychoanalysis and Psychoanalytic Psychology) of APA.

Christine A. Courtois, PhD, ABPP, a board-certified counseling psychologist retired from clinical practice in Washington, DC, has been an adjunct professor of psychology and social work at several universities and is now an independent consultant, trainer, and author on topics of trauma psychology and treatment. She has authored, coauthored, or coedited a dozen professional books on the dynamics and treatment of child sexual abuse, complex trauma, and posttraumatic stress disorder. Dr. Courtois was chair of the *Clinical Practice Guideline for the Treatment of PTSD in Adults* for the American Psychological Association (2017) and for Professional Practice Guidelines on the Treatment of Complex Trauma in Adults (forthcoming jointly from the APA Division 56 [Trauma Psychology] and the International Society for the Study of Trauma and Dissociation) and previously for the International Society for Traumatic Stress Studies (2012). Dr. Courtois is past president of APA Division 56 and founding associate editor of the division's journal, *Psychological Trauma*. She is the recipient of numerous professional awards from several organizations.